SECOND EDITION

MANAGEMENT IN PHYSICAL THERAPY PRACTICES

SECOND EDITION

MANAGEMENT IN PHYSICAL THERAPY PRACTICES

Catherine G. Page, PT, MPH, PhD

Adjunct Professor
Nova Southeastern University
Tampa, FL

F.A. Davis Company • Philadelphia

F. A. Davis Company
1915 Arch Street
Philadelphia, PA 19103
www.fadavis.com

Printed in the United States of America

Last digit indicates print number: 10 9 8 7 6 5 4 3 2 1

Editor in Chief: Margaret Biblis
Senior Acquisitions Editor: Melissa A. Duffield
Manager of Content Development: George W. Lang
Developmental Editor: Lisa Consoli
Design and Illustration Manager: Carolyn O'Brien

As new scientific information becomes available through basic and clinical research, recommended treatments and drug therapies undergo changes. The author(s) and publisher have done everything possible to make this book accurate, up to date, and in accord with accepted standards at the time of publication. The author(s), editors, and publisher are not responsible for errors or omissions or for consequences from application of the book, and make no warranty, expressed or implied, in regard to the contents of the book. Any practice described in this book should be applied by the reader in accordance with professional standards of care used in regard to the unique circumstances that may apply in each situation. The reader is advised always to check product information (package inserts) for changes and new information regarding dose and contraindications before administering any drug. Caution is especially urged when using new or infrequently ordered drugs.

Library of Congress Control Number: 2014945713

To all physical therapists who as the voices of the profession in healthcare organizations take on managerial responsibility for quality patient care.

The content of most textbooks is perishable, but the tools of self-directness serve one well over time.

Albert Bandura

Like the authors of many texts, I was driven by my professional experiences to write the first edition of this book. Particularly challenging in my broad range of clinical experiences as a physical therapist and department head, mixed with academic experiences as teacher and program director, were my managerial responsibilities. Equally challenging has been teaching management courses to physical therapy students. The management course is rarely considered the highlight of one's professional education. Sparking students' interest in the course is often an important first step.

I used the first edition of this text to teach a newly created management course and as a new text in a well-developed course. As expected, there were things that I thought should be improved in the format and organization of the text, and there were things that already needed to be updated because of the rapid changes in the healthcare policies and organizations in the United States. The need for a second edition was evident so that the content could be presented more effectively and clearly. A second edition is also an opportunity to bring the content up to date, and to provide new resources for accurate and relevant information for current managers and students of physical therapy management.

Since the first edition, some things have *not* changed. Many physical therapists continue to transition easily and successfully from clinical to managerial positions. More often than not, however, other physical therapists (and many students) seem to be willing to go to any means to avoid management because of their commitment and interest in direct patient care, or perhaps a fear of the unknown. The second edition continues to recognize that management responsibilities are complex, not for everyone, and remain important for clinicians to understand their work beyond the direct patient care they provide.

The second edition continues to provide an introduction to the physical therapist as manager for those whose career plans are to intentionally seek management positions in any healthcare setting. It also provides the reluctant manger or student an opportunity to view the broad range of possibilities for physical therapists as managers that they might not consider otherwise. As clinicians they will be better prepared to see work-related issues from the perspective of the boss or corporate demands.

This text is intended to serve as a springboard for the discussion of the physical therapist as manager across all healthcare settings rather than a "how-to" on management. Ideally, the text will provoke conflicting opinions and opposing views so that readers practice making important management decisions with no clear, black-and-white guidelines. The management activities are based on my real-life experiences in a wide variety of healthcare settings—either direct work experiences or discussions with other managers who have shared their experiences. Some of the actual decisions made in these situations had positive outcomes; others did not. Through discussions with others while working on these activities, readers have the opportunity to reflect on the decisions they would make in these situations from different perspectives. There are no hard and fast correct answers. The objective is to develop the ability the weigh the pros and cons of important decisions that impact the care of patients through the management of the work in physical therapy practices.

In addition to the management activities, in this edition, Web resources have been organized into lists at the ends of the chapters. These resources present the opportunities to add depth and breadth to topics during learning activities. They are also the tools for self-directed investigation and up-to-date information for learners after the course is completed so that their practices may remain current.

Although reorganized, the chapters in Section 1 of the second edition continue to lay the foundation for understanding the complexity of healthcare organizations, the culture and business of healthcare, the role of managers and leaders in these organizations, and managerial challenges for the physical therapy profession. Selected contemporary healthcare issues are presented, which include workforce diversity, the culture of physical therapy, the leadership-management continuum, the Affordable Care Act, and reimbursement for payment for physical therapy services. Readers are asked to examine their current views on management as a career goal. Appendix 1 was added to present a brief history of theories of management, leadership, and organizations.

Each chapter in Section 2 addresses one of the core areas of responsibility of healthcare managers, which include vision, mission, goals; policies and procedures; marketing; staffing; patient care; fiscal; legal, ethical, and risk management; and communication. A simplified model for strategic planning is presented and employed throughout the text to develop managerial decision-making skills. For example, in one of the activities, students are asked: *What should the team do? Consider: Where are they now? Where do they want to be? What do they have to work with? How will they get there?* The activities in these chapters provide opportunities to explore each area of managerial responsibility in more depth. These chapters may stand alone with activities to apply concepts. The *"Time-Out for . . ."* activities in Section 2 chapters serve as the tools needed for the potential development of a business plan, feasibility study, or program proposal. To assist learners, new outlines for the preparation of these documents are found in Appendix 2.

Each chapter in Section 3 addresses management of physical therapy in a different setting—long-term care, outpatient centers, special education units in schools, home health agencies, and hospitals. The importance of the management of multidisciplinary rehabilitation units is addressed. Each chapter in Section 3 is divided into two parts. Part 1 addresses contemporary issues found in a particular setting. Part 2 identifies issues in each of the eight areas of managerial responsibility presented. At the end of each chapter are numerous activities that provide the opportunity to develop managerial decisions using a strategic planning tool to guide readers in their decision-making.

The style of the text is to present complex management concepts in a user-friendly, interactive format that reflects the real world of contemporary physical therapy practice through interesting activities. I would be pleased if these learning experiences lead to physical therapists who seek for themselves the latest and most important information about healthcare organizations, policies, and the responsibilities of managers. My hidden agenda is that the number of physical therapists who are eager to seek out management positions increases. It is important to their careers and it is important to our profession that we expand this aspect of professional practice. I hope that readers have the same wonderful career that I have had because I have been a manager.

Catherine G. Page, PT, MPH, PhD

REVIEWERS

Jacob Francis Brewer, PhD, PT, DPT, NCS
Associate Professor
Physical Therapy
Hardin-Simmons University
Abilene, Texas

Mary Dockter, PT, PhD
Associate Professor & Chair
Department of Physical Therapy
University of Mary
Bismarck, North Dakota

Clifton Ford Frilot II, PhD, MBA, PE
Associate Professor
Rehabilitation Sciences, Physical Therapy
    Program
Louisiana State University Health Sciences
    Center Shreveport
Shreveport, Louisiana

John Duane Heick, PT, DPT, OCS, NCS
Associate Professor
Department of Physical Therapy
A.T. Still University of Health Sciences
Mesa, Arizona

Peri J. Jacobson, PT, DPT, MBA
Assistant Professor & Director of Clinical
    Education
Physical Therapy Program
Bellarmine University
Louisville, Kentucky

Nancy R. Kirsch, PT, DPT, PhD
Professor
Physical Therapy
Rutgers University
Newark, New Jersey

Steven G. Lesh, PhD, PT, SCS, ATC
Department Chair of Physical Therapy
Southwest Baptist University
Bolivar, Missouri

Renee Mazurek, PT, DPT
Clinical Assistant Professor
Academic Coordinator Clinical Education
Physical Therapy Program
University of Wisconsin-Milwaukee
Milwaukee, Wisconsin

Ann Noonan, PT, EdD
Associate Professor
Physical Therapy
Lynchburg College
Lynchburg Virginia

Jeffrey Rothman, PT, EdD
Chair & Professor
Department of Physical Therapy
College of Staten Island/Graduate Center CUNY
Staten Island, NY
Executive Officer
Doctorate in Physical Therapy Programs
The Graduate Center of The City University of
    New York
New York, New York

Robert Sandstrom, PhD PT
Associate Professor
Physical Therapy
Creighton University
Omaha, Nebraska

Olaide Sangoseni, PT, DPT, MSc, PhD
Assistant Professor
Physical Therapy Program
Maryville University
Saint Louis, Missouri

Anthony Sarola, PT, GCS
Associate Faculty
Doctor of Physical Therapy Program
Touro College, Manhattan Campus
New York, New York

Ralph Russell Utzman, PT, MPH, PhD
Associate Professor & Academic Coordinator of
    Clinical Education
Division of Physical Therapy
West Virginia University School of Medicine
Morgantown, West Virginia

CONTENTS

4

Introduction to Healthcare as a Unique Insurance-Based Business   51

RESPONSIBILITIES OF THE HEALTHCARE MANAGER   65

5

Responsibilities for Vision, Mission, and Goal Setting   68

6

Responsibilities for Policies and Procedures   78

7

Marketing Responsibilities   84

12

Communication Responsibilities   157

SECTION **3**

MANAGEMENT IN SPECIFIC HEALTHCARE SETTINGS   167

13

Management Issues in Long-Term Care   169

14
Management Issues in Outpatient Centers   192

15
Management Issues in School-Based Services   216

16

Management Issues in Homecare
Organizations   234

17

Management Issues in Hospitals
and Health Systems   254

Appendix 1

A Brief History of Organizations,
Leadership, and Management   281

Appendix 2

Outlines for Three Strategic Plans   284

CONTEMPORARY ISSUES IN HEALTHCARE MANAGEMENT

The two ultimate responsibilities of mid-level healthcare managers are:

1. Identifying and implementing the means for professionals to provide quality care to each of their patients.
2. Contributing to the goals and protecting the interests of their organizations so that necessary resources for providing that care are available.

The balance and coordination of these responsibilities depend on the ability of managers and leaders to grasp the fundamentals of organizations, leadership, and management and to appreciate the unique business of healthcare.

The four chapters in this section of the text provide the context for the contemporary challenges facing physical therapists who are managers or who seek to become managers in any type of healthcare organization. First, the potential opportunities and career paths that can lead to mid-level and executive management positions in healthcare are defined. Questions about the roles of physical therapists as managers in healthcare organizations are raised for consideration by the physical therapy profession.

Next, with these possibilities and questions in mind, the management of the complex, changing nature of healthcare organizations in the United States is introduced. The cultures of different types of healthcare organizations and systems are explored in the context of their responsibilities to, and the expectations of, the communities they serve. Clarifying the differences between healthcare leaders and managers assists readers in understanding how the goals of healthcare organizations are achieved.

The third chapter introduces healthcare as a unique business that requires every manager to develop a comprehensive view of the interactions of the stakeholders in the U.S. healthcare system and their influence on the access, quality, and costs of patient care. The types of health insurance and the regulation of insurance are presented in Chapter 4.

For health professionals who are not managers, Section 1 provides information that may facilitate discussions between physical therapists and their managers as important questions are raised about work ethics and healthcare organizations.

Becoming a Healthcare Manager

LEARNING OBJECTIVES

- Compare and contrast the qualifications of healthcare managers with prior clinical experience with those having academic degrees in some branch of management and no clinical experience.
- Discuss the pros and cons of career ladders that include formal managerial responsibilities.
- Determine the role of mentoring physical therapists (PTs) as they transition from clinical to managerial roles.
- Discuss the relationship of direct patient care skills and management skills of physical therapists, regardless of their job titles.
- Determine the typical responsibilities of mid-level and executive managers in healthcare settings.
- Determine the types of managerial opportunities across different types of healthcare organizations.
- Discuss the need for new managers to possess communication skills, a sense of perspective, and industriousness.
- Determine the need for and appropriateness of delegation.
- Distinguish between a manager's horizontal and vertical communication skills.
- Discuss contemporary issues presented to healthcare mid-level managers that affect patient care outcomes including the nature of work, a diverse workforce, planning, and financial reporting.
- Discuss the challenges to the physical therapy profession in defining and promoting the managerial role of physical therapists in healthcare organizations.

Management Opportunities

All healthcare organizations provide physical therapists with many opportunities to pursue a range of management roles. For example, physical therapists may:

- assume *all* managerial roles in businesses they own
- become frontline supervisors of a single practice within a large, national rehabilitation corporation
- manage several practices as area or regional managers in a large rehabilitation corporation
- manage units of large healthcare organizations
- manage rehabilitation field operations of staff who are not physically in the same locations in home-care organizations and school systems

As part of their professional development, physical therapists may rise through the levels of management in healthcare organizations. In all types of healthcare settings, even new graduates often take on the duties of a unit supervisor or a team leader soon after graduation. Often, success in these positions quickly leads to promotions to mid-level management (positions that are typically defined as one level above the line workers and professionals and two levels below the CEO[1]).

Physical therapists may move from their professional roles in patient care to their first managerial positions without much preparation for their new duties. It is certainly common for many organizations to identify "rising stars" from among their ranks for direct, front-line supervisory roles. These new supervisors are often expected to automatically transfer their strong patient care skills to practice management. They are typically successful because even novice physical therapists are prepared to solve unique problems, implement plans, and communicate effectively.

With this experience and additional managerial training or education, many supervisory physical therapists seek to move up to mid-level management. Healthcare organizations typically require that some mid-level managers, and their upper-level managers, have degrees in management rather than clinical experience In fact, many of them offer in-house training or tuition deferment programs to encourage promotion from within their ranks of healthcare professionals.

Novice Physical Therapists as Managers

Recent research efforts have contributed new information about the healthcare managerial skills required for new physical therapist graduates. In one study, hospital-based, private practice, and academic physical therapists were asked to rank 75 managerial activities. All groups identified communication, financial control, resource allocation, entrepreneur, and leadership skills as the five most important categories for physical therapists in managerial positions. However, the groups differed significantly in their ranking of the activities.[2]

Another study was based on the finance, information management, networking, human resource management, operations, and planning and forecasting (FINHOP) model of administration and management. The model was derived from previous work called the leadership, administration, management, and professional (LAMP) model,[3] and the six categories of administration

and management identified by Luedtke-Hoffman.[4] The study, using the FINHOP model, determined the level of importance of 121 administration and management skills for new physical therapist graduates in 2010.[5] Respondents were physical therapists in academic programs and in hospital-based and private clinical practices. There were no statistical differences among the responses of these subgroups.

Three expected levels of independence in the FINHOP management skills were identified. Expectations were that graduates would be most independent in those managerial skills that related most to direct patient care responsibilities, moderately independent in those skills related to organizational management, and least independent in skills related to the management of the organization within the larger environment.[5]

This study seemed to reflect the typical physical therapist career ladder of the past. New graduates have traditionally practiced managerial skills on a small scale within their zone of safety of direct patient care. Even with very little clinical experience, some PTs were then promoted to line supervisory positions with responsibility for small units in organizations or small freestanding practices within large corporations. As this group gained experience some PTs then moved into mid- and upper-level management positions with responsibilities reaching beyond physical therapy in healthcare organizations. Perhaps the only changes in this career path over the years have been the result of changes in healthcare organizations. For example, even line supervisory positions are more likely to include responsibility for interdisciplinary teams. Over the years, it also seems that more non-clinical managers have joined clinicians in mid-level and upper-level management positions in healthcare.

Health Leadership Competency Model (HLCM)

At the same time the FINHOP model was developing, the Healthcare Leadership Alliance (HLA) began an effort to define contemporary healthcare managers across clinical and non-clinical disciplines. The HLA is a consortium of six major professional membership organizations that offered certifications in management. A consensus process was used to agree on the following five competency domains as common among all practicing health-care managers:[6]

1. Communication and relationship management
2. Professionalism
3. Leadership
4. Knowledge of the healthcare system
5. Business skills and knowledge

To take this effort a step further, an evidence-based, behavioral approach was taken to develop the Health Leadership Competency Model (HLCM).[7] The HLCM begins with three major domains—transformation, execution, and people. The 26 competencies within the domains are listed in Sidebar 1.1. Like the FINHOP model, each HLCM competency has three to five levels for development and assessment of managers as they progress on their career ladders.

The individual physical therapist interacting with the individual patient remains the foundation of the profession, so it is reasonable that managerial expectations for new graduates also lie with direct patient care. Anecdotally, however, it appears that even within a year of graduation, new physical therapists face challenges that demand skills to address demands of a healthcare organization beyond patient interactions that are presented in the HLCM model.

Many health professionals ask themselves why anyone would want to be a healthcare manager. The complexity and challenges of the position can be daunting, but managers see the rewards in having a positive influence on the lives of many more patients and on the community at large. The work of managers is like multiplying the satisfaction of direct patient care a thousand-fold. Mid-level managers essentially influence a broader spectrum of patients and patient care as they accomplish the organization's goals through the work of others.

Adapting the work of others to anticipate or react to ongoing changes seems to be *the* standard operating procedure for healthcare. These ongoing work adaptations are often provoked by new market demands and technological advances, which challenge mid-level managers and make their work exciting and unpredictable.

An opportunity to demonstrate that there may be a better way to handle matters motivates many

---

SIDEBAR 1.1

HLCM Competencies[7]

Transformation—Visioning, energizing, and stimulating a change process that coalesces communities, patients, and professionals around new models of healthcare and wellness.

Achievement Orientation

Analytical Thinking

Community Orientation

Financial Skills

Information Seeking

Innovative Thinking

Strategic Orientation

Execution—Translating vision and strategy into optimal organizational performance.

Accountability

Change Leadership

Collaboration

Communication

Impact and Influence

Information Technology Management

Initiative

Organizational Awareness

Performance Measurement

Process Management and Organizational Design

Project Management

People—Creating an organizational climate that values employees from all backgrounds and provides an energizing environment for them. Also includes the leader's responsibility to understand his or her impact on others and to improve his or her capabilities as well as the capabilities of others.

Human Resources Management

Interpersonal Understanding

Professionalism

Relationship Building

Self-Confidence

Self-Development

Talent Development

Team Leadership

people who are often mystified by the decisions made by "upper-level management." Other people may reach a point in their careers at which they are ready for new responsibilities and new skill sets. Rather than continuing to narrow their work within a clinical specialization, a transition to management responsibilities presents opportunities in a broader sphere of influence. See Activity 1.1.

Transitioning From Patient Care to Management

Some healthcare professionals find themselves formally and deliberately seeking management positions in healthcare organizations or through the development of independent (private) practices. Others find themselves in managerial roles that they often reluctantly accept because no

one else among the ranks of frontline workers is willing to assume other responsibilities. These successful professionals may remain in the dual role of clinical specialist and manager in their new supervisory positions or while they transition to management as a second profession.

In today's healthcare organizations, the dual clinician-manager role may be less common than in the past. Healthcare systems now rely more on merging clinical and support services under fewer and fewer mid-level managers. The discipline-based leader exclusively managing others with the same clinical skills and responsibilities (i.e., a physical therapist who manages only other physical therapists) is no longer the standard operational model. Instead, healthcare managers from any discipline are expected to have generic managerial skills that can be applied across organizational units that include a mix of health professionals.

McConnell cautioned healthcare organizations to avoid assuming that people suddenly become managers because they received a promotion or assuming that a clinical specialty is critical to healthcare management. Rather, he emphasizes that the appointment of new managers should depend on the important management skills that are truly transportable across the traditional departments or units in healthcare organizations. Those skills include proper delegation, clear and open two-way communication, budgeting and cost control, scheduling, handling employee problems, and applying disciplinary action.[8]

Regardless of their clinical disciplines, people who are promoted from within face the same challenges in making career transitions to management roles. Several years ago, Lombardi identified these transitions that remain relevant in today's healthcare system:[9]

- *Self-direction to selfless service.* Managerial work depends on highly variable and unpredictable factors rather than on the more specific professional needs and desires that drive professional performance.

- *Autonomous control to circumstantial control.* The work of managers depends on unpredictable circumstances and situations rather than on assigned caseloads and productivity expectations. Flexibility is much more critical.

- *Quantitative to qualitative outcomes.* The outcomes of a manager's efforts are more dependent

---

ACTIVITY 1.1
WHAT WOULD YOU DO?

Tina Thompson is a recent physical therapy graduate who accepted her first position as a staff physical therapist in a large healthcare system. She was assigned to one of four outpatient rehabilitation centers that are staffed with a supervisor, another physical therapist, a physical therapist assistant, a rehabilitation technician, and a part-time occupational therapist. Several other physical and occupational therapists are available to work per diem (by the hour as needed) if there are spikes in the number of patients or to replace people on vacation or on sick leave.

After being on the job for only 2 months, Tina and the staff are told by their supervisor that he has been reassigned to open the system's fifth center. Privately, he tells Tina that he would like to recommend that the Vice President of Rehabilitation Services promote her to take over his position. It means about a 20% salary increase and Tina will be expected to devote about 20% of her time to her new duties while maintaining a reduced patient load.

What questions should Tina ask? Whom should she meet with? What are the pros and cons of accepting the promotion?

on perceptions than on clearly defined measures. The immediate gratification that healthcare professionals receive through patient outcomes and the financial rewards for reaching productivity goals are diminished.

● *Definitive clinical criteria to overall comprehensive goals.* The performance criteria for managers are often gray and flexible as organizations change, and managers' responsibilities fluctuate with the needs of the organization. The clear job descriptions of clinicians are replaced with expectations that are more ambiguous.

Put another way, clinical professionals focus on making independent decisions about individual patients based on the continued development of their technical skills for quality direct patient care. As managers, they are one step removed from patients and individual outcomes. Instead, their focus is on facilitating others and building networks in the broader healthcare organization. The rewards of helping patients accomplish their goals are replaced with the less concrete managerial rewards of helping others achieve their work performance goals.[10] They find more variability and a need for more flexibility in their daily work in these new positions.

The transition to management certainly provides exciting opportunities for the acquisition of a new skill set for new duties. At the same time, there is that period of discomfort that comes from leaving behind the structure and familiarity with patient care to take on the uncertainties of management. Managerial opportunities and possibilities can be intimidating, but they enrich and challenge even those new managers who reluctantly assumed their new roles.

Formal Graduate Management Education

Whether managing by choice or by fiat, healthcare professionals may choose to explore graduate degrees to prepare for management positions, or they may learn the skills by immediate necessity of experience, self-study, or in-house training. Typically, it is some combination of all of these strategies. Determining the value of formal programs is an important decision. Activity 1.2 offers

---

ACTIVITY 1.2
MANAGEMENT EDUCATION/PREPARATION

1. What should someone look for in a formal management degree program?
2. What are all of the graduate degree possibilities? Is the master of business administration (MBA) or master of public administration (MPA) the degree of choice for healthcare managers? Are there other choices? Defend your preferences.
3. What do the following organizations say about healthcare management?
   American College of Healthcare Administrators http://www.achca.org/
   Occupational Outlook Handbook of the U.S. Department of Labor's Bureau of Labor and Statistics http://www.bls.gov/oco/ocos014.htm
   American College of Healthcare Executives http://www.ache.org/
   Commission on Accreditation of Healthcare Management http://www.cahmeweb.org/
   Association of University Programs in Health Administration http://www.aupha.org/i4a/pages/index.cfm?pageid=1

   Institute for Diversity in Health Management http://www.diversityconnection.org/
   American Association of Healthcare Administrative Management http://www.aaham.org/

4. Identify at least two graduate programs in management. Compare and contrast their curricula, costs, and graduate placement information. Are they accredited? By whom? Which one is most attractive? Why?
5. Identify a healthcare corporation or system that has an internal management development program. Find out about it. Talk with a physical therapist who has experience with one. What is good about the program? What is its downside? Determine whether the emphasis of the program is developing people management skills or developing financial management skills. Does it matter? Why?

some ideas for exploring management degree programs.

Mentoring

Another important consideration in transitioning from clinical care to management responsibilities is the identification of mentors who can help in the process. Morton-Cooper and Palmer identified the importance of mentoring in healthcare careers and suggested that it should begin with the very first clinical position. In their model, the person who seeks mentoring must initiate it as a long-term intimate, personal, and enabling relationship. The mentor does not formally assess the person, but rather provides unstructured support for learning and for facilitating access to the important social and political networks needed for continued career socialization.[11]

Mentoring, when a person is taking on new managerial responsibilities, may be even more critical than having a clinical mentor. The changing needs within healthcare organizations make the roles and expectations of managers much more volatile than the roles of clinicians. The support of a mentor or mentors as a new manager "thinks out loud" is very important in meeting day-to-day managerial challenges and for long-term career development.

A different model of mentoring places the responsibility for mentoring on the organization. In this model, assigned mentors are responsible for introducing new employees to the organization's culture and the technical and functional aspects of their positions. Such a formalized program is believed to improve the retention of employees because they develop emotional ties to the organization through their mentors. Increased job satisfaction and productivity are the results.[12] This model does not preclude a person from personally initiating mentoring relationships from within or beyond his or her organization. See Sidebar 1.2 for more information on mentoring.

Transitioning to new roles and mentoring, like most management issues, are found in all types of businesses. Healthcare requires special manager skills because of the nature of the business—the provision of efficient and effective healthcare for people in the communities while controlling ever-increasing costs with ever-decreasing reimbursement. Larger and more complex healthcare

---

SIDEBAR 1.2

Roles of a Mentor

Novice managers should identify what they need in a mentor(s) to ensure smooth transitions from health professional to manager. Identifying which of the following types of mentors is most important is a critical first step:[10]

- Sponsor: to open doors for the new manager
- Coach: to show "the ropes" of the new position
- Protector: to buffer negative experiences
- Exposer: to create new opportunities
- Challenger: to stretch the manager's new skills and scope of work
- Role model: to develop new behaviors by example
- Counselor: to accept and confirm efforts and to offer friendship

---

organizations require more levels of management to run their special businesses.

Managers in Large Healthcare Organizations

The day-to-day healthcare worker in a large healthcare organization or system has very little direct interaction with upper-level managers including the chief executive officer and a cadre of vice presidents who are responsible for organizational units such as finance, purchasing, human resources, marketing, facilities management, and medical services. The larger the organization becomes, the more divided the executive functions become. The division of labor enables organizations to keep current with the complex changes in healthcare reimbursement, rules and regulations, new technology, and other demands. It often appears that upper-level management is top-heavy because the number of mid-level management positions often decreases as healthcare organizations flatten their bureaucratic structures.

Mid-level managers today in healthcare have a direct influence on the coordination and delivery of patient care through frequent interactions with the personnel they supervise and other managers. This level of management may be organized by departments such as rehabilitation, pharmacy, nursing, housekeeping, dietary, and business office; or they may be organized into multidisciplinary teams with a focus on the delivery of specialized patient care such as a heart institute or a stroke team. Many large healthcare organizations are a hybrid of the two models.

Management in Other Healthcare Settings

In smaller healthcare organizations, all levels of employees may interact with upper-level managers almost every day. For example, in a long-term-care skilled nursing facility the finance, purchasing, human resources, marketing, facilities management, and medical services requiring many vice presidents in hospital systems are typically all the direct responsibility of a single nursing home administrator. These administrators work in concert with their directors of nursing and rehabilitation who lead the direct patient care clinical services. They also rely on business office managers who typically handle human resources, payroll, reimbursement, and billing. Both the clinical and business managers report directly to the administrator. Some administrators may have "home office" corporate support if the nursing home is part of a larger chain of many buildings.

The solo private practitioner physical therapist is another kind of healthcare manager who performs all business roles as both the executive and mid-level manager of the business, while concurrently having all responsibility for direct patient care. These physical therapists may have other staff to supervise in the provision of physical therapy care to patients, and they may contract services such as billing, accounting, and reimbursement contract negotiations.

Examples of other healthcare organizations include home health agencies, physician practice groups, and special education services in school systems that may have a different range of managerial expectations. For instance, a physical therapist may be the countywide coordinator for all rehabilitation services in a school system or the supervisor of an interdisciplinary team that provides rehab services in several schools in a district. The unique challenges for managers in different types of healthcare settings are presented in Section 3. However, regardless of the type of healthcare setting, efforts to meet an organization's goals depend in a large part on the people management skills of supervisors and mid-level managers. Their personal career success is also driven by people management.

People Management Skills

The good news for physical therapists and other healthcare professionals is that unlike other businesses, mid-level healthcare managers spend a great deal of their time—about 65%—on people management, which is already a strength of successful practitioners. With only about 10% of their time spent on financial analysis, the rest of the time is spent dealing with special projects and "administrivia."[9] The emphasis on people management responsibilities may make a move to a management position more attractive, or less threatening, for many physical therapists. A shift of their already well-developed people skills to a different level of interaction with others often comes naturally.

The challenge, of course, is that most people are very resistant to being managed. The best employees know enough and care enough to manage themselves—especially healthcare professionals. We all prefer *not* to be told what to do. In reality, managers *cannot* force people to care about patients, or expect them to know all there is to know about patient care, or demand that they create new approaches to accomplish patient goals. What managers *can* do is to sustain the best interests and qualities of individuals in their work performance so that the organization can then sustain its collective purpose and interests. The more successful that mid-level managers are in developing these employee/employer bonds, the more likely it will be that everyone in an organization will share the same values.[12]

Several managerial perspectives have led to lists of knowledge and skills required of mid-level managers in contemporary healthcare as they do the important work of resolving the tension between the needs of the healthcare organization as a whole and the needs of the individuals who work within it.

Keeping People Happy

Anecdotally, physical therapy managers often describe their job as "keeping everyone happy." *Everyone* means the staff they manage, the upper-level managers they report to, and the shareholders with their attention on outcome. Several authors have explored people management skills in healthcare. First, Kane-Urrabazo identified the importance of nursing managers having the following important characteristics and skills:[12]

- Integrity and trust
- Empowerment and delegation
- Consistency in decisions and mentorship

The actions of managers that result from these important qualities must be consistent with those broader values and beliefs of the organization. Their consistent decisions and mentoring that empower people in a trusting work environment are most likely effective when they are also embedded in the culture of the organization.

Integrity and Trust

The work of Garman, Fitz, and Fraser reinforces this perspective with a similar argument that demonstrating integrity and engendering trust are critical qualities of managers.[14] They extend the generally accepted definition of *integrity*, which is the adherence to ethical standards. They believe the decisions and actions of managers with the highest levels of integrity are consistent, methodical, and backed by clear explanations for them. Input from others who are impacted by those decisions and actions increases the level of integrity.

The authors give equal weight to the importance of a manager's ability to engender trust. Often, earning the trust of another person is easily done, but also easily diminished. Only one negative action or decision can destroy trust. Like integrity, trust in the workplace also depends on consistency, but the focus is on consistent follow-through on commitments made. To be trusted, managers must do what they say they are going to do. Employees expect managers to respect their needs or wants and to make a commitment to meet them. Managers also need to provide an explanation if they cannot keep a commitment or that trust will be diminished.

From a slightly different perspective, Magretta and Stone reinforce the need for integrity and trust. They suggest that managers who know what employees really want ("keep them happy") are at an advantage. Their words of wisdom for managers listed here appear to embody the qualities of trust, empowerment, mentoring, and consistency. These hints also appear applicable to patient care interactions—simply another form of people management, after all:[13]

- Be kind and respectful.
- Be fair.
- Do as you say and mean what you say.
- Guide and give inspiration to people.
- People yearn to be loyal.
- People want to be trusted.
- Foster "know thyself" so people can self-manage.
- Ask this important question often: "Why do you work?"
- Focus on the results of work rather than on how hard someone is working.
- Hang together even if there is disagreement.
- Managing is about trade-offs, not compromise.
- Managers can't be all things to all people.
- Stay the course of the organization.

Embertson bases her view of mid-level managers on five important roles they play. These roles reinforce the need for people management skills in the reaction to change and achievement of the goals in healthcare organizations.[15]

1. *Communicators* who customize the organizational message for the individual by often relying on informal networks.
2. *Entrepreneurs* who recognize the problems on the frontlines of operation and who are able to find solutions faster than managers higher up on the organizational ladder.
3. *Stabilizers* who juggle the organization's goals and budgets while balancing work to please employees and senior managers. They also balance continuity and change in the organization.
4. *Therapists* as they help employees cope with stress about work, particularly during periods of change. Often on a daily basis, mid-level managers may support and encourage

employees who may be anxious about the uncertainty of the organization or feel alienated. Removing emotional barriers to work enables the highest levels of performance.

5. *Future leaders* as they gain the experience and training needed for upper-level management positions.

Finally, in Lombardi's view, what employees really want is a fair wage, work direction, respect, and recognition for their level of performance. Managers who can provide that for people are bound to be successful and feel good about their managerial efforts.[9] Lombardi has also given thought to the characteristics of new managers that relate to people management. He suggests that there are only three: a sense of perspective, industriousness, and communication skills, which are discussed in more depth in the following sections. See Activity 1.3.

A Manager's Sense of Perspective

Lombardi believes that mid-level managers need to consider the perspectives of all stakeholders to take the action that is most likely to be successful when problems arise. Gathering the important points of view on a particular issue—What does the boss think? What do my team members think? What do the other managers think?—is a critical first step in this data-gathering process. The next step for managers is to make an analysis of the reasons that each stakeholder holds a particular perspective, followed by an honest examination of their own self-interests. Then managers face the challenge of synthesizing all of these perspectives to take action.

Perhaps identifying *which* stakeholders' perspectives are salient for any important decision may be a more important skill than the ability to reconcile every possible perspective. No one likes to be left out, yet attempts to be all inclusive may be futile. However, of all possible stakeholders, those consistently seeking, considering, and integrating the perspectives of patients may be key to decisions that positively impact an organization's goals.

A Manager's Industriousness

Industriousness is the second skill in Lombardi's model. Industriousness does not necessarily mean working 80 hours per week to accomplish all of the work for which healthcare managers are responsible. None of the organizational goals can be accomplished by, nor should they be dependent on, one person. Industriousness involves taking initiative while learning to delegate effectively. Why and how often tasks are delegated are major factors in the determination of managerial effectiveness and a mirror of industriousness. The ability to take a worry-free extended vacation depends on a manager whose staff has passed the test for performing delegated responsibilities—a staff expected to cover the duties of absent managers and readily accept the responsibility.

Arnold and Pulich suggest that the key to the success of new managers is based on the avoidance of three common delegation mistakes:[16]

1. Delegation by dumping—automatically passing on whatever needs to be done.

2. Delegation only to good performers—often results in anger if repeatedly asked to step up.

3. Delegation only to ineffective performers—keeps good performers from becoming rivals of the manager.

Delegation based on any of these strategies may lead to excessive work for the manager and diminished work effectiveness for everyone. See Sidebar 1.3 for suggestions for proper delegation.

ACTIVITY 1.3
GIVING THEM WHAT THEY WANT

Sam Thompson is the new Manager of Rehabilitation Services that includes a staff of three physical therapists, three physical therapist assistants, three occupational therapists, three occupational therapy assistants, and one speech-language pathologist. There is also a pool of four physical therapists and two occupational therapists who work as contract, per diem employees. Because he is new to this healthcare system and the person he is replacing was ineffective, Sam wants to wipe the slate clean and get to know his employees. What should his plan be for doing so? How long should it take? What information does he need to gather from his staff? What questions should he expect his staff to ask? What should Sam anticipate as being most important to his staff?

SIDEBAR 1.3

Things to Delegate and Not to Delegate

DELEGATE WHEN . . .

- All necessary information is available for the task to be delegated.
- The responsibilities are more about operations than about planning and organizing.
- Others are more qualified or have the necessary skills that are not your strengths.
- Responsibilities can be provided that allow people to grow and challenge them.
- Assignments require evaluation and recommendations.
- The tasks are more routine, requiring only minor decisions.
- There are clear job descriptions and work expectations.
- A follow-up plan upon completion is in place.

DO NOT DELEGATE WHEN . . .

- The team needs leadership in determining priorities and setting goals.
- The task involves planning and solving new problems.
- The task is developing teams.
- Coaching and motivating are needed.
- Subordinates' performances are being evaluated.
- Personnel are being rewarded or disciplined.
- The assignment was given directly to you to complete.
- The work had already been assigned to someone else; do not overlap assignments.

Industriousness is an important characteristic of mid-level managers for another reason. If managers are the role models for industriousness through their hard-working, conscientious, and energetic behaviors, employees are more likely to incorporate the same behaviors in their patient care. Achieving balance through time management and priority setting also establishes guidelines for clinicians who are responsible for their own work schedules.

It may seem that the entire weight of the organization falls on mid-level managers caught in the crosshairs of the organization's aims to achieve its mission. Often, it is not the amount of work but rather the unpredictable nature of the work that creates stress for managers. An urgent meeting or a new deadline, which was not even considered when the manager arrived at work, often challenges the best laid plans for completing a day's work.

As a result, rather than time management, crisis management is the skill required. Everything that comes up seems to be someone's crisis. Taking care of "it," the sooner the better, and as simply as possible, can require time that was intended for anticipated or scheduled work. Therefore, industriousness is more about fitting things in than blocking time out. Avoiding the temptation to continue expanding the time devoted to work rather than fitting the work into a given block of time is perhaps one of the management skills required for success—and sanity.

The third of Lombardi's essential skills for managers is communication. Because of their position in systems, mid-level managers are at the crossroads of horizontal lines of communication with other mid-level managers and vertical communication with those above and below them in the chain of command.

A Manager's Horizontal Communication

Determining which other mid-level managers are most important to their work is a concern for new managers. The importance of other managers may be variable and dependent on several factors. These factors include the time spent with each other, common management goals to be accomplished, and shared responsibility for a particular patient population.[9] Directly related to perspective and time management, this horizontal interaction is often both the formal and informal means for managers to stay well informed of daily organizational events.

In well-structured organizations, mid-level managers have time for planning and reflecting because they are not caught up in an ongoing, never-ending eruption of daily challenges and problems that must be dealt with or prevented. To accomplish this, organizations need to find the perfect number of mid-level managers—not so many that communication and coordination among them to accomplish the organization's goals are impossible, but not so few that each one is overwhelmed with daily responsibilities so that tasks are left undone or done ineffectively. The fewer mid-level management positions there are, the more important it is for those managers to be prepared to, and permitted to, solve problems for themselves and empower their work groups to make decisions for themselves.[17]

Finding that perfect number of mid-level managers has led healthcare systems to adopt a variety of management models. Many of them take a hybrid approach to mid-level management of services. A hybrid model is a combination of centralized and decentralized management. For instance, mid-level managers of non-clinical services (e.g., physical plant, housekeeping, dietary, maintenance, IT) may have responsibility for centralized services with clearly defined responsibilities across an entire healthcare system. Even with multiple buildings and locations, healthcare systems often centralize those services to control costs by standardizing policies and procedures for consistency in these support services.

Concurrently, the same healthcare system decentralizes its clinical services into units with specialized teams, which allows for more immediate decision-making and for the flexibility required to meet current regulatory and reimbursement demands. For example, one clinical manager may lead an interdisciplinary team in one of the specialty services such as organ transplantation. Another manager may lead the services for patients with diabetes that span inpatient, outpatient, and home-care services in a comprehensive, long-term program.

The responsibilities of managers and the lines of responsibility in these matrix clinical models are much more complex than the management of the traditional silos of healthcare disciplines that were common in the past.[18] For example, the position of director of physical therapy seems to be outdated in large healthcare organizations. Instead, a physical therapist may be the manager of all of the staff from different disciplines in a rehabilitation unit of a hospital or nursing home or lead a specialty team for patients with joint replacements or with open-heart surgery.

Agencies that accredit and license healthcare organizations are responsible for this trend. They demand a demonstration of teamwork as evidence for increased efficiency and quality control. However, some authors fear this focus on intra-team collaboration results in a neglect of the equally important cooperation across healthcare departments.[18] They suggest that healthcare managers must also be responsible for the cooperative, coordinated, and collaborative relationships across departments and programs for the parts to fit within the whole organization. Healthcare teams depend on this interdependence because patient treatments often require multiple inputs from specialty teams and support services during the course of a hospitalization. For example, a patient may require that the output of the care received from Team A becomes the input for Team B that continues the next phase of that care. In turn, Team B's output may be needed again by Team A or even by Team C. The ability to provide this complex patient care and to resolve conflicts is largely dependent on the ability of managers to communicate effectively and efficiently. See Activity 1.4.

A Manager's Vertical Communication

Vertical communication skills are equally important for mid-level managers. First, communication with their immediate superiors and subordinates *must* include a clear understanding of responsibilities, priorities, and level of authority for all duties that each of them is assigned. Second, feedback from

---

ACTIVITY 1.4
HORIZONTAL COMMUNICATION

Rebecca Levin is the Manager of Rehabilitation Services in a Good Shepherd Healthcare System. She wants to analyze her interactions with all of the other managers in the system to determine whether she is concentrating her efforts effectively. Create a list of all of the managers (clinical and support services) with whom Rebecca can expect to interact. Estimate how frequently she would communicate with each manager. What mode of communication would be most likely? Would you expect the communication to be more about planning or more about crisis management?

superiors and subordinates on managerial performance is essential. Establishing the method for, and the frequency of, communication is vital. The determination of what needs to be reported, to whom, and when is critical.

The mid-level manager may have to take the initiative and be persistent for this communication to happen. After all, many people want the same limited amount of one-on-one time with the boss. Consistent communication with upper-level managers is important because of the volatile nature of healthcare and the effect that any change has on the daily operations of patient care. Constant clarification of managerial duties and responsibilities and consistent feedback are essential activities to problem-solving and proactive action that ensure an organization's growth and success.

The same communication needs cascade down from the mid-level manager to the people whom they supervise. Managers must clearly communicate clinical and reporting responsibilities to each employee and consistently provide performance feedback. This communication includes establishing work assignments, giving feedback on productivity and patient outcomes, and realigning responsibilities as needed.

Unlike the stability of a routine schedule for communication with mid-level managers' bosses, the frequency of communication that mid-level managers have with each employee or contingency worker may change as each person's work stabilizes. This need for communication may not be the same for all employees or the same over time for each employee. In all cases, again, the mid-level manager must assume responsibility for initiating and sustaining this communication.

As the go-between for the organization and the employees they supervise, mid-level managers also are the filter for both formal and informal information about the organization as a whole. Knowing what information to share and when to share it is a delicate process. On one hand, no one likes to be the last to know, but on the other hand, too much information can be distracting and disruptive. Managers want to dispel the distrust that may arise if people suspect that there are upper-level management secrets being kept from them. They also should prevent employees from becoming so overwhelmed with information that they no longer listen.

Mid-level managers make similar decisions about what and how much information they should relay to their superiors. What are the small issues that a manager has the authority to handle without reporting? What are the big issues that need to be reported? The ability to be selective about what is important is the art of mid-level management. See Activity 1.5.

ACTIVITY 1.5
THE PERSON IN THE MIDDLE

Scenario One: Jackie Janowitz is the Director of Rehabilitation Services in a large medical center. Jackie has a standing meeting with Paula Johannson, the Vice President for Clinical Services, every Monday at 3 p.m. for about 15 minutes. They call it the "debriefing." They consistently devote some of that time each week to discussing patient care and staffing issues. The rest of the time provides Paula the opportunity to notify Jackie of pending projects or reports, and Jackie reports on any informal "hallway" talk she thinks Paula needs to know about.

This formal weekly process of communication has been effective for the past year or so. However, this is now the third week that Paula has cancelled the meeting because of other things that have come up. Jackie is unsure what to make of this. What do you think? What should Jackie have done over the past 3 weeks? What should Jackie do now?

Scenario Two: Jackie has received an unexpected memo by e-mail from the Vice President for Facilities Management. Effective the first of the month, a little more than 2 weeks from now, the staff office for the rehabilitation team is to be relocated to the basement to expand their current space for outpatient radiology services. How should Jackie react? What should she do next?

Scenario Three: Jackie has all of her staff block out 11:30 a.m. to 12:00 p.m. every other Wednesday so that she may hold a staff meeting if necessary. She is very good about communicating items that the staff needs to know and giving them kudos every day. The meetings are for staff input into decisions, projects, and so forth. She is trying to decide whether the move to a new space, the second time this year, should be communicated by e-mail, whether she should wait until next week's meeting, or whether she should hold an emergency meeting this week. What should Jackie do?

Other Contemporary People Management Issues

This section briefly introduces three issues that demand the attention of contemporary mid-level healthcare managers. These issues include the nature of work, the diversity of healthcare workers, and the reporting of revenue and expenses that affect the most important responsibility of healthcare managers—patient care.

The Nature of Work

There are fewer people than there were in the past who fill the traditional full-time employee role dedicated to one organization for an entire career. Rather, it is more common for health professionals to have several employers during the span of their careers for a variety of reasons, such as job dissatisfaction or promotions. It is now common to have healthcare workers who are assigned to work in organizations by employment agencies for temporary, brief periods. Other healthcare professionals may be independent contractors who accept only assignments attractive to them on a part-time or intermittent basis. At the same time, healthcare employers often limit an individual's work hours to avoid the high costs of benefits packages they are required to offer to full-time employees.

The shift to this contingency workforce of per diem, temporary, short-term, and part-time workers means that healthcare managers are responsible for creating and facilitating teams whose members may not all have a long-term commitment to the organization's goals. These management challenges are intensified because of the 24/7 nature of the business of providing patient care within the demands of third-party utilization requirements. For instance, the rehabilitation process for patients cannot be delayed or interrupted, for even a day without a potential negative impact on discharge plans and reimbursement. The demand for managers to provide 7-day coverage of efficient and effective patient care has significantly increased as a result. It is easy to understand how in times of labor shortages, the human resources manager is likely to be the most critical horizontal connection for mid-level clinical managers.

Workforce Diversity

Another consideration in managing workers in contemporary healthcare is the issue of diversity. Although organizations may direct much attention to the need for cultural competency to meet the needs of diverse groups of people, the actual effect of a diverse staff on the outputs of healthcare organizations remains unclear. One view is that a diverse workforce is desirable because a variety of perspectives is invaluable for solving management problems and for meeting the needs of a wide range of cultures represented by the patients served in any community. Not only has this view not been supported, but also diverse groups of workers have been found to be less communicative and less integrated. This distancing results in increased levels of conflict among workers.[19]

Racial/Ethnic Diversity

The challenge for predominantly white, male upper-level management in healthcare organizations is to see beyond minority hiring in lower-level positions as the answer to diversity challenges. They need to understand that any racial and ethnic tensions in their communities spill over into their organizations. Aries explored these challenges for an understanding of the effect of diversity on healthcare workers and the patient populations they serve. The conclusions of this qualitative study included the following:[19]

- Different groups viewed cultural competence and the effectiveness of organizational interventions to achieve it differently.
- The focus of upper-level managers was managing diversity at the broadest level rather than at the level of patient care.
- Mid-level managers had a great deal of freedom to manage diversity at the departmental level, which resulted in a perception of inconsistent and mixed messages among employees and patients about the institution's commitment to cultural competence.
- Mid-level managers were aware of diversity problems, but felt that the problems were those of particular individuals rather than a systemwide issue. They felt that workers should focus on the demands and competence of coworkers rather than these distracting concerns.

- Frontline workers resented the responsibilities for addressing the needs of diverse patient populations. They felt that cultural stereotyping and racism were embedded in the institution and affected their work.
- For patients, their impression of the quality of care they received was rooted in the way they were treated as members of racial or ethnic groups. They were not sensitive to the effect of the diversity of the staff who cared for them.
- Available translation services were inadequate and relied on informal systems. Bilingual employees were often called on for translation, taking them away from their assigned duties.
- Staff and patients saw biases embedded in the day-to-day operations regardless of the organization's official position on diversity.

The potential for others to perceive managers as playing favorites with staff who are of the same racial or ethnic group may become an issue if they do not communicate job descriptions, performance criteria, and other requirements clearly and consistently to everyone. The more diverse the work group is, the more important it becomes to demonstrate actions and decisions that provoke reactions of fairness and trust. Employees need to be reassured that any new emerging group will not threaten established personnel policies. Managers need to spend time observing and discussing coworker interactions to determine whether the inevitable conflicts that arise in any workplace are individual differences or a broader cultural issue that demands broader systemwide attention.[19]

Generation Gaps

Another source of diversity for consideration is the diversity of different generations of workers. Also controversial, generational differences have received a great deal of recent attention in the popular press. For instance, based on the definitions of generations defined by Zemke, Raines, and Filipczak[20] as Veterans, Baby Boomers, Generation Xers, and Nexters, Arsenault studied how each group viewed the characteristics of leaders. Briefly summarized, the results for each generation were:[21]

- Veterans (born 1922–1943): Value loyalty; believe in authority and hierarchical relationships.
- Baby Boomers (born 1944–1960): Prefer participative, collegial workplace with shared responsibility and respect.
- Generation Xers (born 1961–1980): Expect diversity and change, informality and fun, and question authority.
- Nexters (born 1981–2000): Prefer a polite relationship with authority and want leaders to pull people together. Believe in collective action and a will to change things. They are optimistic, confident, and take pride in civic duty.

Managers need to determine the potential value of recognizing generational differences and their effects on work in healthcare. Identification of ways to build on the strengths of each group may be the key to reducing another source of potential conflict among coworkers. See Activity 1.6.

Financial Issues for Mid-Level Managers

A potential misconception about mid-level managers is that they need a master of business administration (MBA) to function effectively because of their financial responsibilities. It is more likely that their financial responsibilities are limited to completion of reports and requests for data during the organization's budgeting process. This process requires more negotiation than financial skills to influence budget decisions that are not really the responsibility of mid-level managers. Typically, for example, requests for capital equipment, and maybe even supplies, must be approved by, at the least, the next person in command.

Perhaps more important, mid-level managers *are* expected to track and understand income and expenses for their units. They need a level of math proficiency to identify and analyze trends in daily patient care data that must be explained to their bosses. Justification of bonuses and other performance rewards for their employees may be driven by the ability to translate the numbers into action vertically in both directions. Solo practitioners who also are the executive managers for their own businesses normally rely on accountants or business financial experts to assist them with the money management of their businesses. These practitioners need enough knowledge to have discussions for productive decision-making with these experts.

ACTIVITY 1.6
STAFFING

As the only physical therapist at Shady Pines Nursing Home, Bob Crawford has been called to a meeting by the administrator with the Director of Nursing, the occupational therapist (OT), and the part-time speech-language pathologist. The agenda is to brainstorm ideas to address the increasing tensions among the staff about patient schedules, responsibilities for patient care, cooperation between nursing and rehabilitation, and what are perceived to be unfair management decisions about salaries and vacation scheduling.

About 85% of the certified nursing assistants (CNAs) are Haitian. About 60% of the LPNs are African American, and the RNs and all of the therapists and the administrator are white. The PT assistant is Puerto Rican and the two OT assistants are Jamaican. The administrator is in her early 30s but everyone else at the meeting is in their 50s.

The patients who are permanent residents represent a wide range of ethnic groups, but less than 10% are people of color and only 1% speak Spanish. The short-term residents, who are admitted for rehabilitation and typically discharged after a few weeks, are predominantly of the Jewish faith.

How much attention does this management team need to devote to the diversity of their employees to reduce the workplace tensions?

Managers and Patients

The financial bottom line of an organization must be considered in the context of the *real* bottom line—the health and satisfaction of the community it serves. Mid-level managers share responsibility for the implementation of the organization's plans for the delivery of patient care. Most managers in healthcare are at least one step removed from the direct patient care provided by the practitioners they supervise. This creates an important patient–practitioner–manager triad that may be viewed from Anderson's framework for understanding service organizations.[22]

For instance, one of Anderson's propositions is that an employee's perception of being treated unfairly and unjustly may lead to poor work performance, which then leads to less than satisfactory customer satisfaction. When the manager–employee relationship is good, so are work outcomes, and so, it follows, are positive patient outcomes. Any small change in the manager–practitioner relationship may have a huge influence on the employee's relationship with a patient. In other words, the patient-provider relationship mirrors the provider–manager relationship.

When things are not going well, an employee's frustration and dissatisfaction may be sensed as discomfort by the patient. Healthcare is emotional labor in which workers perform the work and manage the work processes as well. Unlike other industries, the patient is part of the production. This uniqueness requires a complex linkage among patients, providers, and managers.[22]

Mid-level managers often find their interactions with their staffs positive and rewarding, but it is the result of those interactions—their indirect influence on patient care—that often remains the true source of their job satisfaction. It is with the mid-level manager that all of the communication, coordination, and collaboration efforts come together to provide efficient and effective services to patients. This manager–practitioner–patient triad makes healthcare managers different from managers in other industries. An important measure of healthcare quality for patients is their perception of how well those services are delivered, rather than the actual interventions included in their care. The patient does not say, "Wow, that was a great IV!" Rather, a patient says, "Wow, everyone really took good care of me." Because these services are intangible, unstandardized, and produced/consumed simultaneously, it is difficult to measure managerial success. Therefore, establishment of the measures of management success is important. Performance evaluation that depends only on the things that can be directly measured fails to provide meaningful information about this complex work. See Activity 1.7.

Executive Managers in Healthcare

Many managers who come from clinical disciplines may feel that mid-level management is as far as they would like to reach beyond patient care. Others may aspire to executive positions, but hesitate as they realize that these career moves create such a huge gap between them and patients that they no longer feel part of their professional

ACTIVITY 1.7
MANAGING PATIENT CARE

Pat Fletcher is an occupational therapist who is the Manager of Rehabilitation Services at Oakmont Medical Center. He makes daily rounds on each of the three floors of his hospital to check on how things are going with his interdisciplinary staff. Pat has had some encounters with a few of the physical therapists who seem resentful that an occupational therapist is checking up on their patient care because he is not a PT. In terms of the manager–practitioner–patient triad, analyze this situation. What action should Pat take?

disciplines. To address the recruitment demands for executives in today's volatile, complex, and expanding world of healthcare systems, the creation of executive leadership development programs has been on the rise since 2003. Fifty percent of healthcare systems now have ongoing programs to meet their specific needs for strategic planning for their organizations while planning for a succession of leaders.[23] These programs provide opportunities for those aspiring to executive positions.

Typically, staff in healthcare organizations know who the executives and executives-in-training are, although they do not interact with them on a regular basis. Employees perceive the executive office to be isolated, or at least distant, from the real work of patient care. Contrary to popular opinion, these hidden executives are not the ultimate decision makers. Rather, they are the agents of their governing boards, which are discussed in Chapter 3. They design the structures and implement the processes needed to support the actions and impressions of all stakeholders in the organization.

Perhaps an even more important executive responsibility is running the collateral organization—that group of task forces, committees, and ad hoc groups that are formed to bring different perspectives on issues. The purpose of this organization-within-an-organization is to address common problems in the accountability chains so that conflict and confusion are defused. Some of these groups are formed to address a particular problem and others are formed as long-standing committees. Executives are responsible for identifying membership in these groups to work out the details of implementing strategic decisions.[24]

The challenges for many executives in healthcare arise because they are typically *not* health professionals yet they manage health professionals who have their own ideas of how healthcare should be run from a clinical rather than business perspective. Clinicians may become resentful because of their perception that non-health-professional bosses do not know how patient care works. Whether this perception is accurate or not, the ability of executives to see and react to the big picture of healthcare may be a far more important skill set than clinical skills.[10] Because healthcare has become a complex business, it is no surprise that the selection of executives in all types of healthcare settings has shifted from physicians and nurses to professional managers without patient care experience.

Conversely, at the least, there needs to be some type of executive partnership with clinical professionals because of the nature and importance of this unique business. This relationship is typically dependent on a physician who is elected or appointed as Chief of Staff. This person is often described as the buffer between physicians and the executive team in a healthcare organization. Depending on this relationship, executives may relate to physicians as customers of the organization. In other hospitals, physicians act as equal partners in the business of healthcare. The reality is that regardless of the organizational relationship between executives and physicians, patients often think hospitals and the physicians treating them are the same entity. Although there may be internal conflicts and tension, it is the melding of the clinical and business components of healthcare organizations that leads to this patient perception and to the organization's ability to provide the right care at the right place at the right time.

In a recent study of the competencies required of the people in three levels of managerial positions (executives/"chiefs," vice presidents, and managers/directors), the researchers recognized the range of the work and the shift in focus of clinical and administrative managers[25] that are consistent with the FINHOP and HLCM models. Based on a review of eight competency models, they identified the following 10 competency domains:

1. **Governance** (boards) and one's own organizational structure.
2. **Healthcare** environment, how it functions as a system, and interactions of healthcare workforce and patients.

3. **General management principles** for healthcare delivery and day-to-day operations.

4. **Business** skills of planning, marketing, and so forth applied to healthcare.

5. **Professionalism and ethics** to align personal and professional behaviors.

6. **Human resources** to recruit, retain, and develop clinical and non-clinical staff.

7. **Finance** to understand costs, payment mechanisms, and the interactions of providers and payers.

8. **Healthcare technology and information management** to plan, implement, and monitor health information systems.

9. **Quality and performance improvement** to understand benchmarks, implement performance improvement, and provide high-quality patient care.

10. **Laws and regulations** to understand the role of government in payment, regulations, and the rights of patients and employees.

Although common to all levels of managers, where a manager's position falls in an organization's hierarchy changes the focus of these competencies. For example, executives and vice presidents are more likely to need competencies related to long-term planning and external relationships in healthcare systems and communities, while managers and directors need those competencies required for daily operational issues.[25]

Regardless of the size or type of healthcare setting, Ross and his coauthors argue that executive management boils down to three basic duties that do not change despite the challenges at any given time in healthcare, although the degree of responsibility may change from setting to setting. These duties include the following:[26]

- Increasing efficiency and financial stability through human resources, financial management, cost accounting, data collection and analysis, strategic planning, marketing, etc.

- Providing a basic social service—care of dependent people when they are most vulnerable.

- Maintaining the moral and social order of their organizations by advocating for patients, serving as arbitrator when there are competing values, and acting as the intermediary for the various professional groups.

These duties often conflict and contradict each other in a continually changing environment. Costs that increase as funding decreases and patient demands that increase while the supply of healthcare workers diminishes are part of the ongoing balancing act of healthcare executives. However, the payoff for executives is that all of their hard, complicated work results in the satisfaction of helping individuals and their communities as a whole, albeit from an indirect, distanced, invisible, and often unappreciated position within healthcare.

The Future of Physical Therapists as Managers

Given the challenges managers experience in healthcare organizations, the role of a professional organization such as the American Physical Therapy Association (APTA) requires some investigation. APTA official documents, such as *The Guide to Physical Therapist Practice* and the Normative Model for Physical Therapist Professional Education, describe the administrative and managerial roles of physical therapists in general terms that are consistent with traditional perspectives of management. The APTA Standards of Practice for Physical Therapy also address some organizational components of physical therapy practice. See Sidebar 1.4.

Although these resources have provided a long-needed clarification of the responsibilities of physical therapists, they lack specificity and continue to

---

SIDEBAR 1.4

American Physical Therapy Association's Standards and Criteria of Practice

STANDARDS OF PRACTICE FOR PHYSICAL THERAPY

http://www.apta.org/uploadedFiles/APTAorg/About_Us/Policies/HOD/Practice/Standards.pdf

CRITERIA FOR STANDARDS OF PRACTICE FOR PHYSICAL THERAPY

http://www.apta.org/uploadedFiles/APTAorg/About_Us/Policies/BOD/Practice/CriteriaforStandardsofPractice.pdf reflect only one model in which a physical therapist is the manager of other physical therapists. Except perhaps for a private physical therapy practice, this model of management does not seem to reflect current trends in teams of interdisciplinary healthcare professionals. The clinical discipline of a manager seems relatively unimportant in organizations with matrix or hybrid management models that include specialized clinical programs.

We do not know a great deal about physical therapists who are currently managers in healthcare organizations, and we know even less about managers of physical therapists who are *not* physical therapists. A potential concern is that unless physical therapists hold managerial positions in which they can influence decision-making in organizations, the broader impact of the physical therapy profession on the business of healthcare may be lost. Important questions remain unanswered as the dynamic nature of healthcare challenges managers and the physical therapy profession, including the following:

- At what point do physical therapists identify more with their managerial roles than their clinical roles?
- What is the most effective means for preparing physical therapists for managerial responsibilities?
- When should physical therapists begin to prepare for managerial responsibilities?
- Are the knowledge and experience of healthcare managers transferable from one healthcare setting to another?
- Should there be parallel tracks for preparing entrepreneur physical therapists and physical therapists who seek managerial roles in other healthcare organizations?
- What is the effect of having a non–physical therapist manager on the professional duties of physical therapists?
- What is the significance of physical therapists managing the work of other professionals?
- What should be the relationship between the knowledge and skills of managers in private practices and those in other healthcare organizations?
- How do the managerial roles of physical therapists impact the vision of the profession?

- What technical, economic, social, and political trends impact the management of physical therapy services?

These questions may require the profession to take a broader perspective on the management of physical therapy practices and to take a closer look at preparing physical therapists for these positions. Physical therapists tend to *plan for* careers in academia or as clinical specialists and *fall into* careers as managers in healthcare. A more clearly defined structure for planning a management career might shift the balance of these three career tracks in the profession. New graduates might feel different if there were a more formal managerial career path in physical therapy for their consideration, or they may seek opportunities presented by healthcare organizations rather than the profession.

It often seems that many physical therapists have left healthcare management positions as the system flattened by reducing the number of mid-level management positions. These organizational changes were missed opportunities for physical therapists to secure a prominent role in new management models in all healthcare settings. By taking a broader view and devoting the same level of commitment to management as it has to other goals, the profession as a whole and physical therapists individually may find themselves at a significant advantage in influencing today's healthcare.

Establishing the current positioning of physical therapy services in healthcare organizations and private practices in communities is another important goal for the profession. Positioning is not the same as demonstrating strong outcomes data with a focus on patient care. It is about the respect and importance of physical therapy services and the profession collectively in a changing healthcare system. Identifying the skills that physical therapists in organizations need to possess to contribute to the positioning of the profession is as important as their ability to practice autonomously in those organizations. See Activity 1.8.

ACTIVITY 1.8
PROFESSIONAL REFLECTION

Take time to reflect on a management track as a possible career path.

Conclusions

Physical therapists and other health professionals may easily identify opportunities for managerial development and advancement in any type of healthcare organization. Many of the communication and people skills that are required for patient care form a strong foundation for the responsibilities of healthcare managers. This realization may be the first step for clinicians in determining their interest in shifting from patient care to broader managerial responsibilities for patient care. This chapter has introduced some of those roles and responsibilities and identified challenges for the physical therapy profession as its position in healthcare organizations continues to be defined.

REFERENCES

1. Huy QN. In praise of middle managers. *Harvard Business Review*. 2001;79(8):72-79, 160.
2. Schaefer DS. Three perspectives on physical therapist managerial work. *Physical Therapy*. 2002;82:228-236.
3. Lopopolo RB, Schaefer DS, Nosse LJ. Leadership, administration, management, and professional (LAMP) processes in physical therapy: a Delphi study. *Physical Therapy*. 2004;21:137-150.
4. Luedtke-Hoffman KA. Identification of Essential Managerial Work Activities and Competencies of Physical Therapist Managers Employed in Hospital Settings [dissertation]. Denton, TX: Texas Women's University; 2002.
5. Schaefer DS, Lopopolo RB, Luedtke-Hoffman KA. Administration and management skills needed by physical therapist graduates in 2010: a national survey. *Physical Therapy*. 2007;87:261-281.
6. Stefl ME. Common competencies for all healthcare managers: the healthcare leadership alliance model. *Journal of Healthcare Management*. 2008;53(6):360-373.
7. Calhoun JG, Dollett L, Sinioris ME, et al. Development of an interprofessional competency model for healthcare leadership. *Journal of Healthcare Management*. 2008;53(6):360-373.
8. McConnell CR. The health care professional as a manager: balancing two important roles. *The Health Care Manager*. 2008;27(3):277-284.
9. Lombardi DN. *Handbook for the New Health Care Manager: Practical Strategies for the Real World*. San Francisco, CA: Jossey-Bass/AHA Press Series; 2001.
10. Haddock CC, McLean RA, Chapman RC. *Careers in Healthcare Management: How to Find Your Path and Follow It*. Chicago, IL: Health Administration Press; 2002.
11. Morton-Cooper A, Palmer A. *Mentoring, Preceptorship, and Clinical Supervision*. 2nd ed. Malden, MA: Blackwell Science Ltd; 2000.
12. Kane-Urrabazo C. Management's role in shaping organizational culture. *Journal of Nursing Management*. 2006;14:188-194.
13. Magretta J, Stone N. *What Management Is: How It Works and Why It's Everyone's Business*. New York, NY: The Free Press; 2002.
14. Garman AN, Fitz KD, Fraser MM. Communication and relationship management. *Journal of Healthcare Management*. 2006;51(5):291-294.
15. Embertson MK. The importance of middle managers in healthcare organizations. *Journal of Healthcare Management*. 2006;51(4):223-232.
16. Arnold E, Pulich M. Inappropriate selection of front-line managers can be hazardous to the health of organizations. *The Health Care Manager*. 2008;27(3):223-229.
17. Griffith JR, White K. *The Well-Managed Health Care Organization*. 5th ed. Chicago, IL: Health Administration Press; 2002.
18. Carson KD, Carson PP, Yallapragada R, Roe CW. Teamwork or interdepartmental cooperation: which is more important in the health care setting? *Health Care Manager*. 2001;19(4):39-46.
19. Aries NR. Managing diversity: the differing perceptions of managers, line workers, and patients. *Healthcare Management Review*. 2004;29:172-180.
20. Zemke R, Raines C, Filipczak G. *Generations at Work: Managing the Clash of Veterans, Boomers, Xers, and Nexters in Your Workplace*. New York, NY: AMACOM; 2000.
21. Arsenault PM. Validating generational differences: a legitimate diversity and leadership issue. *The Leadership and Organization Development Journal*. 2004;25. http://www.emeraldinsight.com/0143-7739.htm. Accessed January 30, 2013.
22. Anderson JR. Managing employees in the service sector: a literature review and conceptual development. *Journal of Business and Psychology*. 2006;20:501-523.
23. McAlearney AS. Executive leadership development in US health systems. *Journal of Healthcare Management*. 2010;55(3):206–222.
24. Corrigan JM, Eden J, Smith BM. *Leadership by Example: Coordinating Government Roles in Improving Health Care Quality (Quality Chasm Series)*. Washington, DC: National Academies Press; 2003.
25. Landry AY, Stowe M, Haefner J. Competency assessment and development among health-care leaders: results of a cross-sectional survey. *Health Services Management Research*. 2012;25(2):78-86.
26. Ross A, Wenzel FJ, Mitlyng JW. *Leadership for the Future: Core Competencies in Healthcare*. Chicago, IL: Health Administration Press; 2002.

CHAPTER 2

Managers and Leaders in Contemporary Healthcare Organizations

LEARNING OBJECTIVES

- Discuss the key milestones in the development of organization, leadership, and management theories.
- Establish the location of organizations on the mechanistic–organic continuum of organizations.
- Discuss the leader–manager continuum in terms of organizational characteristics.
- Link leaders, lateral leaders, managers, and followers to the mechanistic–organic model of organizations.
- Apply the four perspectives of leaders and the Global Leadership and Organizational Behavior Effectiveness (GLOBE) leadership dimensions to a selected leader.
- Discuss women in leadership roles.
- Examine the influence of innate managerial skills on personal and professional development.
- Relate the spans of control of managers to types of organizations.
- Discuss the influence of leaders and managers on an organization's culture.
- Relate personal work experiences to organizational socialization, in-groups, and levels of cultural interaction.
- Apply the roles of managers in the competing-values framework to contemporary healthcare organizations.
- Consider Peter F. Drucker's management concepts in terms of professional development of healthcare managers.

Introduction

Organizations are social arrangements in which collective goals are pursued through accepted roles and responsibilities that are controlled within a set boundary. Every organization is a unique culture—not all organizations are the same, nor have organizations always been the same, nor does any organization always remain the same. The introduction to the theories of organizations, leadership, and management lays the foundation for looking at the uniqueness of healthcare organizations.

As organizational theories have evolved to explain the complex relationships of people at their work, new theories of leadership and management have developed to align with them. Arising from sociology and psychology, theories were added by academics who led new schools devoted to management. This wide range of perspectives of organizations and work has evolved from Weber's and Taylor's work on the bureaucracies and the control of work in factories at the beginning of the 20th century, to Senge's learning organizations in the 1990s, and the emerging theories of social networks as we have moved into the 21st century. A brief summary of these theories is presented in Appendix 1. Some combination of these ideas continues to drive the leading and managing of contemporary healthcare organizations. See Activity 2.1.

An Organizational Continuum

Olden asks leaders and managers two major questions about work in healthcare organizations: (1) How should the thousands of tasks that make up the work to be done be divided into jobs and departments? (2) How should jobs and departments be coordinated to achieve the organization's goals? Depending on the answers to these two questions, organizations, and each of the units within them, can be placed somewhere along a continuum of mechanistic to organic arrangements for that work.[1]

At the mechanistic end, work is organized through clear job descriptions, rigid vertical chain of command for decision-making, centralized control and standardization, written communication, many rules, and specialized tasks and departments (a traditional bureaucracy). Mechanistic models are more likely to be effective when the environment in which the organization sits is stable and predictable. Conversely, at the organic end of the spectrum organizations have flexible structures for quick adaptation to a turbulent environment, vague job descriptions with less specialization, and fluctuating divisions of labor and authority. Tasks are assigned to teams that determine the means and assume responsibility for the outcomes. Information technology becomes more important, and horizontal communication takes the form of committees, task forces, and teams with liaisons that function across all of these units (an open system).

Leaders and managers are more likely to implement and adjust their organizational models to reflect some combination of the two extremes at any point in time. They may slide more toward one end of the continuum than the other, but they take advantage of the characteristics of both arrangements. For example, mechanistic-leaning organizations tend to be more efficient and result in a lower cost per unit. Fewer mistakes are made because more protocols are implemented through highly specialized workers. As a result, little horizontal coordination occurs although many people must work together. Mechanistic models slow down innovation and change, and their adaptation to external forces is weak.

To overcome these weaknesses, organizations begin to slide a little toward the organic work arrangements. This melding of the extremes allows quicker responses through reliance on interdepartmental coordination and the empowerment of employees to make immediate decisions to address matters such as reimbursement changes, patient requests, and the need for new technology while controlling what is predictable and stable in an organization. However, too much organic structure may lead to less predictability, lower efficiency, and increased costs. Leaders and managers must then readjust to keep their organizations in balance with internal and external demands.

Determination of the right place along the mechanistic–organic continuum at any point in time and for each unit within a large organization is linked to the values, goals, and size of an organization. Olden gives the example of an organization that highly values compassion in which organic work arrangements might be expected to prevail, except the organization also needs mechanistic arrangements to control costs, ensure patient safety, and adopt new technology.[1]

The bigger an organization becomes, the more likely it is to rely on mechanistic work arrangements because of the sheer volume of tasks to be completed. Yet separate departments within the organization may incorporate many aspects of organic models. For example, predictable tasks that are simple and routine or complicated and dangerous

---

ACTIVITY 2.1
ONE HUNDRED YEARS OF THEORIES

Do you think more leaders and managers make decisions based on these theories, or do you think theorists make observations and offer explanations for what they see? What are your general impressions of large organizations such as Walmart and small organizations such as a bike shop? Which do you think is more important: managers and leaders who are concerned with people, or managers and leaders who are concerned with the financial bottom line?

are managed mechanistically through standardized tasks that reduce risks and costs. More unpredictable tasks require organic processes that allow flexible problem-solving with input from workers rather than top-down standardized policies and procedures.

This mechanistic–organic continuum model of organizations reinforces the need for a comparable leader–manager continuum model. At the leader end, an organic set of skills is desirable to collaborate with others, plan work, and develop new ideas for services. At the manager end, organizations need a mechanistic skill set to control costs, provide direction, and keep work on track. The roles of leaders and managers support this management paradox.

Leaders and Managers

The study of organizations has been well founded and scrutinized, but an overload of information on leadership and management may raise concerns about its quality. Determining the value of the latest studies and trendy approaches makes it difficult to decide whom or what to believe. It sometimes appears that everyone who has managed or been managed or who is declared a leader writes a book about it. Readers must be cautious about books that focus on only one piece of the leadership–management puzzle. Pfeffer and Sutton urge people who aspire to healthcare leadership and management responsibilities to commit to the same level of expectations for evidence in business decisions that health professionals are expected to value in healthcare. Reliance on facts, rather than conventional wisdom (e.g., to-do lists or rules of thumb), to determine the preferred solutions to organizational problems is no less important than is basing clinical decisions on the best evidence.[2]

Physical therapists and other health professionals, all of whom are educationally prepared for evidence-based practice, may be at an advantage in assuming leadership and managerial roles. Having people in both clinical and managerial roles who can find and analyze information is vital for the successful running of contemporary healthcare organizations. The ability to present and support facts may be a key to success for new managers if thinking and analyzing take precedence over how-to strategies and slogans.

Assuming that leaders and managers possess these rational decision-making skills, organizations still struggle with understanding the other characteristics and skills expected of them and debates continue. For instance, can a leader and a manager be the same person? Is everyone, at some level, a manager? Is everyone a potential leader? Are leaders born or made? There seems to be general agreement that leaders guide, set the overall course, and determine the major goals of organizations. Managers implement the plans to accomplish those goals through the oversight of the combined efforts of others on a day-to-day basis. Administrators, another commonly used title, apply or formally impose rules and standards. However, the general public, as well as scholars, have used these terms interchangeably or inconsistently throughout the years to describe the people who run organizations.

Leader–Manager Continuum

In the face of the confusion and interchangeability surrounding these terms, efforts to differentiate leaders and managers have become the norm. These differences between leaders and managers are found in Figure 2.1, in which leader and manager characteristics or roles are presented as

LEADER ←→	MANAGER
Purpose Driven	Objectives Drive
Emotional	Rational
Fulfill Mission	Fulfill Contracts
Do Differently	Do Better
Inspire Risk	Avoid Risk
Seek New Systems	Tweak Existing System
Look Outward	Look Inward
The Big Picture	Day-to-Day Routine
Take Initiative	Seek Control
Confront Order	Maintain Order
Set Organizational Context	Plan and Execute
Transformational	Transactional
Innovative	Stable
Flexible, Supportive	Well-Ordered
Open Systems	Bureaucracies
Do the Right Thing	Do Things Right
Change Things	Keep Things Running
Coordinate and Cultivate	Command and Control
The Future	The Present

FIGURE 2.1 The leadership–management continuum.

anchors on continual dimensions rather than as "either-or" qualities. For example, the more a person's responsibilities are controlling and executing to reach specific objectives in a bureaucratic organization, the more the person manages rather than leads. Although people may have the management job title, in a more open system, they may be considered leaders rather than managers. Particularly when their attention is directed to fulfilling the mission of the organization, identifying opportunities for new approaches, and pursuing opportunities through greater interaction with outside stakeholders, they may consider themselves, or be considered by others, as leaders. This leader–manager continuum illustrates the grayness and fluidity of these roles.

Followers

Regardless of the abilities of people to be effective in management or leadership roles, the context (organizational culture) is critical to determining where they fall along the leader–manager continuum and their success in either role. The hierarchical level of the position, the national culture, and leader–follower generational gaps may give rise to, or may inhibit, the behaviors and skills of leaders and managers.[3]

Followers, in the end, may really determine whether someone is a leader or manager by assigning that person the designation regardless of actual job title or job description. Leaders are effective only when other people recognize them as leaders, and people expect their managers to be in charge, know what is best, and tell them the right thing to do. They become disappointed and confused when these expectations are not fulfilled.[4]

Kellerman has taken a different view of followership that emphasizes the importance of the relationships between leaders and followers. Even in more organic organizations in which who is following and who is leading is not always clear, there is some sort of dominance and deference.[5] She defines followers as people who do what others want them to do and are lower in the hierarchy of organizations. But subordinates don't always see themselves as subordinates with less power and influence than superiors. For example, in some organizations expertise

trumps position in leadership. To assist managers and leaders in understanding followership, Kellerman categorizes followers into five groups:

1. **Isolates** are completely detached, alienated, and unaware of their leaders. They just do the job and maintain the status quo.

2. **Bystanders** are aware of what is happening, but choose not to get involved. They do as expected but do not care about the work or organization.

3. **Participants** are engaged and try to make an impact, which may be positive or negative. They are good junior partners when they agree with leaders, but act as independent agents when they don't agree.

4. **Activists** feel strongly about their organizations. They work very hard on behalf of the leader as part of the inner circle of allies, or they may work just as hard to undermine a leader.

5. **Diehards** are prepared to "die for the cause." They have an all-consuming devotion that emerges only under dire situations in which they put the interests of others before themselves. These followers may be assets to leaders or lead to their downfall. Whistleblowers are considered diehards.

Kellerman suggests that leaders should not devote too much attention to isolates and bystanders who do little to contribute to the organization's goals, and identify the good and bad followers in the other three groups. Good followers actively support a leader who is effective and ethical and oppose a leader who is not by making informed judgments before taking any actions. Conversely, bad followers oppose a leader who is good or actively support a bad leader.[5]

This model may be a useful tool for leaders as they attempt to understand their effectiveness in achieving their personal and professional goals. It may also be helpful to understand that followers, like leaders and managers, fall along a continuum. Whether an employee moves from being one type of follower to another over time or is a different type of follower for different organizational goals remains unknown. The model provides ideas to be considered as leaders and managers are explored in more depth. See Activity 2.2.

ACTIVITY 2.2
LEADER? MANAGER? FOLLOWER?

At this point in your professional development, consider your skills and interests.

● Where do you fall on the leader–manager continuum? Why?
● If you had only one wish, would you choose to be the best possible leader or the best possible manager? Why?
● What kind of follower have you been? Explain.

What Do Leaders Do?

Although leadership is not easily defined, there have been leaders as long as there have been groups of followers who need one to reach a common goal. Leadership in society appears to be vital, yet the contributions of individual leaders to the outcomes of particular organizations are nebulous. Getting a handle on leadership is a little more difficult than grasping the roles of managers because *leader* really is not a job title with a clear job description. Announcements for managerial or administrative positions typically do not say, "Leader Wanted," although what the employer really wants is someone who can lead.

Defining those leader responsibilities and measuring the effectiveness of the ability to lead when hiring and evaluating performance are critical. Developing in-house programs to prepare leaders from within is a strategy used by some organizations, while others continue to rely on an "I-know-it-when-I-see-it" approach to identifying potential leaders for organizations. Depending on the circumstances, leaders may come and go, or they may assume varying levels of leadership over a given time span. They may function effectively and without much fanfare, performing many managerial duties until an occasion arises that moves them along the continuum to a leadership role—they rise to the occasion.

Lateral Leaders

Rather than the notion that leaders are at the head of organizations, the idea of leadership that is distributed throughout an organization—lateral leadership—has gained acceptance, particularly in more organic organizations. Leading from alongside people rather than leading them from above, lateral leaders function as mentors and consultants to teams of workers who are typically enmeshed with several outside vendors or contractors to achieve the goals of an organization. Members of these teams may be reassigned as the needs of the organization demand, which means that people have different leaders for different projects. Lateral leaders rely more on teaching and persuasion than they do on directing and controlling. These are leaders who are neither controlled nor controlling, and, in fact, may have no formal authority over others.[6]

Advances in communication technology have played a major role in facilitating lateral leadership. With technology, more people have more information more quickly. The freedom created by access to information enables people to work harder and more creatively in reaching decisions. The more creative, flexible, and self-motivated people need to be, the more decentralized—lateral—leadership needs to be.[7]

The idea that no leadership is the best leadership is derived from these concepts. However, larger, more complex organizations need more than lateral leaders to reach their full potential. They also need a leader or leaders whose roles are to innovate, to communicate the vision, and to challenge the status quo.[6] Some type of executive unit has to have global responsibility for an organization, yet even the most rigid bureaucracy devotes some effort to seeking input from others.[8]

The secret to leadership success seems to be the balance of these contradictions rather than choosing one or the other.[9] As organizations are moving along the mechanistic–organic continuum, this balance becomes particularly important, which further contributes to the complexity and the confusion about leadership. For instance, Pfeffer suggests that leaders must:[2]

● Be in control and project confidence yet realize their limitations because of organizational realities.
● Be wise yet modest to avoid self-enhancement.
● Lead, yet get out of the way—no leadership may be the best leadership.
● Build systems and teams yet take little direct credit for their successes.

See Activity 2.3.

Who Are Leaders?

If someone said, "Take me to your leader," to whom would you go? What position does this person hold? Does this position automatically mean leader? To address these questions, Grint adds four more questions in his perspectives of leaders:[10]

● Person Perspective. Is it who leaders are that makes them leaders?
● Results Perspective. Is it what leaders achieve that makes them leaders?
● Position Perspective. Is it where leaders operate that makes them leaders?
● Process Perspective. Is it how leaders get things done that makes them leaders?

Leaders may have a large impact, albeit potentially more negative than positive, on the accomplishment of the organization's goals. Although a direct link between organizational culture (and its subcultures) and leadership is uncertain, if what a leader proposes works, it continues to work because it becomes a shared assumption (a major factor of culture) among followers. Leaders are highly symbolic of the beliefs about the goals of an organization and they create the culture that drives management.[11]

This influencing process is typically defined as leadership and reflects the characteristics and behaviors of leaders, as they are perceived by their followers, to accomplish organizational outcomes in a particular context.[3] This definition is similar to the one proposed in the second phase of the Global Leadership and Organizational Behavior Effectiveness (**GLOBE**) research project. In this project leadership was defined as the ability of an individual to influence, motivate, and enable others to contribute to the effectiveness and success of the organizations of which they are members. Based on a study conducted with 1,996 leaders in 62 countries, the GLOBE group developed an instrument to measure the degree to which selected leaders held the values of the leadership dimensions. Their identified leadership dimensions are the following:[12]

● Charismatic/value-based (visionary, inspirational, integrity, decisive)
● Team-oriented (collaborative, integrative, diplomatic)
● Participative (non-autocratic, allow participation in decision-making)
● Autonomous (individualistic, independent, unique)
● Humane (modest, tolerant, sensitive)
● Self-protective (self-centered, status-conscious, face-saver)

Whether it is the GLOBE model or not, it is important to have a framework for determining what it is that makes leaders successful and how much leaders are really contributing to the overall expected outcomes of an organization. For instance, it is impossible to determine how much and what kind of development leaders may need to become more successful if the organization does not define and measure the roles and efforts of leaders. Consideration also has to be given to women in leadership roles.

Female Leaders

Lantz reports on the surveys of executives that were conducted by the American College of Healthcare during the course of 16 years. In the study, women in healthcare organizations were more likely to hold positions as department heads or some other mid-staff positions and much less likely than men to be the chief executive officer (CEO), chief operating officer (COO), president, or vice president—only 12% of healthcare CEOs in these surveys were women in 2006. Although there was a steady improvement in these numbers leading up to 2006, Lantz concluded that women were underrepresented in leadership positions, given that 78% of the healthcare workforce are women.[13]

She identified several potential barriers that organizations need to address to overcome this underrepresentation. First, the organization failed in some ways because mentoring for women and other minorities was lacking, they failed to include women in plans for succession, and women were not offered opportunities to serve on hospital boards and board committees. Second, in addition to making gender-based compromises and sacrifices within two-career families, women also faced stereotypes about gender differences in social roles, personality traits, and leadership capabilities.[13]

Meanwhile, Eagly and Carli suggest that the expectations for leaders have become more feminine as organizations lean toward organic work arrangements. For instance, democratic principles, work teams, participatory decision-making, delegation, growth, and more diversity in the workforce demand more sharing of information, fairness, and the enhancement of self-worth. All of these demands and strategies are considered more feminine skills.[14] Gergen believes that women leaders see themselves as the center of a circle with two-way spokes reaching out in many directions rather than at the head of a command-and-control hierarchy. Women are expected to become the future leaders of leaders because of this softer approach, which is based on openness, transparency, consensus, and relationships. They tend to be more successful at leading themselves, leading within organizations, and partnering with other organizations.[15]

See Sidebar 2.1 and Activities 2.4 and 2.5.

Who Is a Manager?

Despite the importance placed on leadership, management is considered one of the most transforming innovations of civilization.[17] It will continue to play a major role in our lives because, regardless of the configurations of current and future organizations, management goals can only be accomplished by the process of affecting groups of people and manipulating resources that are beyond the scope of individual effort. Any time the needs exceed the resources available, things need to be managed—whether they be prehistoric hunters and gatherers, family budgets, or generating profits for shareholders. Because humans have always had needs that exceeded their resources, management is considered a generic, innate ability rather than specialized knowledge.

SIDEBAR 2.1

Understanding Influence[16]

- Influence is the mechanism for using power to change behaviors or attitudes. Influence produces an effect without direct command or force.
- Influence is more powerful than direct power because it is a process of acceptance and mutual agreement that results in commitment and good work.
- When influenced, people feel that decisions made are their choices.
- Direct commands typically result in discontent and take more effort because employees need to be constantly supervised to ensure their compliance.
- People would rather not be told what to do unless the circumstance has become dire; then they welcome the fact that someone takes control.
- Influence is a two-way rather than top-down process.
- To exert influence, a person must be willing to be influenced by others and be open to new information. Of course, to be influential a person has to "walk the talk."
- People need to be taken seriously by the influencer, or the influencer will be quickly discredited.

ACTIVITY 2.4
LEADERSHIP PERSPECTIVES

Which of the following perspectives best explains that person as a successful leader?

- Person Perspective. Is it who that person is that makes him or her a leader?
- Results Perspective. Is it what that person achieves that makes him or her a leader?
- Position Perspective. Is it where that person operates that makes him or her a leader?
- Process Perspective. Is it how that person gets things done that makes him or her a leader?

To reinforce this innate human nature, consider that each of us manages our everyday lives although only some of us hold managerial positions. We even form mini-organizations when it takes more than one person to accomplish some set of tasks such as planning a class reunion, or preparing a holiday dinner, or holding a church bazaar. Regardless of what is being managed or the type of organization, it is helpful to consider three sources of power for managers—affiliative, personal, and institutional—which are defined as:[16]

- *Affiliative Power Managers:* They want to be liked more than they want to get the job (patient care) done so they make decisions based on what makes people (staff) happy. They are the mothers who deep-fry the Thanksgiving turkey because that is what everyone likes, although they know it is not the healthiest choice.
- *Personal Power Managers:* These are strong bosses who make employees feel strong. They are democratic but depend on turf building and self-aggrandizing, so friction among units of an organization (e.g., physical therapy versus occupational therapy versus speech-language pathology) results. They are competitive, but they are not team players because decisions are based on "me" first. They are the bossy aunts

who make all of the arrangements for a family reunion cruise without taking a vote on the available options.

- *Institutional Managers:* These are managers who are of service to the organization (healthcare system or rehabilitation team). Because they are mature and self-confident, they easily and eagerly reward performance. They put the organization before themselves in decision-making. They are the parents who put hours into fund-raising drives without receiving much notice for their efforts.

Although a big part of who we are, management itself is a misunderstood concept. We all have more direct contact with managers of businesses and organizations than we do with leaders. Our experiences may be less than pleasant because we are often already emotionally charged as we approach the "person in charge" when things go wrong at the grocery store, a bank, or restaurant. When things are going well, we do not really pay much attention to how a business is managed and may often wonder what a manager really does.

Experiences at work with bosses also lean toward the difficult. On one hand, in any organization, 60% to 75% of people report that the worst (or most stressful) part of their jobs is their immediate supervisors.[4] On the other hand, the great managers who take care of our complaints and the great bosses who make us better than we thought we could ever be are the ones who make great organizations, often without much notice. See Activity 2.6.

Magretta and Stone suggest that despite the naysayers who predict the death of management and are not sorry to see it go, organizations will always need managers in some form. The more complex an organization becomes and the more specialized work becomes, the larger the role management plays to effect an integrated outcome. Although there is an expectation that individuals will take more initiative and assume more responsibility at work and that more and more of us will become independent contractors, organizations and managers are still needed to get things done.[17] Perhaps in purely organic, high-tech, virtual organizations that are driven by self-organizing teams with lateral leaders, the traditional middle manager position may be eliminated or alternative positions may be created. Even in extremely mechanistic models, managers will be needed as the processes for turning complexity and specialization into performance continue to change.

What Do Managers Do?

The importance of managers and organizations was the life work of Peter Drucker, who is credited with developing the foundation of management's body of knowledge, which includes his 25 books. Both practical and theoretical, his contributions have endured for more than 60 years.[18] According to Drucker, managers who understand the following seven principles and manage themselves accordingly will build successful, productive, and achieving organizations all across the world by establishing standards, setting examples, and leaving a legacy of a greater capacity to produce wealth and a greater human vision:[19]

1. Management's task is to make people capable of joint performance so that their strengths are effective and their weaknesses are irrelevant. We depend on management for our ability to contribute to society and achieve our personal goals.

2. Management is deeply embedded in all cultures. What managers everywhere do is the same, but how they do it is very different.

3. Management's job is to think through and exemplify an organization's objectives, values, and goals so that people are committed to them. Without this commitment, there is no enterprise (organization); there is a mob.

4. Training and development that never stop must be built into every aspect of an organization.

5. Every organization is built on communication and individual responsibility because people have many different skills and knowledge to do many different types of work that must be pulled together.

6. Just as we need a diversity of measures to determine human performance, we need a diversity of measures to determine the performance of an organization and its continuous improvement.

7. The results of organizations are not within its walls. Results only exist on the outside in the satisfied customer, the healed patient, and the student who learned something and puts it to work 10 years later.

Competing-Values Framework

To help new managers synthesize ideas to meet their important responsibilities, Quinn and his associates developed a competing-values framework of management that unifies the four major historical stages of management (organization) theories. These are the rational goal, internal process, human relations, and open systems models.[20] See Figure 2.2 for a representation of the relationship of these models.

This competing-values framework has received a great deal of attention from researchers and consultants. Managers also find it compelling in their everyday duties because this framework provides a synergistic, dynamic, and logical approach to their work in modern, complex organizations.

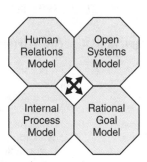

FIGURE 2.2 Quinn and associates' competing-values framework of management. (Adapted from Quinn RE, Faerman SR, Thompson MP, McGrath MR. *Becoming a Master Manager: A Competency Framework*. 2nd ed. New York, NY: John Wiley & Sons; 1996.)

No one of the four models alone is adequate to keep an organization running, and the rejection of even one of the competing values jeopardizes an organization's effectiveness. This model is also valuable for integrating the concepts in the mechanistic–organic and leader–manager continua.

Historically, each of the four models in the framework was developed as *one* perspective of a very complex construct—the management of organizations. Rather than completely replacing the product orientation of the rational goal model for the processes of the internal process model, focusing on people management in the human relations model, and then using open systems to drive decisions, the competing-values framework model demonstrates that all four models are needed simultaneously by contemporary managers in complex organizations.

The arrows in Figure 2.2 reflect the paradoxes of managing with all four models through the crossovers created by them. The arrows represent the need for managers to balance the relationships among internal processes while in an open system and balance their human relations (people) responsibilities with their rational, fiduciary responsibilities.[20] Even as new systems approaches to organizations evolve, the age-old need to balance these relationships will endure.

The strength of this all-inclusive framework is its usefulness as a tool for understanding the competition among the four models for the attention of a manager. It applies to large, complex bureaucracies and small businesses, such as solo practitioners in physical therapy practices. Managers must be prepared for all of the roles derived from the competing-values framework perspective presented in Table 2.1 in comparison with Fayol's classic list of the traditional managerial goals. This comparison demonstrates how management roles have evolved and the shifting required of managers as they move among the competing-values framework models to meet the salient, value-laden goals of an organization at any point in time.

It is not hard to understand why many people are reluctant to assume managerial positions. These positions seem daunting and overwhelming to outsiders and often confusing and unclear to insiders. It is hoped that the competing-values framework as seen in Figure 2.2 is a helpful tool for demystifying management so that the rewards and advantages of these important responsibilities are realized by more people. Transitioning from a clinician to a manager is not as unrealistic or unattractive as many people think. Many clinicians find themselves pushed (coerced by higher management or driven by a sense of responsibility to step up when no one else is available) to move from patient care to management positions because they are good at what they are currently doing. Why do so many of them, despite initial reluctance, like their work once they are in a management position? As suggested before, it may be because management skills are innate, and clinicians have already developed the softer management skills through their patient care experiences.

All managers assume every one of the eight management roles defined in the competing-values framework. Consider, for instance, how even a physical therapist serves as producer, director, coordinator, monitor, facilitator, mentor,

---

TABLE 2.1 Traditional and contemporary views of managerial roles in the competing-values model

TRADITIONAL FUNCTIONS[17]	CONTEMPORARY ROLES[20]	RELATED COMPETING-VALUES MODELS[20]
Organizing	Producer: task-oriented, driven, time management	Rational Goal Model
Leading	Director: clarifies goals and visions, plans, delegates	Rational Goal Model
Planning	Coordinator: scheduling, logistics, designing work, projects	Internal Process Model
Controlling	Monitor: checks on compliance of individuals and groups, facts and figures, details	Internal Process Model
Coordinating*	Facilitator: builds teams, manages conflict	Human Relations Model
	Mentor: helpful, open, fair development of others	Human Relations Model
	Innovator: adaptation, creates change, trend analysis	Open Systems Model
	Broker: external resources, image, reputation, negotiator, liaison, presents ideas to others for acceptance	Open Systems Model

*Coordinating has been deleted in revisions of Fayol's work.

innovator, and broker in patient care. The actual day-to-day duties associated with these roles may differ from one level of management to another, and the emphasis on particular roles may shift within the same managerial position. Effectiveness as a manager at any level lies with the ability to integrate and balance these competing roles—to deal with the paradoxes that are the result of four different models of management. See Activity 2.7.

Span of Control

In addition to the specific responsibilities of managers presented in Section 2, another aspect of what managers do is related to their spans of control. A manager's span of control (SOC) is defined as the number of subordinates that can be effectively supervised. The SOC becomes important as organizational models change. Hard-and-fast rules about how many people each manager manages are less acceptable in large healthcare organizations with ongoing expansion and shifting of work units. Instead, Liebler and McConnell recommend consideration of the interaction of the following factors that impact the SOC:[21]

- Type of work: the more routine and homogeneous, the larger the SOC can be
- Degree of training of the worker: the better trained and motivated, the larger the SOC can be
- Organizational stability: the higher the turnover and frequency of changes, the smaller the SOC must be
- Geographical location: the broader the dispersion of work units, the smaller the SOC must be
- Flow of work: the more work needs coordination, the smaller the SOC must be
- Supervisor's qualifications: the more training and experience, the larger the SOC can be
- Availability of staff specialization: the more available others are to assist, the larger the SOC can be
- Value system of the organization: the greater the need for conformity, the smaller the SOC must be

---

ACTIVITY 2.7
CASE STUDY

Jordan Janko has been a physical therapist for 4 years. She has been focused on her patient care responsibilities, and she is in the final stages of preparing to sit for the board certification examination in neurology. Since her graduation, she has worked in the same large medical center. Her performance evaluations have been outstanding, and she has enjoyed her role as clinical instructor for the past 2 years. Her patients love her. She is very satisfied with her position and the organization as a whole, although there have been several periods of major organizational changes. For instance, she has reported to four different people in 4 years because of changes in the organization or changes in the people in those positions. From her perspective, some of these changes have been good while others have not.

Jordan is flattered when the Vice President of Clinical Services (VPCS) approaches her with a new opportunity. She has heard the rumors about yet another impending reorganization, so she is not surprised that four new management positions are being created in the rehabilitation services department. The VPCS is offering her one of the new positions—Coordinator of Adult Neurorehabilitation. The position involves the management of a new interdisciplinary team that will include approximately 20 people who will report to her. Many of the coworkers with whom she has enjoyed working will be on the team and there will be some new hires. The VPCS tells Jordan that management wants rehab to become an exemplary model for patient outcomes and satisfaction, and it is agreed that she is the only one who can lead the neuro unit to excellence.

What manager and leader qualities do you think Jordan displayed in her patient care to make her such a strong candidate for this new position? Where on the leader–manager continuum would you place this new position? Where does the new neuro unit fit on the mechanistic–organic continuum? What models and roles in the competing-values framework will she need to focus on? What will be her span of control? Should Jordan take the job? What pros and cons should she consider?

Organizational Culture

Because an organization's culture is based on its values, culture is now explored in more depth. Many clinicians accept healthcare managerial positions by investigating motivational factors, such as high starting salaries and good benefits, perfect location, and interesting job assignments. Fewer people may attempt to compare the crux of each organization—its culture—when making these important career decisions. Culture is a deep, pervasive, yet abstract and vague essence of an organization that is often expressed as "This is just how we do things around here." An organization is a culture unto itself. We become part of an organization's culture by learning the "rules of the game." Joining a new organization may be compared with moving away from home and learning to make one's way in new territory. Or a major shift in an organization's mission or business model may provoke a mild angst that is similar to living in a country that experiences a major political or social upheaval. Leaders and managers bear responsibility for their unique work cultures and developing the means for socialization of all workers into them.

Edward Schein's classic definition of *organizational culture* is "the pattern of shared basic assumptions learned by a group as it solved its problems of external adaptation and internal integration which has worked well enough to be considered valid, and, therefore, to be taught to new members as the correct way to perceive, think, and feel in relation to those problems."[22]

This culture drives all aspects of an organization's decisions about operations and relationships to its external stakeholders. Priorities and problem-solving approaches employed depend on culture. The subtlety and power of culture as it unifies and controls the behavior of a group or sub-group should not be underestimated.[23]

Because culture is an abstraction with the qualities of structural stability, depth, breadth, and integration, Schein advises caution in assuming or defining it only by that which can be observed.[22] He advises that culture is more than the typical list of human-made objects. Culture is also defined by observed interactions of people and their group norms; publicly announced values and policies; organizational climate (the feeling conveyed by physical layout and the way people interact);

embedded skills; thinking habits; rituals; and shared meanings and symbols. The stability of culture provides comforting meaning and predictability to its members, which also makes it so difficult to change. It survives even when the members of an organization leave. Culture is also so deeply embedded in organizations that it is unconscious, or at least not observable, and it is ubiquitous. Finally, culture is the integration of all of those shared basic assumptions and artifacts into a whole that is bigger than the sum of their parts.

Despite difficulties with definitions and measurement of both the abstraction and the artifacts of healthcare organizational culture, it continues to be perceived as an important factor in the delivery and outcomes of patient care. The following basic assumptions seem to be agreed upon:[24]

1. Healthcare organization cultures affect quality and performance.
2. Although resistant to change, cultures are malleable and manageable.
3. Strategies to change cultural attributes that positively or negatively impact organization performance are possible.
4. Benefits accruing from cultural changes outweigh any dysfunctional consequences.
5. A toolbox of concepts, tools, and methods is needed for robust insights into the complex, multidimensional aspects of culture.

Research on Organizational Culture

Culture is of interest to a wide spectrum of scholars such as sociologists, psychologists, anthropologists, and managers. To demonstrate the range of perspectives about healthcare organizational culture, a summary of a few recent studies is provided:

- Carney asked clinical and non-clinical healthcare managers in Ireland to identify and rank the cultural determinants of quality care. They concluded that quality care was most likely to prevail in organizations whose cultures promoted excellence in care delivery, ethical values, and involvement of clinicians in planning strategies.[25]
- The Children's Mental Health Services Research Center engages in organizational culture and climate studies. It determined that

100 mental health clinics across the country included all three types of organizational culture defined in its Organizational Social Context (OSC) tool. It determined a relationship between the type of organizational profile (rigidity, proficiency, and resistance) and work attitudes, staff turnover, and service quality. Rigidity in this tool refers to control and regulations. Proficiency implies highly competent staff who place the clients first. Resistance cultures show little interest in change and react with apathy at attempts to change.[26]

- The same researchers conducted an experimental, controlled study of 36 state-run child welfare clinics. One half of the clinics engaged in the Availability, Responsiveness, and Continuity (ARC) program for 1 year while the control group clinics conducted business as usual. The organizational climate scores of the ARC centers improved significantly, and staff turnover was significantly reduced when compared with the control clinics. The findings suggest that organizations can change with planned interventions.[26]

- Top-level managers were typically the subjects in 12 studies on hospital culture that were analyzed. One conclusion of the analysis was that there is indeed a hospital culture, although not consistently defined and measured. The primary goals of the studies were to relate hospital culture to factors such as safety and patient and employee satisfaction. Hospitals (more typically private than public) with strong cultures have higher employee satisfaction and are likely to show improved clinical outcomes. Culture strength is derived from consistent, visible role modeling and leadership and is certainly something observed as consistent employee behavior.[27]

Although the current science of healthcare organizational culture may not be decisive or even clearly understood, leaders and managers have the challenge of sorting through a large toolbox to better understand their responsibility for culture. See Activity 2.8.

To explore organizational culture in more depth, three particular aspects of organizations are introduced here.

ACTIVITY 2.8
HEALTHCARE ORGANIZATION CULTURE

Identify the shared basic assumptions that characterize a typical healthcare organization.

Where do these assumptions place the typical healthcare organization on the mechanistic–organic continuum?

When should these assumptions be changed?

Discuss how leaders and managers would facilitate the passage of these basic assumptions to new employees.

Intercultural Communication in Organizations

Gudykunst's approach to the study of intercultural communication includes a useful three-level model for understanding the many communication interactions that are at the heart of healthcare organizational culture. Moving from broad, general topics to personal information, data generated in all three levels of communication help determine how well individuals fit the stereotype of a given sub-group and how well that group matches the assumptions of the whole organization.[28] The three levels are:

- Level 1 Interactions. Communication based on the broad foundation of assumptions about values, beliefs, norms, and so forth within an organization.
- Level 2 Interactions. Communication influenced by information regarding social groups or roles within the culture. Each sub-group has a unique set of embedded skills, thinking habits, and rituals. This level also includes communication based on categorizing people by job title, gender, or age.
- Level 3 Interactions. Communication based on personal information about the individuals who make up the Level 2 social sub-groups.

Figure 2.3 shows the three levels applied to healthcare organizations and their patients. People in healthcare organizations rely on Levels 1 and 2 communication (interactions) as the tool for coping with the large amount of data that they need to process in their work. In short-term circumstances

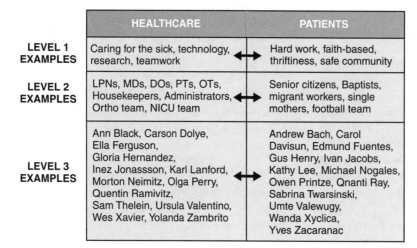

	HEALTHCARE		PATIENTS
LEVEL 1 EXAMPLES	Caring for the sick, technology, research, teamwork	⟷	Hard work, faith-based, thriftiness, safe community
LEVEL 2 EXAMPLES	LPNs, MDs, DOs, PTs, OTs, Housekeepers, Administrators, Ortho team, NICU team	⟷	Senior citizens, Baptists, migrant workers, single mothers, football team
LEVEL 3 EXAMPLES	Ann Black, Carson Dolye, Ella Ferguson, Gloria Hernandez, Inez Jonassson, Karl Lanford, Morton Neimitz, Olga Perry, Quentin Ramivitz, Sam Thelein, Ursula Valentino, Wes Xavier, Yolanda Zambrito	⟷	Andrew Bach, Carol Davisun, Edmund Fuentes, Gus Henry, Ivan Jacobs, Kathy Lee, Michael Nogales, Owen Printze, Qnanti Ray, Sabrina Twarsinski, Umte Valewugy, Wanda Xyclica, Yves Zacaranac

FIGURE 2.3 Levels of interaction in healthcare.

particularly, interactions based at Levels 1 and 2 are often adequate for predicting most behaviors of others and for responding appropriately. For example, Level 1 value-driven interactions apply to issues such as patient confidentiality. Level 2 interactions deal with stereotypical ideas about physical therapists, elderly patients, and so on. The point is that these two levels of communication may suffice for most day-to-day communication needed to achieve good healthcare outcomes.

However, when relationships are long term or when problems are complex, more knowledge about the individuals involved in decisions becomes important and Level 3–based interactions that delve deeper into what others feel and think become increasingly necessary. Level 3 communication between patients and providers and among a team of healthcare providers may be common in healthcare organizations that lean toward organic arrangements of work.

Managers must be aware of which level of communication is needed as they guide the work of others. Level 1 interactions may be needed when staff do not value maintaining schedules or others fail to follow the expected norm of offering unsolicited assistance. Team communication may be disrupted if nurses rely on Level 2 interactions that reinforce social stereotypes about physical or occupational therapists. The over- or underutilizing of the expertise of therapists in team decision-making may result. Identifying opportunities for Level 3 interactions among work teams in order for them to get to know each other may be critical to increasing the effectiveness of patient care and job satisfaction. Managers in organizations that rely heavily on

contingency workers need to pay particular attention to the interactions of this subgroup at all three levels because of the potential influence that they have on the work of organizations. At the same time, the influence of in-groups and out-groups is another manifestation of culture that demands the attention of managers.

In-Groups and Out-Groups

In larger organizations, there may be several subgroups (subcultures) that are influenced by the unique nature of their work and the roles of the members in it. For example, in a large hospital, the business office subculture is different from the nursing subculture, which is different from the marketing department's subculture, which is different from the medical staff's subculture. These healthcare in-groups are like all in-groups. Their members are expected to behave and think alike and to cooperate with no expectation of equitable return on effort. People derive their social identities from their membership in groups whose values and norms are internalized.

They find comfort in the group because of their united view of out-groups—which are all other groups who present no emotional concern to the in-group and from whom an equitable return for cooperating *is* expected by the in-group. Dividing into in-groups and out-groups is universal to human nature, and individuals belong to many in-groups based on religion, social status, job roles, and so on. The influence of an in-group is so powerful that separation or alienation from an in-group may be anxiety producing.[28,29]

In some cases, physical therapists as a whole may be an in-group. In other cases, there may be in-groups and out-groups of physical therapists in one organization's subculture of physical therapy. Consider physical therapists who work in the outpatient center of a hospital who may consider the therapists who work in the inpatient units as an out-group. They may be reluctant to work in the other setting and minimally interact with each other. The outpatient team may be very willing to assist each other with patient load demands because of their commitment to each other and patient outcomes. They are likely to agree on many aspects of care and how they do their work. The very same physical therapists, however, may be less willing to assist physical therapists working in the inpatient units unless there was some form of additional reward for doing so. They are less likely to agree on approaches to patient care and patient outcomes. The reverse scenario is also true.

In both cases a healthcare manager who disrupts the in-group/out-group dynamics may provoke a great deal of animosity and anxiety among the staff. Creating opportunity for all of the physical therapists in an organization to be of one in-group may become important for accomplishing the goals of physical therapy practice within a large healthcare organization. More likely, attending to in-groups composed of a variety of professionals may be the new managerial challenge.

Organizational Socialization

Like all newcomers, physical therapy students and recent graduates experience reality (culture) shock. They have a strong basic need to belong and three things can happen when the shock wears off. They learn the rules of the game to fit in, they never fit in, or they may accept some of the culture and reject other parts as they attempt to change the organization. The attempts to change it are not necessarily a bad thing for an organization.[30] However, if the organization they want to change is their only potential source of income (or they need to receive a good grade), some people may face difficult decisions about bucking the system. They may face what seems to be overwhelming odds to change the culture. If there are no other job opportunities to turn to, failed attempts to change may create a very negative work experience.

Culture shock and fitting in are referred to as *organizational socialization*—a dynamic, ongoing process that passes along the correct ways to perceive, think, and feel about the organization's problems of external adaptation and internal integration. This process is like culture itself—subtle, difficult to understand, yet powerful and important. It is helpful to consider this socialization process as a continuum with *totally socialized* anchoring at one end and *no socialization at all* found at the other end.[30] The degree of socialization at any point in time may be anywhere along this continuum. Even when promoted from within an organization, people must be re-socialized. Not only do their roles change, but their views of the organization are adjusted as well.

Socialization is like a spiral that continues to twist and expand as people change, their social roles change, and the organizational culture changes. Employees, therefore, may have ongoing phases of reality shock, reorientation, and resettling as their organizations change, or as they change jobs. Employees also bring their own personal and professional values and norms to a job that concurrently influence the organizational culture. Reciprocal balancing of these major influences is at the heart of managerial work.

Formal and Informal Socialization

It is not surprising that actually doing one's job is typically complicated by the difficulty and frustration a person feels when grasping for these non-tangibles of organization culture that underlie all work.[31] Connecting the implementation of concrete policies and procedures with the underlying reason or value—the why—that drives that work may be troubling or confusing. Guiding the process of socialization is the responsibility of middle managers in most organizations. It may be very structured and formalized, or it may be a casual afterthought.

The larger the organization, the more formal the process for socialization becomes. New employees take part in individual and group orientation sessions, as well as ongoing employee development programs. The orientation sessions typically include presentation of the mission, policies and procedures, and safety regulations. The development courses are typically conducted to address some particular customer service or program issue.

Mentors may be assigned to guide new employees formally as well. In either case, the underlying "whys" of the way work is done may be presented simply as the mission of the organization, and the opportunity to discuss potential conflicts of values and norms is rare. This type of socialization through orientation sessions is more about learning the formal rules of the organization, but the responsibility for their implementation lies with managers guiding people to behave accordingly.

The other component of socialization is informal. In larger organizations, informal socialization is sporadic and hit or miss. Responsibility for this socialization process lies more with coworkers as new employees take initiative to learn how to fit in with each other. This informal process more often occurs among peer employees, rather than between a boss and an employee, as the need for information arises, or when seasoned employees feel the need to set the new person straight (regardless of what they heard from the boss or during orientation sessions).

This informal socialization may be inconsistent with, if not counter to, the information gained in the formal sessions when a particular subculture emerges or loyalty to an in-group overwhelms loyalty to the organization. It may be a truer reflection of the norms and values of the organization than are presented as the written mission and goals.[30] Managers who understand the importance of informal socialization, and encourage it, are at an advantage in both large and small organizations.

In smaller organizations, formal socialization methods may be minimal. Employees may find themselves just thrown into the work as they learn the ropes on their own, or they may find the informal socialization intermingled in their day-to-day work. Here are two examples of possible scenarios in small organizations:

- Scenario 1: A physical therapist, who has never worked in a skilled nursing facility before, accepts a position as the only physical therapist in one. Challenges may result because the formal socialization mechanisms are nonexistent or directed toward nurses rather than the needs of physical therapists. In this case, informal socialization will be through other healthcare providers in the nursing home who may not relate to the norms and values the physical therapist brings to the organization.

- Scenario 2: A novice physical therapist accepts a position in a small private physical therapy practice. Socialization to the practice—and to the profession—is likely to be more intense and more integrated into the day-to-day work because the entire organization is the in-group.

Importance of Socialization in Organizations

Formal and informal socialization processes are vital to the organization as it attempts to meet its goals. For instance, the socialization of employees imparts the following aspects of work:[30]

- Cooperation and cohesion of employees needed by employers to get the job done
- Job satisfaction and job turnover
- Morale and productivity of individual employees
- Interactions among employees and with their supervisors

Managers cannot overestimate the power of individuals to do their own thing and their reluctance to change. Understanding the success or failure of an organization and the success or failure of a person in the organization often boils down to the ability to align the values, personal as well as professional, of individuals with the organization's way of doing business. A reciprocal willingness to compromise becomes necessary.

However, the relationship between the depth of identity with an organization and an employee's health and well-being may not always be positive or linear. Although the socialization of employees strengthens the ability of an organization to meet its goals, when identification with the organization becomes too strong, managers need to address the potential negative effects on employees and the organization. Commonly called *workaholism*, over-identification to the point that the organization's or in-group's goals become *personal* goals often leads an employee to underestimate job demands and/or overestimate coping skills and resources. Managers must be alert to employees who always seek to work harder and provide them opportunities to recover from their efforts.[32]

Socialization is often expressed as clichéd phrases—*get on board, join the club, fit in, get with it, get in the groove, toe the line,* or *go along to get along.* Although it may be hard to define how this happens, employees know that it does happen with varying degrees of comfort and ease. One of the major factors in the comfort level that healthcare professionals experience as they join organizations is their concurrent professional socialization, which may either facilitate or impede organizational socialization. Novice physical therapists who are still defining their professional roles may find they are more heavily influenced by the culture of an organization than experienced physical therapists who are more likely to have strongly developed professional roles. This may serve a healthcare organization well, but it may not be good for the future of the profession.

See Activity 2.9 and Activity 2.10.

Conclusions

The success of any organization depends on balance—the balance of leaders and managers, the balance of focus on human and financial factors, the balance of the importance of internal and external processes, the balance of mechanistic and organic arrangements of work, and the balance of formal and informal socialization—to facilitate the achievement of goals. This chapter has attempted to identify, explain, and clarify these often conflicting perspectives of organizations and the roles of leaders and managers in them.

ACTIVITY 2.9
BECOMING SOCIALIZED

Consider your personal experiences (volunteer, student, employee) in a particular organization. What components of that organization's culture were most striking as you became part of it?

How were you socialized into that organization?

ACTIVITY 2.10
SUMMERVILLE PHYSICAL THERAPY

Summerville Physical Therapy has been the only physical therapy practice in a small town for 15 years. The owner, Judy Jiminez, PT, and her staff (Susan Solomon, PT, and Andrew Bilirakis, PTA) have prided themselves on their commitment to serving the community, especially their flexibility in scheduling and office hours to meet the transportation needs of their rural patients who travel great distances to town for their healthcare.

Judy decides to retire and sells her practice to National Physical Therapy Corporation (NPTC). It is an offer she cannot refuse and she is relieved to be told by NPTC that all of her good, hard work will continue. She has agreed to stay on until a physical therapist from another NPTC office relocates and takes over the practice. Susan and Andrew will become employees of NPTC and are pleased to learn that their salaries and benefits will increase as a result, although they will miss Judy.

Six months later, Susan and Andrew invite Judy to lunch to "catch up" because she has been traveling since her retirement. They report the new "outsider" boss is very difficult in his demands on their hours and imposed productivity goals. They report that many people are going to the hospital in the next town for their physical therapy although it is farther away. They feel that nothing is the same.

If you were Judy, what would you say to Susan and Andrew? Are their reactions to the changes in Summerville Physical Therapy typical? How has the organizational culture changed? How have things moved on the leader–manager continuum? Has the organization moved on the mechanistic–organic continuum? How would the changes be explained in the competing-values framework? What formal and informal socialization processes may have occurred or may need to occur? At what level of communication may problems lie? Identify the in-groups. What do you expect the outcome for Susan and Andrew to be?

REFERENCES

1. Olden PC. Managing mechanistic and organic structure in health careorganizations. *The Health Care Manager.* 2012;31(4):357-364.

2. Pfeffer J, Sutton RI. *Hard Facts, Dangerous Half-Truths, & Total Nonsense: Profiting From Evidence-Based Management.* Boston, MA: Harvard Business School Publishing; 2006.

3. Antonakis J, Cianciolo AT, Sternberg RJ. Leadership: past, present, and future. In: Antonakis J, Cianciolo AT, Sternberg RJ, eds. *The Nature of Leadership.* Thousand Oaks, CA: Sage Publications; 2004:3.

4. Bellman GM. *Getting Things Done When You Are Not in Charge.* 2nd ed. San Francisco, CA: Berrett-Koehler Publishers; 2001.

5. Kellerman B. What every leader needs to know about followers. *Harvard Business Review.* 2007;85(12):84-89.

6. Harvard Business School. *The Results Driven Manager: Getting People on Board.* Boston, MA: Harvard Business School Press; 2005.

7. Malone T, Ancona D, Bailyn L, et al. *What Do We Really Want? A Manifesto for the Organizations of the 21st Century.* Cambridge, MA: Massachusetts Institute of Technology; 1999.

8. Schwaninger M. *Intelligent Organizations: Powerful Models for Systemic Management.* New York, NY: Springer; 2006.

9. Lucas JR. *Broaden the Vision and Narrow the Focus.* Westport, CT: Praeger; 2006.

10. Grint K. *Leadership: Limits and Possibilities.* New York, NY: Palgrave Macmillan; 2005.

11. Den Hartog DN, Dickson MW. Leadership and culture. In: Antonakis J, Cianciolo AT, Sternberg RJ, eds. *The Nature of Leadership.* Thousand Oaks, CA: Sage Publications; 2004:249.

12. The GLOBE Foundation. *Syntax for GLOBE National Culture, Organizational Culture, and Leadership Scales.* Glendale, AZ: Thunderbird School of Global Management; 2006.

13. Lantz PM. Gender and leadership in healthcare administration: 21st century progress and challenges. *Journal of Healthcare Management.* 2008;53(5):291-330.

14. Eagly AH, Carli LL. Women and men as leaders. In: Antonakis J, Cianciolo AT, Sternberg RJ, eds. *The Nature of Leadership.* Thousand Oaks, CA: Sage Publications; 2004:279.

15. Gergen D. Women leading in the twenty-first century. In: Coughlin L, Wingard E, Hollihan K, eds. *Enlightened Power: How Women Are Transforming the Practice of Leadership.* San Francisco, CA: Jossey-Bass; 2005:1.

16. Harvard Business School. *Harvard Business Essentials: Power, Influence, and Persuasion; Sell Your Ideas and Make Things Happen.* Boston, MA: Harvard Business School Press; 2005.

17. Magretta J, Stone N. *What Management Is: How It Works and Why It's Everyone's Business.* New York, NY: The Free Press; 2002.

18. Harvard Business School. *Classic Drucker.* Boston, MA: Harvard Business School; 2006.

19. Drucker P. Management and the world's work. *Harvard Business Review.* 1988;66:65.

20. Quinn RE, Faerman SR, Thompson MP, McGrath MR. *Becoming a Master Manager: A Competency Framework.* 2nd ed. New York, NY: John Wiley & Sons; 1996.

21. Liebler JG, McConnell CR. *Management Principles for Health Professionals.* 6th ed. Sudbury, MA: Jones & Bartlett Learning; 2012.

22. Schein EH. *Organizational Culture and Leadership.* 4th ed. San Francisco, CA: Jossey-Bass; 2010.

23. Ott JS. *The Organizational Culture Perspective.* Chicago, IL: Dorsey Press; 1989.

24. Scott T, Mannion R, Davies H, Marshall M. The quantitative measurement of organizational culture in health care: a review of the available instruments. *Health Services Research.* 2003;38(3):923-945.

25. Carney M. Influence of organizational culture on quality healthcare delivery. *International Journal of Health Care Quality Assurance.* 2011;24(7):523-539.

26. Glisson C. Assessing and changing organizational culture and climate for effective services. *Research on Social Work Practice.* 2007;17(6):736-747.

27. Siourouni E, Kastanioti CK, Tziallas D, Niakas D. Health care provider's organizational culture profile: a literature review. *Health Science Journal.* 2012;6(2):212-233.

28. Gudykunst WB. *Bridging Differences: Effective Intergroup Communication.* 3rd ed. Thousand Oaks, CA: Sage Publications; 1998.

29. Iyengar MR, Lepper MR, Ross L. Independence from whom? interdependence with whom? cultural perspectives on ingroups versus outgroups. In: Prentice DA, Miller DT, eds. *Cultural Divides: Understanding and Overcoming Group Conflict.* New York, NY: Russell Sage; 1999.

30. Klausner M, Groves MA. Organizational socialization. In Farazmand A, ed. *Modern Organization: Theory and Practice.* 2nd ed. Westport, CT: Praeger; 2002:207.

31. Mooney M. Professional socialization: the key to survival as a new qualified nurse. *International Journal of Nursing Practice.* 2007;13(2):75-78;.

32. Avanzi L, Van Dick R, Fraccaroli F, Sarchielli G. The downside of organizational identification: relations between identification, workaholism and well-being. *Work & Stress: An International Journal of Work, Health & Organisations.* 2012;26(3):289-307.

Healthcare Organizations

LEARNING OBJECTIVES

- Discuss the challenges for healthcare organizations and strategies for meeting them.
- Discuss the potential of accountable care organizations and patient-centered medical homes to ensure quality and decrease healthcare costs.
- Analyze the complexity of U.S. healthcare from the perspectives of stakeholders.
- Compare private and public healthcare organizations and their boards of directors.
- Analyze the relationship of healthcare executives, physicians, and boards of directors.
- Discuss the development of healthcare ethics.
- Discuss the consulting efforts of outside organizations to influence healthcare access, quality, and costs.
- Predict the future of healthcare organizations.

Introduction

Some facts are necessary to set the stage for this chapter. Healthcare in the United States has evolved from a scattering of healthcare providers and hospitals that met local needs to a major industry that continues to expand and evolve. In 2011 about 7.5 million people were employed as healthcare practitioners and technicians[1] in 5,724 hospitals,[2] and national healthcare expenditures in the United States totaled $2.7 trillion. Because 20% of these expenditures went to physicians and clinics and another 31% paid for hospital care,[3] hospitals and physicians are the focus of this chapter. Other healthcare organizations and services are addressed in Section 3, Management in Specific Healthcare Settings.

The Healthcare Challenge

Contemporary healthcare systems are challenged to show the value (quality divided by cost) of the services that they deliver for that $2.7 trillion. This value is linked to the three long-standing goals of healthcare policy—improve access to care, improve the quality of care, and reduce cost and cost acceleration. Healthcare organizations can influence their value by either delivering a higher level of quality at the same or lower cost or by delivering the same level of quality at a lower cost. Although important to the fiscal bottom lines of healthcare organizations, their broader social responsibility to contribute to the well-being of the communities they serve also depends on quality and cost of the services they provide. However, controlling the acceleration of costs is no small challenge because of the following characteristics of the business of healthcare:[4]

- The development of new healthcare technology increases the demand for services. In response, insurance premiums are raised to pay for those services.
- New technology increases competition among healthcare systems and does not decrease the need for healthcare workers.

- Consumers cannot easily assess quality, but they expect it.
- Consumers use other products and services more consistently and more often than they use healthcare services.
- There is a tendency to practice defensive medicine (use of medical testing and treatments to safeguard against malpractice lawsuits rather than to meet the needs of patients).
- There is poor communication among providers and with their patients, sometimes resulting in duplication of services.
- There are wide geographical variations in the costs and availability of healthcare.
- Moral hazard may result from consumer isolation from the actual costs of healthcare (because health insurance is a tax-free employee benefit and third-party payers make payment decisions, consumers fail to consider the cost of their decisions to seek healthcare services).
- Healthcare continues to be driven by acute care and physician practices, although chronic conditions are the predominant problems of the population.
- In addition to increased demands for accountability, healthcare organizations face challenges such as the rise of new diseases, keeping patients safe as the complexity of care increases, decreased federal and state budgets, and the sharing of patient information while protecting patient privacy.

Meeting the Challenge

McConnell provides a chronological picture of how today's healthcare organizations have responded to these value challenges along with increased regulation, unbridled costs, and raised consumer demands for quality with decreased revenue. The first cost reduction response for many healthcare organizations was to partner with other organizations to share services such as purchasing, laundry, business office services, blood banking, and diagnostic radiology. These shared services relationships developed into cooperative ventures and networks in a variety of integrated delivery systems. Hospitals began to contract with external corporations for management services, and the corporate development of for-profit hospital "chains" followed. The next evolutionary

step was the centralized ownership of healthcare organizations characterized by mergers (two organizations become one) and acquisitions (one absorbs another).[5] This progression of reorganization reflects the complex private–government relationship in healthcare policy and funding. For example, Title XVIII, Health Insurance for the Aged and Disabled Act (Medicare) of 1965, offered incentives for hospitals to develop multi-unit chain operations through the 1980s, and the Health Security Act in 1993 encouraged the trend of healthcare mergers and acquisitions that continues today.[6]

Although evolving, the role of managers remains consistent in these new healthcare organizations. Managers continue to get things done through people; however, their methods for adding value to organizations have changed. For instance, many mid-level healthcare managers now split their reporting responsibilities, which means they may answer to several bosses in several different locations. Managers have also been impacted by new organizational models such as the "hospital within a hospital" and the "center of excellence" that have been created in response to very specific purposes and certification demands.

Because healthcare organizations are so much larger, the managers' span of control (the number of people supervised) may significantly increase while their visibility and availability to employees decrease.[5] At the same time, managers may find that today's unstable healthcare environment creates greater demands. They are guided by a few simple rules rather than detailed plans to achieve an even more careful balance of just enough structure to support innovation and new learning, but not so much that new ideas are stifled.[7]

As these organizations have evolved into large healthcare systems, they have been able to adopt strategies to control costs. All under more powerful boards of directors, some of these strategies are increased buying power because of sheer volume, replacement of permanent employees with contingency workers, elimination of duplicate services, and the outsourcing of many other services.[5] These mega-healthcare systems have such a powerful competitive advantage that freestanding hospitals are almost a thing of the past.

However, a potential problem has been identified. Reviewers of recent studies of healthcare organizational models were unable to conclude that these systems provide the solutions once hoped for to improve healthcare delivery. Many have begun to decentralize control of their component organizations as a result.[6] Because the learning curve of organizational change is steep, it may be premature to draw conclusions about organizations that will continue to be in transition long after full implementation of the 2010 Patient Protection and Affordable Care Act in 2014.[6]

Accountable Care Organizations

Many healthcare organizations have already transformed the way they deliver care to *all* of their patients in anticipation of their participation in accountable care organizations (ACOs). In one part of the 2010 Patient Protection and Affordable Care Act (ACA or Obamacare), Congress empowered the Centers for Medicare & Medicaid Services (CMS) to recognize the voluntary formation of ACOs. CMS rewards ACOs financially if they slow the growth of Medicare Parts A and B expenditures and also maintain or improve the quality of care in seamless models of care.

By 2012, CMS had approved 153 ACOs that provide services to 2.4 million Medicare recipients. These patients remain free to choose any approved Medicare provider regardless of the provider's participation in an ACO.[8] They may not even know whether the doctor or hospital is a member of an ACO. Other people may have already noticed some effects of these efforts for seamless care that suggest an ACO is in place.

For example, one expected advantage of ACOs is increased communication among providers with a decrease in duplication of services and a seamless continuity of care. Patients may notice the physician or nurse sitting at a computer. They are able to review old medical records, information from an emergency room visit, notes on visits to other providers, and lab test results that can be easily compared with previous tests, medications, and so on. Computer prompts may appear for scheduling recommended preventive screens based on the patient's age and condition. Hospital patients may now rely on caregivers to access records in the physician's office if they are part of the same ACO. Upon discharge, a nurse may offer to phone in a patient's prescriptions to the pharmacy across the street (because it is part of the same ACO) for convenient pickup on the way home. The risk of alterations in drug regimens may be reduced while pharmacists and nurses have the opportunity to check for drug interactions and adverse effects.

The plan is for all providers in an ACO to be electronically and seamlessly connected, which is expected to reduce costs, reduce risks, increase savings, and, therefore, increase profits. The sponsoring ACO organization decides which groups of physicians, pharmacies, freestanding outpatient centers, home-care agencies, and other providers are included in their initial application. The ACO may later decide to include other Medicare providers (perhaps a skilled nursing facility or physical therapy practice) to round out the care continuum, control costs, and improve quality. Those organizations that are not part of an ACO may be at a financial disadvantage as a result. Other smaller organizations may not be able to participate because the expenses for connecting to common documentation and billing systems may be prohibitive. Patients may decide that there are advantages to choosing providers that are part of the same ACO such as increased consistency and communication about their ongoing healthcare. Such consumer choices may also negatively impact non-ACO organizations.

CMS uses 33 measures of quality through data collected in four broad areas: care coordination and patient safety, use of appropriate preventive health services, improved care for at-risk populations, and patient and caregiver experience of care. Based on the scores on these measures, an ACO receives payment based on one of CMS's cost-saving models. In one model, the ACO providers share in savings only, or they may choose a model with higher risks because it includes a share of the losses if costs go up. They receive a higher share of profits if costs go down.[8] Many healthcare organizations anticipated the development of ACOs and took the lead; many others appear to be considering ACO membership. It may be too early to determine the impact of ACOs on healthcare costs and quality of care. Readers are encouraged to monitor the local impact of ACOs on healthcare delivery and their personal healthcare.

Patient-Centered Medical Homes

Patient-centered medical homes (PCMHs) are another new type of healthcare organization that has the potential to provide seamless, longitudinal care at the level of the patient in the community. A PCMH is a panel (group) of primary care physicians (and perhaps other health professionals such as pharmacists) who organize to coordinate and review the care of patient groups they are accountable for. By January 2013, a total of 5,198 organizations had received recognition as PCMHs by the National Committee on Quality Assurance (NCQA).[9] This recognition is required to qualify for the financial incentives offered by insurers and the federal government to PCMHs for their efforts to coordinate and improve the quality of community-based primary care. One requirement for NCQA recognition is that the PCMH use standardized electronic data collection on care delivery and patients that is shared among providers and submitted to NCQA for annual analysis.

The success of this new model for primary care is heavily dependent on patients who are able to actively engage in their own care and share ongoing information about their conditions. Patients with complex, chronic conditions who do not have social advantages may present the greatest challenges to the ability of PCMHs to achieve their quality goals. ACOs are expected to include PCMHs. By building on the primary care they provide, the expectation is that the ACO will improve the quality of care and reduce their costs of the care of people with chronic conditions. The appropriateness of hospital admissions and a decrease in the need for expensive inpatient episodes are other expectations as primary healthcare is integrated more effectively in healthcare systems.

U.S. Healthcare Complexity: The Players

To understand the complexity of U.S. healthcare requires going beyond broad healthcare policies, new organizational models, and the actual buildings that house healthcare organizations—hospitals, nursing homes, home-care agencies, retail clinics, community pharmacies, outpatient centers, and so on. A list of the many stakeholders in healthcare presents an expanded view of the diverse interests of people and organizations that impact every healthcare organization.

Beginning with patients, of course, the list of stakeholders includes:

- PATIENTS
- MEDICAL PRODUCTS MANUFACTURERS (prosthetic devices, surgical tools, pharmaceuticals, hospital beds and other furniture, other capital equipment, durable medical equipment, information technology, etc.)
- MEDICAL SUPPLIES MANUFACTURERS (intravenous solutions, blood banks, enteral feedings, needles, syringes, bandages and dressings, sutures, ointments, disinfectants, etc.)
- WHOLESALERS AND DISTRIBUTORS OF THE SAME PRODUCTS AND SUPPLIES
- HEALTHCARE EXECUTIVES, MANAGERS, AND OUTSIDE CONSULTANTS
- HEALTHCARE PROFESSIONALS AND TECHNICIANS
- RECRUITING AND TEMPORARY STAFFING AGENCIES
- SUPPORT SERVICE WORKERS (housekeeping, food service, maintenance, human resources, etc.)
- EMPLOYERS
- INSURANCE COMPANIES AND BROKERS
- STATE DEPARTMENTS OF INSURANCE REGULATION
- MEDICAID PROGRAMS—one for each state
- STATE AND LOCAL DEPARTMENTS OF HEALTH
- U.S. DEPARTMENT OF HEALTH AND HUMAN SERVICES (regulatory, direct patient care, and research responsibilities through Administration on Community Living, Agency for Healthcare Research and Quality, Centers for Disease Control and Prevention, Food and Drug Administration, Health Resources and Services Administration, Indian Health Services, National Institutes of Health, Substance Abuse and Mental Health Services, Centers for Medicare & Medicaid Services, U.S. Public Health Service Commissioned Corps, Bureau of Prisons, Department of Defense, Veterans' Administration, etc.)
- MEMBERS OF THE U.S. SENATE AND HOUSE OF REPRESENTATIVES

- STATE AND LOCAL ELECTED OFFICIALS
- LOBBYISTS AND POLITICAL ACTION COMMITTEES REPRESENTING HEALTHCARE ORGANIZATIONS AND PROFESSIONALS

Given this mix of private and government entities, the difficulty in grasping the idea of U.S. healthcare as a "system" is not surprising. It is not difficult, however, to understand how challenging it is to make dramatic changes in healthcare. Change is particularly hard when stakeholders do not have equal status, which further complicates dealing with conflicting needs and perspectives. For example, the medical profession drives healthcare spending while patients remain on the edges of decision-making. Healthcare legislation is often piecemeal and based on the needs of those with special interests rather than on the good of the public. Healthcare delivery is a local process, which encumbers data collection required for the rational decision-making in forming national healthcare policy. See Sidebar 3.1.

More Complexity: Public and Private Healthcare Organizations

Another aspect of U.S. healthcare complexity is its mix of public (governmental) and private healthcare organizations. Regardless of their public or private status, healthcare organizations share a common history of theories and models of organizations with other businesses. However, collectively, they are different from other businesses because of particular organizational dynamics that set them apart, such as:[10]

- Their mission of service to alleviate pain and suffering and restore patients to health
- The complex, highly regulated environment—internal and external—under which they operate
- Professional cultures (physicians, nurses, healthcare managers)
- The rapidly changing healthcare market

The typical consumer may not be aware of how much healthcare is like other businesses. They may understand how they are different organizations, but not find differences among healthcare organizations obvious or interesting, especially at times of crisis when they have an immediate need for healthcare. For example, most people are not aware of the type of a hospital or who owns it—unless it is a military or veterans' hospital. Except for differences in direct patient care experiences, all hospitals seem to be more or less the same to most people who often have little choice in selecting one. There are, however, differences.

The American Hospital Association classifies the 5,724 hospitals into several groups. The two major groups are Community Hospitals and Other Hospitals. The group of 751 Other Hospitals that are *not* generally accessible to the public include federal government hospitals (208), psychiatric hospitals (421), long-term acute care hospitals (112), and hospitals embedded in other institutions such as prisons and colleges (10). The much larger group of 4,973 Community Hospitals are generally accessible to anyone choosing to enter one. Community Hospitals may be general or specialty and include academic health centers. They may be rural (1,984) or urban (2,989). They may be part of a larger healthcare system or network (4,542). They may be not-for-profit (2,903), state and local hospitals (1,045), or investor-owned/for-profit (1,025).[2]

Both for-profit and not-for-profit hospitals (typically within broader healthcare systems) may be present in any large community. Based on these data, about 80% of all hospitals are not-for-profit organizations. The reason for a preponderance of not-for-profit hospitals lies with their history.

SIDEBAR 3.1

Shareholders and Stakeholders

A *shareholder* (stockholder) is a person or organization that owns shares of a for-profit corporation through the purchase of stock holdings in that company. Shareholders may be able to vote for the members of the board, take part in other decisions of the company, and share the profits.

Stakeholders are a much broader group because the term includes *anyone* who has a legitimate interest (stake) in any type of organization. A stakeholder is anyone who may influence an organization or be affected by it. All shareholders are stakeholders, but not all stakeholders are shareholders.

They began as charitable institutions, often with religious affiliations, to care for the indigent people who had no other means to receive healthcare. Many of these small, basic service hospitals have evolved into large healthcare systems, such as Florida Hospital (Seventh Day Adventists); Catholic Health System in Buffalo, New York; and KentuckyOne Health (the 2012 merger of Jewish Hospital, St. Mary's Healthcare, and St. Joseph Health System).

These pioneer faith-based hospitals were granted income tax–exempt status in return for their contributions to the poor and needy. As healthcare needs increased over the years, other not-for-profit healthcare corporations were created that had no religious affiliations. The tax exemptions continue to apply to all of them. Discenza explains that these large, business-oriented healthcare organizations continue to keep their not-for-profit status because they meet the following criteria: they are self-sustaining from revenues for the care they provide, they have no owners, and they may accept tax-deductible contributions to achieve their missions. They may also access bond markets to raise capital, but they may not engage in political activity or influence legislators. Individuals cannot benefit from revenues beyond reasonable salaries in not-for-profit organizations.[11] Because of these legal characteristics, not-for-profit does not mean that an organization does not intend to make money. Contrary to popular opinion, not-for-profit organizations may actually generate enormous profits, *but* the profits may only be used to sustain and grow their organizations.

In the public sector, government-owned organizations and public corporations are also exempt from taxes, but they are subject to political decisions for funding to meet the unique needs of special populations. A similar movement to a system or network model has also evolved in these healthcare organizations:

- The Veterans' Administration's VISN (Veterans' Integrated Service Network) has 23 regions in which healthcare services for veterans are provided in 1,700 units (hospitals, clinics, community living centers, etc.)[12] (see Web Resources).
- Combined, all branches of the military have 59 hospitals and 600 clinics around the world to provide healthcare for enlisted men and women and their families. These military units appear to be virtually connected through the latest health information technology.[13] (See Web Resources for Military Health System information.)
- On a much smaller scale, the U.S. Public Health Service includes hospitals within the Indian Health Service and Bureau of Prisons (see Web Resources for the U.S. Public Health Service).

Conversely, the few remaining for-profit hospitals are corporations that focus on profits that are distributed as dividends to individual investors (shareholders). Shareholders are often physicians, but may be anyone, including employees, who is offered stock options as an employment benefit. For-profit hospitals also contribute indirectly to the good of the community through the payment of taxes like any other corporation does and through their limited obligations to provide care to people who are indigent. They also may engage in political campaigns and influence legislators.[11] See Activity 3.1.

Even More Complexity: Executives, Physicians, and Boards

Griffith and White suggest that, essentially, all healthcare systems are open systems that transform resources into services to meet the demands of their communities while earning income. They are more likely to meet these goals by clearly answering

---

ACTIVITY 3.1
YOUR HEALTHCARE SYSTEM

1. What surprises you about the healthcare organizations in your community? What reputations do they have? Who are the healthcare stakeholders in your community?
2. Are there ACOs in your area? What do you know about them? What is in the news about your local healthcare organizations?
3. What are your impressions about the culture of healthcare organizations in your community? How do you expect the cultures of different types of hospitals to differ? How are for-profit and not-for-profit organizational cultures different? How are they the same?

three important questions: Why are we here (or what is our purpose)? Why did we select this purpose? What strategy is the best to achieve our purpose?[14] The chief executive officer (CEO), the chief medical officer (CMO), and the chairperson of the board of directors (BOD) of a healthcare organization each are likely to answer these questions differently because of their unique responsibilities and duties. The challenge is for these decision makers to reach some point of agreement on their answers.

The CMOs are generally responsible for all clinical components of a healthcare system. They function as the intermediary for physicians and the executive team, and they monitor the quality of all patient care. They may hold other titles such as vice president of medical affairs, medical director, or chief of staff. Emerging new executive positions held by physicians include chief quality officer and chief medical information officer.

Chief executive officers may see the purpose of a healthcare organization a little differently from the way that CMOs do. Chief executive officers must take a much broader view in their responsibilities for the *total* management of all components of a healthcare organization, including patient care. Often in organizational charts, the line leading from the CMO to the CEO is a dotted line to demonstrate that many aspects of patient care are beyond the expertise of the CEO, who nevertheless remains accountable for it. That dotted line is extremely important as these two executives attempt to reconcile their values and goals to agree on purpose.

Although they are responsible for all clinical and support services, often CEOs are not the final authority. They answer to BODs, whose members may perceive an organization's purpose from the more externally driven viewpoint of its role in society. This three-part organizational structure, perhaps more than anything else, makes healthcare organizations unique and complex. The application of traditional organizational theories and models to these special places is often confusing as a result.

Boards of Directors

Large for-profit and not-for-profit corporations have boards of directors (BODs) that represent either the stockholders (for-profit) or the public (not-for-profit) as they govern an organization. Boards are comparable to the legislature, county commissions, or city councils in public (governmental) institutions. Boards are responsible, in varying degrees of formality and direct responsibility, for defining an organization's purpose and all aspects of ensuring that its purpose is accomplished. They hire the CEO and may have input into the election or appointment of the CMO. How a BOD is appointed, how it is organized, and how it conducts its work are reflected in a variety of models that are just as complex as the organizations themselves. Boards are all legal entities with fiduciary responsibilities, but there are differences.[15]

For instance, board members of for-profit corporations are more likely to be paid for their services. They direct their efforts to dispersing the organization's profits to stockholders, and may rely on lobbying efforts to advance their business agendas with public policy makers. Not-for-profit board members are less likely to be paid, represent the public stakeholders in the organization, and direct their efforts to fundraising through charitable donations, grants, and the like.[15]

Boards of directors differ because of the varying degrees of responsibility they really have, and their relationships to CEOs and CMOs. Some boards may be intimately involved in the day-to-day management of an organization while others may be widely separated from management. Instead, they devote their energy to broader, long-term strategic planning and the development of strong relationships with external stakeholders. Some BODs serve simply to rubber-stamp decisions of CEOS. Other CEOs rely heavily on boards for management decisions.[15] See Activity 3.2.

ACTIVITY 3.2
MORE IMPRESSIONS

1. Select an organizational chart of any healthcare system from its webpage. Analyze its components and their relationships.
   • Who sits on its board of directors?
   • What are your impressions of the CEO and CMO?
2. Summarize your impression of this organization.
3. How can you become a member of a board of a healthcare organization?
   • Why would you want to be a member?

Healthcare Organizational Ethics

The actions of the CEO–CMO–BOD triad of decision makers in healthcare organizations present many ethical challenges as well. Although the field of healthcare organizational ethics appears to be in its infant stage, its increasing importance should not be underestimated. In their review of 56 research studies on healthcare organizational ethics, researchers confirmed the lack of a theoretical healthcare ethics framework, a wide variety of ethics measurement tools, and poorly defined topics and terminology.[16]

The researchers also emphasized that in today's delivery of patient care, the codes of ethics for individual professions are often insufficient.[16] Multidisciplinary care may require a multidisciplinary code of ethics to address the disparities between patient needs and organizational demands that professionals face. A better framework is also needed to guide healthcare organizations as they negotiate their place in the broader social context of relationships with other organizations.[16] One response to this need in all types of organizations was the passage of the Sarbanes-Oxley (SOX) Act in 2002. Although applicable to for-profit corporations, many hospitals adopted the accountability and reporting requirements of this law, such as CEO certification of financial reports, public reporting of executive salaries, and independent internal auditors.[17]

Boyle believes all stakeholders face ethical challenges that arise when decisions of complex healthcare organizations are inconsistent with their common values. He identifies these values as integrity, honesty, fairness, respect for others, promise keeping, and prudence. Boyle recognizes that the risk of unethical actions increases when the eye of the organization is on its tangible, monetary goals rather than goals related to the care and health of the community. Examples of actions that suggest that a healthcare organization may be unethical include misleading advertising, cover-up of errors, acceptance of poor quality care, favoritism, suppression of rights, nondisclosure, and corruption. If employees feel that they are unsupported, undermined, or discouraged from pursing good works because of these actions, then cynicism, poor morale, and even shame may result.[10]

Pearson and his coauthors suggest that a healthcare organization must set its moral compass so that the importance of caring for the sick and injured is an unshakeable value. Organizations must also clearly identify who is responsible for monitoring this moral compass and establish processes to deal with the inevitable conflicts that arise.[18] Since the 1960s, hospital ethics committees have had an education and consultation role in biomedical issues such as end-of-life care and other patient treatment issues. Pozgar suggests that ethics committees need to move beyond this role to address equally important organizational issues such as staff cover-ups when errors occur, reimbursement schemes, and kickbacks.[17] Some people argue that if an organization has successful processes that address its moral obligations, all other successes, will follow. (See Activity 3.3.)

Access, Quality, and Costs

Regardless of the type of healthcare organization, even those exclusively devoted to physical therapy services, each one faces the challenges of access

---

ACTIVITY 3.3
GOOD VERSUS GOOD

At a recent meeting of the stroke team in a large healthcare system, one of the occupational therapists shared her concern with the group about the quality of the medical devices that were recently delivered to the rehabilitation unit from Allgood Medical Suppliers. The rest of the group agreed with her, pointing out that many of the walkers were very cheap and unsteady, and some of the wheelchairs seemed used or repaired. Many of the staff felt that this was related to the hospital's efforts to control costs by buying the cheapest equipment and supplies possible. The speech-language pathologist, Harry Hughes, said that he suspected something more was taking place. A friend of Harry's who works for Allgood told him that the hospital receives a kickback for doing business with them. They turn to their manager, Laura Lancer, and demand action.

Why should Laura take action?

Where should Laura look for guidance?

What action should she take?

(discussed in Chapter 4), quality, and costs of healthcare. Many non-government organizations lead the efforts to address these challenges from a wide range of perspectives and responsibilities. The following brief descriptions explore the functions and roles of some of them. Links are provided to delve into these organizations in more detail.

The National Coalition on Healthcare (NCHC)

The NCHC is a watchdog group of more than 100 organizations that seeks to improve healthcare in the United States. This coalition includes organizations as diverse as AARP, American College of Surgeons, CVS Caremark, Duke Energy, the Episcopal Church, and the International Brotherhood of Teamsters. Their mission is to bring together key stakeholders in order to achieve an affordable, high-value healthcare system for patients and consumers, for employers and other payers, and for taxpayers. With their political action committee (PAC), this diverse group is united in supporting efforts for healthcare that include coverage for all, cost management, improvement of quality and safety, equitable financing, and simplified administration.

Institutes of Medicine (IOM)

The IOM is a component of the National Academy of Sciences. It is an independent organization that conducts research mandated by the U.S. Congress or other government agencies and private organizations. It takes pride in the use of consensus to facilitate cross-disciplinary problem-solving. Of particular interest are three important IOM studies that are summarized here.

First, in a 2000 report, *To Err Is Human: Building a Safer Health System,*[19] the IOM discovered that more people die in a given year from preventable adverse events in hospitals alone than die from motor vehicle accidents, or breast cancer, or AIDS. Many of these errors are related to healthcare culture and how healthcare organizations are organized and managed rather than incompetence or carelessness of individuals. These terrible outcomes are linked to: ·

- A fragmented system in which rigid specialization and powerful influences make it difficult to hold people accountable.

- Resistance to the movement toward the implementation of information systems that are coordinated for patient-centered care.
- Limited financial incentives for healthcare organizations to improve quality and safety.
- A medical liability system that is a serious impediment to efforts to uncover and learn from errors.

Next, in 2001, the IOM's Committee on Quality of Healthcare in America prepared *Crossing the Quality Chasm,* in which the committee expressed its concerns about healthcare in the United States. The healthcare provided is not the healthcare that could, *and should,* be provided because of outmoded *systems* of work in healthcare that set employees up to fail.[20] The committee suggested that the only solution requires a total restructuring of healthcare organizations to address both quality and cost concerns through improved administrative and clinical processes. The committee recommended that all stakeholders support an environment for improvement through:

- Creation of infrastructures to support evidence-based practice
- Facilitation of the use of information technology
- Alignment of payment incentives
- Preparation of the workforce to better serve patients in a world of expanding knowledge and rapid change

The Committee on Quality of Healthcare in America also encouraged all healthcare organizations to adopt six simple aims for improvement of the quality of care. Care should be:

- *Safe*—avoiding injuries to patients from the care that is intended to help them
- *Effective*—providing services based on scientific knowledge to all who could benefit and refraining from providing services to those not likely to benefit (avoiding underuse and overuse, respectively)
- *Patient-centered*—providing care that is respectful of and responsive to individual patient preferences, needs, and values and ensuring that patient values guide all clinical decisions
- *Timely*—reducing waiting time and sometimes harmful delays for both those who receive care and those who give care

- *Efficient*—avoiding waste, including waste of equipment, supplies, ideas, and energy
- *Equitable*—providing care that does not vary in quality because of personal characteristics such as gender, ethnicity, geographical location, and socioeconomic status

More recently, the IOM convened a consensus group to address the need for continuous learning and improvement in healthcare. In 2012, that group published *Best Care at Lower Cost: The Path to Continuously Learning Health Care in America.*[21] They argued that available knowledge was too rarely applied, and data generated in patient care were not systematically gathered so that organizations could change in response to new information. Their vision is that the best available evidence, with appropriate consideration for individual preference, will be used to deliver the best results in reliable and efficient care. Their recommendations included the following:

- Improve the capacity to digitally collect and compile clinical data to generate new knowledge.
- Streamline research regulations to ensure privacy and the seamless use of clinical data.
- Make the use of decision support and knowledge management tools routine in healthcare delivery.
- Involve patients and families in decisions that reflect their preferences for health and healthcare.
- Facilitate community–clinical partnerships to improve individual and population health.
- Structure payments to reward communication and coordination among members of the care team.
- Improve systems and processes to streamline healthcare operations and reduce waste.
- Structure payments and contracts to reward effective and efficient care that continuously improves.
- Increase transparency on organizational performance for healthcare decisions.
- Make continuous learning a core priority for all participants in healthcare.

The Joint Commission

According to its website, the mission of The Joint Commission is "to continuously improve healthcare for the public, in collaboration with other stakeholders, by evaluating healthcare organizations and inspiring them to excel in providing safe and effective care of the highest quality and value." Its accreditation and certification of more than 20,000 healthcare organizations and programs in the United States is recognized as a symbol of quality and commitment to performance standards.

In its 2012 annual report, *The Joint Commission's Annual Report on Quality and Safety,*[22] it is reported that 620 (18%) Joint Commission–accredited hospitals achieved the outstanding accountability measure of performance required to be included in the Top Performers on Key Quality Measures program. The seven measure sets were heart attack care, pneumonia care, surgical care, children's asthma care, inpatient psychiatric services, venous thromboembolism care, and stroke care. Although proud of the efforts of this small group of hospitals, The Joint Commission admits that a great deal of work needs to be done to fulfill its mission.

The Commonwealth Fund

According to its website, the mission of the Commonwealth Fund is "to promote a high-performing healthcare system that achieves better access, improved quality, and greater efficiency, particularly for society's most vulnerable, including low-income people, the uninsured, minority Americans, young children, and elderly adults." It supports independent research on healthcare issues and supports grants to improve healthcare practice and policy. Its international program in health policy is designed to stimulate innovative policies and practices in the United States and other industrialized countries.

In 2005, the Commonwealth Fund established a Commission on a High Performance Health System in response to the need for national leadership to revamp, revitalize, and retool the U.S. healthcare system. The commission has broad representation of experts and leaders representing private and public stakeholders in healthcare who are often called on by policy makers at all levels of government to provide expert testimony and assistance. These experts provide the U.S. Congress with information and technical assistance based on their work and that of the Commonwealth Fund. The official documents of this commission generated some of the major ideas in the Affordable Care Act—including new insurance market regulations, the requirement for everyone to have coverage, the availability of premium and cost-sharing subsidies for low- and moderate-income families, and payment and delivery system reforms. Other examples of the work of the Commission on a High Performance Health System include the following:

- In 2011, its *High Performance Accountable Care: Building on Success and Learning From Experience*[23] report provided a set of recommendations for ensuring the successful implementation and spread of the ACO model, which it believes holds particular promise for healthcare delivery to people with chronic or complex medical conditions.

- Other findings were reported in the 2012 edition of its *Rising to the Challenge: Results From a Scorecard on Local Health System Performance*.[24] For example, despite pockets of improvement, the United States as a whole failed to improve on 43 key indicators of healthcare quality when compared with the top-performing countries. The key indicators are grouped as access, prevention and treatment, costs, potentially avoidable hospital use, and health outcomes. The findings also show clearly that where you live matters. There is a two- to threefold variation in the indicators between the leading (Upper Midwest and Northeast) and lagging (southern) communities.

- In another 2012 report, *The Performance Improvement Imperative: Utilizing a Coordinated, Community-Based Approach to Enhance Care and Lower Costs for Chronically Ill Patients*,[25] the Commonwealth Fund presents a strategy for improving the coordination of health services provided to people with multiple chronic health conditions. The report argues that the nation should be able to achieve substantial improvements in care for these patients while saving billions in healthcare costs through coordinated, locally based efforts.

These brief descriptions of the efforts made by important and sophisticated groups suggest that many people and organizations share the same values and aims for healthcare in the United States. Optimistically, because of these interdisciplinary, comprehensive views of healthcare, progress is being made. Alternatively, even with the brightest and best tackling the unique, complex delivery of healthcare in this country, it continues to face many challenges. Impressions of today's U.S. healthcare system and its future may be further influenced by comparisons with the healthcare systems of other countries. See Sidebar 3.2.

Conclusions

Leaders and managers in any healthcare organization do not lack for interesting work as they influence the access, quality, and costs of healthcare. Particularly because this is a period of adjustment as the Affordable Care Act continues to be implemented, opportunities may arise that are currently not even considered. From a personal and professional view, it is critical that physical therapists monitor these changes. The American Physical Therapy Association webpages link to many resources at the Practice and Patient Care, Payment, and Advocacy tabs (see Web Resources). How physical therapy independent, private practices and outpatient corporate practices fit in ACOs and PCMHs is uncertain. Leaders and managers need to monitor the activities of the organizations discussed, the Centers for Medicare & Medicaid Services, and state and local healthcare activity to remain current with the evolving healthcare policies.

SIDEBAR 3.2

Healthcare Systems in Other Countries

The Organizations for Economic Co-operation and Development (OECD)

http://www.oecd.org/health/

The OECD provides comparative data to assist governments in setting social and economic policies including healthcare. Explore their health topics and statistics.

REFERENCES

1. United States Department of Labor, Bureau of Labor Statistics. Occupational Employment and Wages, May 2011, 29-0000 Healthcare Practitioners and Technical Occupations (MajorGroup). http://www.bls.gov/oes/current/oes290000.htm#nat. Accessed July 2013.

2. American Hospital Association. Fast Facts on US Hospitals, 2001. http://www.aha.org/research/rc/stat-studies/fast-facts.shtml. Accessed February 2013.

3. Centers for Medicare & Medicaid Services. The nation's health dollar ($2.7 trillion), calendar year 2011: where it went. Available at: http://www.cms.gov/Research-Statistics-Data-and-Systems/Statistics-Trends-and-Reports/National-HealthExpendData/Downloads/PieChartSourcesExpenditures2011.pdf. Accessed February 22, 2013.

4. Burns LR, Bradley EH, Weiner BJ. The management challenge of delivering value in health care: global and US perspectives. In: Burns LR, Bradley EH, Weiner BJ, eds. *Shortell and Kaluzny's Health Care Management: Organization Design and Behavior.* 6th ed. Clifton Park, NY: Delmar Cengage Learning; 2012.

5. McConnell CR. Managers and mergers: functioning in a blended organization. *The Health Care Manager.* 2008;27(4): 369-377.

6. Burns LR, Wholey DR, McCullough JS, Kralovec P, Muller R. The changing configuration of hospital systems: centralization, federalization, or fragmentation? In: Friedman LH, Savage GT, Goes J, eds. *Annual Review of Health Care Management: Strategy and Policy Perspectives on Reforming Health Systems.* London, England: Emerald Group Publishing Ltd; 2012:189-232. *Advances in Health Care Management;* vol. 13.

7. Weiner BJ, Helfrich CD. Complexity, learning, and innovation. In: Burns LR, Bradley EH, Weiner BJ, eds. *Shortell and Kaluzny's Health Care Management: Organization Design and Behavior.* 6th ed. Clifton Park NY: Delmar Cengage Learning; 2012.

8. Centers for Medicare & Medicaid Services. CMS factsheet: CMS names 88 new Medicare Shared Savings Accountable Care Organizations.http://www.cms.gov/apps/media/press/factsheet.asp?Counter=4405&intNumPerPage=10&checkDate=&checkKey=&srchType=1&numDays=3500&srchOpt=0&srchData=&keywordType=All&chkNewsType=6&intPage=&showAll=&pYear=&year=&desc=&cboOrder=date. Accessed February 21, 2013.

9. National Committee for Quality Assurance. Patient-centered medical homes. http://www.ncqa.org/Programs/Recognition/PatientCenteredMedicalHomePCMH.aspx. Accessed February 26, 2013.

10. Boyle P, DuBose ER, Ellingson SJ, et al. *Organizational Ethics in Health Care: Principles, Cases, and Practical Solutions.* San Francisco, CA: Jossey-Bass; 2001.

11. Discenza S. Managing costs and revenues. In: Buchbinder SB, Shanks NH. *Introduction to Health Care Management.* Sudbury, MA: Jones and Bartlett; 2007.

12. U.S. Department of Veterans' Affairs. Veterans' health care. http://www2.va.gov/directory/guide/division_flsh.asp?dnum=1. Accessed February 26, 2013.

13. Defense Health Services System website. http://www.health.mil/DHSS.aspx. Accessed February 22, 2013.

14. Griffith JR, White K. *The Well-Managed Health Care Organization.* 5th ed. Chicago, IL: Health Administration Press; 2002.

15. McNamara C. Free complete toolkit for boards. http://www.managementhelp.org/boards/boards.htm. Accessed February 22, 2013.

16. Suhonen R, Stolt M, Virtanen H, Leino-Kilpi H. Organizational ethics: A literature review. *Nursing Ethics.* 2011:18(3); 285-303.

17. Pozgar GD. *Legal Aspects of Health Care Administration.* 11th ed. Sudbury, MA: Jones & Bartlett; 2012.

18. Pearson SD, Sabin JE, Emanuel EJ. *No Margin, No Mission: Health-Care Organizations and the Quest for Ethical Excellence.* New York, NY: Oxford University Press; 2003.

19. Kohn LT, Corrigan JM, Donaldson MS, eds. *To Err Is Human: Building a Safer Health System.* Washington, DC: National Academy Press; 2000.

20. Committee on Quality of Health Care in America. *Crossing the Quality Chasm: A New Health System for the 21st Century.* Washington, DC: National Academy Press; 2001.

21. Smith M, Saunder R, Stuckhardt L, McGinnis, JM, eds. *Best Care at Lower Cost: The Path to Continuously Learning Health Care in America.* Washington, DC: National Academies Press, 2012.

22. The Joint Commission. *Annual Report: The Joint Commission's Annual Report on Quality and Safety.* http://www.jointcommission.org/annualreport.aspx. Accessed July 2013.

23. Guterman S, Schoenbaum, SC, Davis K, et al. *High Performance Accountable Care: Building on Success and Learning From Experience.* New York, NY: The Commonwealth Fund; 2011.

24. Radley DC, How SKH, Fryer AK, McCarthy D, Schoen C. *Rising to the Challenge: Results From a Scorecard on Local Health System Performance.* New York, NY: The Commonwealth Fund; 2012.

25. The Commonwealth Fund Commission on a High Performance Health System. *The Performance Improvement Imperative: Utilizing a Coordinated, Community-Based Approach to Enhance Care and Lower Costs for Chronically Ill Patients.* New York, NY: The Commonwealth Fund; 2012.

WEB RESOURCES

American Physical Therapy Association. http://www.apta.org/. Accessed July 23, 2013.

The Commonwealth Fund. http://www.commonwealthfund.org/About-Us/Mission-Statement.aspx. Accessed July 23, 2013.

Federal Bureau of Prisons: An Agency of the U.S. Department of Justice. http://www.bop.gov/about/co/health_services.jsp. Accessed July 23, 2013.

The Federal Health Program for American Indians and Alaska Natives. http://www.ihs.gov/. Accessed July 23, 2013.

Institutes of Medicine of the National Academies (IOM). http://www.iom.edu/. Accessed July 23, 2013.

The Joint Commission. http://www.jointcommission.org/. Accessed July 23, 2013.

National Coalition on Healthcare (NCHC). http://nchc.org/. Accessed July 23, 2013.

U.S. Department of Defense: The Military Health System. http://www.health.mil/About_MHS/Organizations/Index.aspx. Accessed July 23, 2013.

U.S. Public Health Service. America's health responders. http://www.usphs.gov/. Accessed July 23, 2013.

U.S. Department of Veterans Affairs. http://www.va.gov/. Accessed July 23, 2013.

CHAPTER 4

Introduction to Healthcare as a Unique Insurance-Based Business

LEARNING OBJECTIVES

- Discuss the perspectives of patients, employees, employers, providers, and insurers in health insurance.
- Determine the role of employment and employers in healthcare insurance.
- Discuss the regulation of healthcare insurance.
- Compare and contrast types of private and public healthcare insurance.
- Identify the challenges presented to managers by the underinsured and the uninsured.
- Analyze the healthcare insurance issues presented in a case study.
- Identify contemporary challenges in the payment for healthcare services.

Introduction

Healthcare is a business, and, in many ways, its management parallels the management of all businesses. On one hand, finances, human resources, capital equipment needs, the control of costs, and the generation of profits are just as much a part of the business of healthcare as they are the substance of other businesses. On the other hand, the business of healthcare is unique because of its purposes—healing injuries and preventing, managing, and curing diseases—as well as the complex manner in which healthcare is conducted and paid for. A patient (with an employer if applicable), an insurer, and a healthcare provider (person, organization, system) make up the basic unit of healthcare business.

Proceed to Activity 4.1 and take the pre-test to determine your current understanding of health insurance. Refer to the Glossary at the Centers for Medicare & Medicaid Services (CMS) website for definitions of any unfamiliar healthcare terminology as you read this chapter (see Web Resources).

The basic unit of healthcare is considered in a presentation of the key components of the Patient Protection and Affordable Care Act (ACA) of 2010. This analysis adds to the understanding of the complexity of U.S. healthcare through the perspectives of patients, employers, providers, and insurers on healthcare access, costs, and quality.

Patients' Perspective

The business of healthcare places the patient in an unusual consumer position. When receiving

51

ACTIVITY 4.1
HEALTH INSURANCE PRE-TEST

1. Who pays for your health insurance? Who are all of the beneficiaries on your insurance plan? Parents? Spouse? Children?
2. What kind of health insurance plan do you have? Preferred provider organization (PPO)? Health savings account (HSA)? Other?
3. How much is the deductible? How much are the co-payments? What is the maximal annual or lifetime allowance on the policy? Do you have prescription drug coverage? Does the plan include payment for physical therapy services? What other services are covered?
4. On your (or anyone's) payroll stub, which payroll deduction is greatest: Federal Insurance Contribution Act (FICA for Social Security)? Medicare Payroll tax? Your health insurance premium contribution? What is the employer's contribution to your insurance plan?

healthcare services in any setting, or when purchasing medications, durable medical equipment, or other supplies, patients must contend with several intervening influences. The simple exchange of money for goods and services, which is the basis for any other business transaction, becomes complicated in healthcare. Rather than directly getting what they pay for, most patients are removed from the exchange of money for healthcare services.

Patients are familiar with out-of-pocket payments to meet deductible limits or co-payments at the time of service in healthcare. Their providers may have mentioned the need for preauthorization for payment before services can be rendered. Beyond that, patients may not know what the healthcare service they receive actually costs and how much insurers pay providers. Furthermore, patients have to determine how and whether the rules for healthcare change as they move from one type of healthcare setting to another. People often deal with uncertainty as their health insurance plans change from year to year or as they move from one employer to another, or as they move from private to public insurance.

These special business circumstances are often confounded because people who require healthcare are often seeking it when they are most vulnerable

and anxious—at times of sickness or injury. It is understandable that this emotional state often leads to conflicting feelings of helplessness and frustration with "the system" and relief when their health problems are alleviated. For many people, the only choice involved when they are sick or injured is whether to seek healthcare. When they cross over to patient status, most decisions about the details of their care are not in their control. Patients have relied on insurers and providers to determine what they need, how much they need, and where to get it. For instance, a familiar scenario may be the following:

1. A person becomes very ill with a high fever, severe cough, and nausea.
2. That person sees a doctor and becomes a patient. If the patient is insured, the doctor may be one approved by the person's insurer, or the doctor may be "out of network" and not part of the panel of providers included in the insurance plan.
3. The doctor makes decisions about tests, medications, referrals, and so forth. All of the decisions are guided by preauthorization policies and drug formularies in the patient's healthcare insurance plan.
4. The doctor collects money from the patient as required by the insurer (e.g., deductible fees to be met before full benefits take effect or a co-payment at the time of service). Each patient receives a receipt for payment that may not clearly reflect the services received.
5. The doctor then submits a claim (bill) to the insurer for the remainder of the payment due according to the terms of the provider–insurer contract. The insurer pays the doctor's claim for payment of services if all of the rules for submission of the claim are met. The patient may later receive an explanation of benefits from the insurer that includes a list of services paid for and any remaining fees that are the patient's responsibility.
6. More often than not, the patient recovers and is satisfied with the healthcare delivery and the outcome—a return to health.

This relatively straightforward healthcare scenario reflects the roles of the three players. The basic healthcare business unit becomes amplified and very complex if a patient is hospitalized or requires long-term care. Several providers and many modifications in the plans of care over time mean more insurer authorizations and compliance with a myriad of rules. For patients with complex, chronic conditions, tracking a series of simultaneous services with a range of providers over extended periods can be overwhelming.

Employers' and Employees' Perspective

Legally, employers have not been required to offer health insurance benefits. The health insurance industry ballooned during World War II when employers were unable to continue to raise wages by law and compensated workers with benefits such as insurance instead. This shift from wages to benefits also allowed employers to control payroll costs and taxes on wages. Health insurance became the benefit of first choice because it had the potential to reduce the costs of sick day benefits by keeping workers healthy. Over the years, fueled by the demands of collective bargaining units (unions) and the competition for qualified workers, health insurance became a major expense of doing business.

Maintaining employment status to be eligible for health insurance benefits has been an important decision for many people. Decisions about health insurance benefits will remain important to employers and employees with continued implementation of the Affordable Care Act (ACA) through 2014, which is discussed at the end of this chapter.

Employers attempted to reduce some of their healthcare benefit expenses by:

- Reducing the number of employees who are eligible for health insurance benefits.
- Replacing a single, expensive health insurance plan with a "cafeteria selection" of a broad range of benefits for employees within several health insurance plans that are less expensive for the employer and that allow employees to choose a plan most appropriate for their needs.
- Increasing the employees' contribution to pay for health insurance rather than the employer assuming the total cost.

Although some of these strategies may change with enactment of the ACA, *annual* contract negotiations between employers and health insurers are

likely to continue. As a result, during "open enrollment" periods every year, employees sort through complicated information on new healthcare plans selected by the employer. People feel differently about this decision process. For example, a young, healthy, single man may select the health insurance plan that maximizes his take-home pay because it is the choice with the smallest employee payroll contribution for the insurance premium. This type of plan typically means a high deductible with coverage for hospitalizations and major medical problems. Because he is likely to use health care only intermittently, if at all, he saves more money in his paychecks in exchange for paying out-of-pocket for minor healthcare services until he has spent the deductible amount.

In contrast, a single mother with a complex medical history, a chronic condition requiring ongoing medication, and two children who need immunizations and frequent doctor's visits for upper respiratory infections has a much more complicated decision. She may feel overwhelmed by the complexity of the options she faces. She needs to analyze the financial implications of each health plan that the employer presents against the odds of sickness or injury occurring in her family. Having to leave her current physicians who are not in the network of providers in a plan that may be financially better for her is another important factor in her decision.

Other employed people may be eligible for a discounted health insurance policy through membership in a union or some other social organization. Contingency workers (e.g., part-time, temporary contract, per diem) may directly purchase an individual policy, as do people who become suddenly unemployed. Of course, a person may choose to be uninsured and risk paying for all medical expenses "out of pocket." At this time, the decision to hold a health insurance policy has been optional for many people. With full enactment of the ACA, proof of health insurance is expected to be mandatory.

Workers' Compensation

The other related cost of doing business that is important to both employers and employees is workers' compensation (workers' comp). Each state has its own statutes that require employers to establish no-fault insurance programs (compensation is paid without assigning blame) to protect workers who are temporarily or permanently injured or sick because of their work. These statutes must also protect employers from legal action brought by injured or sick employees. The result is employees who have some guarantee of benefits regardless of fault for the injury or sickness, and employers who are able to anticipate payments of mandated benefits rather than risk huge, unpredictable losses from lawsuits.

There is wide variation among workers' comp programs from state to state. Employers may pay their premiums to any insurance company, they may be self-insured, or they may contribute to state-operated funds for workers' compensation as their only option. In some states, all three options are available. Not all employers must carry workers' compensation insurance and how much they must carry is variable. Links for resources and workers' comp information on each state can be found at the U.S. Department of Labor's Division of Federal Employees' Compensation webpage (see Web Resources).

Workers' comp insurance is expensive although states tightly regulate the system. Because the benefits paid to injured workers are high, many insurance companies are reluctant to enter the workers' comp market. This lack of competition among insurance companies creates cost problems for employers who must meet state regulations before obtaining coverage. The benefits are expensive because the first prong of this two-prong program is compensation for lost wages and the loss of potential *future* wages because of injury or illness. Compensation is based on types of injuries and proportional loss of the use of body parts. For instance, the benefits for a worker who loses a limb would be different from those of a worker who is paralyzed from the waist down. The idea is a "partial" person should be able to return to "partial" work. The system does not keep up well with new injuries and illnesses that arise from new types of contemporary work.

The second prong of workers' comp is medical benefits for the treatment and care of these injured or sick employees. It includes rehabilitation to improve the ability to return to work. Each worker who is able to function in any limited capacity is expected to return to some type of work. Healthcare providers are not only challenged by restrictive reimbursement models, but also by workers' comp patients enmeshed in the personal conflicts arising from rehabilitation to return to work as opposed to the promise of compensation for loss of potential wages if they do not return to work. Workers' comp benefits include payment for pain and suffering, as well as payment for any necessary retraining—which are potentially conflicting financial incentives for injured or sick workers.

Although the system was established to avoid work-related litigation, injured workers are often embroiled in lawsuits to increase the values established for particular injuries. The classic example is the loss of a finger. The change in potential earning capacity is different for a renowned concert violinist than it is for a bank teller. Attorneys are also involved when employers contest workers' comp claims as fraudulent or when workers think insurers are taking illegal or unfair action.

There is a parallel workers' compensation program for federal employees and other special categories of workers engaged in interstate commerce types of businesses such as longshoremen, the merchant marines, miners with black lung, and employees of the U.S. Energy Commission (the U.S. Department of Labor, Office of Workers' Compensation Programs; see Web Resources).

Providers' Perspective

The term *healthcare provider* covers a wide range of services. For example, healthcare may happen in a physician's office, a large teaching hospital, a pharmaceutical company, a drugstore, or a home-care agency. Providers may be a physical therapy office with a solo owner, a national chain of corporate-owned outpatient physical therapy centers, or a free-standing, specialized rehabilitation hospital. Each of these providers is regulated differently, provides services differently, is reimbursed differently, and measures success differently. What they have in common is competing for the same limited, ever-decreasing healthcare dollars through their negotiations with health insurance companies.

Healthcare providers may receive different payments for providing the same service depending on which health insurer is buying it and the terms of the contract with that insurer, which may change from year to year. Because of these annual changes in health insurance plans, patients may pay a different amount for their share in deductibles and co-payments. Healthcare providers may have contracts with several different health insurance companies and may need to "adjust" their decisions for each patient with the same condition according to the contract terms and guidelines for the treatment of specific diseases. Because these guidelines seem to be established or adopted by insurance companies inconsistently and arbitrarily, changes have required the constant vigilance of managers. Also, providers have had to "shift" their costs among insurers. In order to cover the cost of care provided to patients whose insurers reimburse less than what it costs to provide that care, the charges to insurers that pay more have increased.

Insurers' Perspective

One source of insight into health insurance companies is through their professional organization, the America's Health Insurance Plans (AHIP), whose members provide health insurance to more than 200 million Americans through employer-sponsored coverage, the individual insurance market, and public programs such as Medicare and Medicaid (see Web Resources for the AHIP webpage). American's Health Insurance Plans advocates for public policies that expand access to affordable healthcare coverage in a competitive marketplace through its lobbying efforts. Like any business, the goals of insurance companies are to increase revenues, control costs, and achieve the largest possible profits. Healthcare organizations and providers have the same goals. The problem is that the two groups can only reach their goals to the potential detriment of the other. Insurers' profits increase with the number of people who have health insurance, regardless of who is paying for it. Insurers' profits also increase when the reimbursements (payments) they make to providers are decreased, when the price of health insurance policies is increased, or when both occur simultaneously. There seems to be nothing wrong with the following basic principle of business for insurers:

REVENUE (selling as many insurance policies as possible and stock to investors)

– **EXPENSES** (administrative costs and reimbursement to providers)

PROFITS divided among insurance company stockholders

For providers, the same basic business principle looks like this—notice the insurers' expenses become the revenue for providers:

REVENUE (reimbursement from insurers that continues to decrease)

– **EXPENSES** (rising healthcare delivery costs and more people with access)

PROFITS that may be inadequate for sustaining not-for-profit organizations

This revenue-expense principle has placed the health insurance industry in the position of negotiating with employers for contracts with the highest possible premiums for health insurance coverage with the fewest possible benefits. At the same time, insurers have negotiated with providers for the least amount of reimbursement for providing the limited services included in the benefit plans negotiated with employers. Although driven by competitive market forces to sell insurance, insurers have played a major role in driving the costs of health insurance, affecting access, and influencing the quality of healthcare through their contract negotiations.

The National Association of Insurance Commissioners (NAIC) is composed of all state insurance regulators, who serve the public interest by regulation of the insurance companies that make up AHIP, promotion of competition in the insurance industry, and facilitation of fair treatment of consumers. The NAIC seeks to coordinate the insurance regulations among states. This becomes important to large, nationwide insurance companies that must comply with different rules in each state where they do business and seek permission for selling insurance across state lines. Other important regulatory issues are variations in premium rates from one part of the country to another and rates among particular groups such as women and older people.

Government-Supported Healthcare Insurance

The U.S. government is heavily involved in the direct health insurance business and the administration of healthcare entitlement programs. The same insurance companies used by employers and individuals administer these government programs. This section includes the health insurance available to government workers, military employees, veterans, other special populations, and Medicare and Medicaid recipients.

According to a 2010 Gallup poll, 17% of workers in the United States are employees of the government—federal, state, and local (see Web Resources for 2010 Gallup poll). Civilian employees of the federal government receive health insurance through the Federal Employees Health Benefits (FEHB) Program, which includes a range of benefits for current employees, retirees, and survivors (see Web Resources for FEHB). Other government employees are insured through programs in each state, county, city, or other municipality. As expected, controlling health insurance costs and benefits is as important to public employers and employees as it is in the private sector.

The federal government also insures military employees and their dependents through the U.S. Department of Defense's Military Health System, which is managed by Tricare (see Web Resources). Healthcare services are provided through the system of military hospitals at home and overseas or through contracts with private healthcare providers that are willing to participate in the program.

As former military employees, some veterans receive federally supported healthcare through the Veterans' Health Administration's (VA) system of hospitals and clinics (see Web Resources for VA website). Eligibility is determined by the need for healthcare, which is based on the level of service-connected disabilities and the veteran's level of income and assets. Through the VA, funds are provided for the salary of medical school faculty who are VA physicians, and medical research.

The U.S. Public Health Service Corps provides direct patient care services through the hospitals and clinics of the Indian Health Service and the Bureau of Prisons (see Web Resources for links to these organizations).

Federal Entitlement Programs

The government collects taxes through employers to offer health insurance in two entitlement programs. In the 1960s, two programs for special populations were created—Title XVIII of the Social Security Act established Medicare for the aged and disabled, and Title XIX established Medicaid for the poor, which has traditionally been linked to Aid to Families With Dependent Children (AFDC) programs in each state. These programs are managed by the Centers for Medicare & Medicaid Services (see Web Resources) within the Department of Health and Human Services. Moving from the original system in which the government ran Medicare itself, the CMS establishes contracts with private insurance companies called intermediaries (for Part A) and carriers (for Part B) to process claims, provide services to providers and beneficiaries, handle appeals, and so on for the Medicare and Medicaid programs. The intent of this transfer of responsibility to private insurers was to open Medicare and Medicaid up to market forces with the expectation that competition among insurers would reduce the costs of these programs. This potential promise has not yet materialized.

Medicare

Medicare beneficiaries include people who are eligible for Social Security and are either 65 years old or older or under the age 65 with certain disabilities, or any age with end-stage renal disease. Medicare has four parts. People are automatically enrolled in Part A of Medicare at no cost when they turn 65 or if they are otherwise eligible. Medicare Part A provides health insurance for inpatient hospital services, short-term nursing home care, and home-based healthcare. Part B of Medicare is voluntary. People may choose to have deductions made from their Social Security benefits each month to pay for Part B coverage. Part B provides insurance for outpatient health services including such things as physical therapy, diagnostic tests, and visits to the doctor. Both Parts A and B may have deductibles and co-payments depending on which Medicare intermediary and carrier a person chooses.

As part of its attempts to reform Medicare, Congress enacted legislation to add Medicare + Choice (also called Medicare Part C and now known as Medicare Advantage). Medicare Advantage plans offer beneficiaries who are already enrolled in Medicare A and B a wide range of alternative coordinated care plan models such as health maintenance organizations (HMOs), preferred provider organizations (PPOs), health savings accounts (HSAs), points of service (POSs), and provider-sponsored organizations (PSOs), among others. These plans may require higher premiums (Social Security deductions), but include expanded benefits—no deductibles, smaller co-payments, no-cost annual physical examinations, preventive diagnostic screens, prescription drug coverage, and health promotion programs at little or no cost. Medicare Part D (the Medicare Prescription Drug, Improvement, and Modernization Act of 2003) includes prescription drug benefits for Medicare Part A and Part B enrollees for the first time.

Other Medicare Beneficiary Expenses

A popular misconception is that Medicare is free; however, beneficiaries contributed to Medicare through payroll taxes while they worked, and a premium (insurance payment) for Medicare Part B is deducted from Social Security each month. Medicare recipients face a wide range of out-of-pocket expenses that are dependent on the Medicare plan and the level of coverage they select. The sicker a person is, the quicker he or she will reach the maximum limits of Medicare insurance coverage, and the more he or she will pay out of pocket as the deductible amount and co-payments for the care received.

Because people may have limited incomes as they age, it should be no surprise that insurance companies market "Medigap" insurance policies to cover those healthcare expenses not covered by Medicare plans, and long-term-care insurance policies for extended care in nursing homes, which is not a Medicare benefit. Another unique aspect of Medicare is that it often involves the coordination of benefits for beneficiaries who may have a concurrent health insurance policy through an employer, a spouse who works, or pension plan benefits. Managers need to know the rules for determination of which insurer is the primary insurer for each dually insured patient. (See Web Resources for CMS's Coordination of Benefits & Recovery Overview information and PDF.)

Medical Necessity

A final important point—Medicare benefits are based on medical necessity, which means that Medicare only covers medical services and treatments that are considered necessary and reasonable according to evidence-based standards of care.

Carriers and intermediaries have had complex mechanisms for determining what services are reasonable and necessary. These determinations have been open to interpretation within an insurance company and among insurers to the chagrin of providers and patients. Because these insurance companies also have divisions for insuring non-Medicare recipients, they have often applied Medicare rules for coverage in these plans as well. For example, a Medicare Part B recipient receives coverage through ABC Insurance Company that preauthorizes outpatient physical therapy services three times a week for 3 weeks to treat her rotator cuff tear. A non-Medicare patient with an ABC health insurance policy may also be limited to the same level of physical therapy services. Although nine treatment sessions may be reasonable and necessary for a 70-year-old woman to return to function after a rotator cuff tear, it may not be an adequate plan of care for a 17-year-old basketball player with the same diagnosis.

Medicaid—A Federal/State Entitlement Program

Whereas age is the eligibility measure for entitlement in the Medicare program, Medicaid is a means-test entitlement, in which enrollment is limited to people below certain limited income and asset levels. Each state creates and manages its own Medicaid program (see Web Resources) with state funds generated by a range of state taxes. In order to qualify for matching federal money, a state's program must adhere to certain guidelines for determining a person's eligibility status. The proportion of money that each state receives from the federal government is dependent on each state's ability and willingness to provide medical care to its needy population. These health insurance policies are a source of ongoing political contention as the roles of states and the federal government are debated.

Medicaid is much more complex than Medicare because of the variety of healthcare services across the life span that each state is willing to pay for. How these programs are paid for and who delivers services are highly variable decisions from state to state. For example, in many states, Medicaid does not pay for outpatient physical therapy services. Within any state, the way the Medicaid program is administered for children and families may be different from the way it is administered for the elderly. One group's Medicaid health insurance may be managed as an HMO and another group's as a PPO, for instance.

Many special needs groups are also eligible for Medicaid. Some of them are mandatory beneficiary groups that each state must include in its Medicaid program to receive federal funds, while the inclusion of other populations is optional for each state.

Other Medicaid Beneficiaries

Over the years, Medicaid benefits were expanded to include people beyond the initial groups of beneficiaries. For example, the federal government approves demonstration projects with waivers of eligibility for Medicaid for some women with breast cancer, people with tuberculosis, and programs to avoid institutional placement of the elderly. Each group eligible for Medicaid may receive different benefits, and people within the same group may receive different benefits from one state to another.

States also must provide Medicaid insurance to anyone who receives Supplemental Security Income (SSI). This program was Title XVI of the Social Security Act, and it provides cash assistance to the aged, blind, and disabled below certain income levels. States may decide to offer Medicaid coverage to other groups, for instance, people who are not eligible for SSI but require nursing home care or people with disabilities who work may have Medicaid benefits in some states.

Finally, some Medicare beneficiaries have such low incomes that they also are eligible for Medicaid. A complicated cost-sharing arrangement is implemented that is presented through the Federal Coordinated Health Care Office (Medicare-Medicaid Coordination Office) for people who have dual eligibility between both Medicare and Medicaid (see Web Resources).

Medicaid is further complicated by the fact that not all people below the poverty level are eligible for Medicaid, and neither do all people who are eligible for Medicaid receive its benefits. People may not know they are eligible or they may not feel a need for health insurance.

Children's Health Insurance Program (CHIP)

Children's Health Insurance Program is another federal/state program (Title XXI of the Social Security Act) that mandates health insurance to children in families whose income and assets are too much to qualify for Medicaid, yet not enough to obtain a private insurance policy (see Web Resources). In some states, CHIP is part of the Medicaid program, in other states it is freestanding, while hybrid models are used in others.

Individuals With Disabilities Education Act (IDEA) and Individuals With Disabilities Education Improvement Act (IDEIA)

Other federal legislation that has a peripheral healthcare component is the IDEA that was revised as IDEIA in 2004 (see Web Resources). This civil rights legislation creates a federal/state program to aid children with disabilities through support of special education and related services in school systems, which include rehabilitation services and medical equipment. This aid also reaches at-risk infants and toddlers through early intervention programs. Because each state implements this program to meet its own needs, it is important for managers to seek specific information on a state's services. See Activity 4.2.

The Uninsured and Underinsured

The uninsured have no health insurance, and the underinsured have insurance that is inadequate to meet their healthcare expenses. Both groups are at risk for unmanageable debt and bankruptcy because of healthcare, according to the National

---

ACTIVITY 4.2
IT'S LIKE AN AIRPLANE TICKET

Mary Jane Olsten, one of the patients at County Healthcare System's Northside outpatient rehabilitation clinic, asks to speak to Carla Simone, the manager of the clinic. Mary Jane is a little upset and wants to let someone know. She tells Carla she has overheard conversations as she sat in the waiting room before her visits. Some patients have no co-payments, others pay less than she does, and nobody pays as much as she does. Mary Jane does not feel as though she is getting any more for her money than others get and she feels she should. As a matter of fact, she has talked to one of the other patients and learned that he gets more attention and longer treatments than she does. She wants to know what Carla is going to do about it. What should Carla say?

Patient Advocate Foundation (NPAF) (see Web Resources). The underinsured may have resources to pay for their contribution to an insurance premium and can often pay the out-of-pocket expenses for co-payments and deductibles as well. They may not, however, be financially prepared to pay healthcare bills when they exceed the maximum allowable amount of a health insurance policy. Ongoing deliberations with collection agencies and significant lifestyle changes made to pay medical bills have been necessary for many people.

Both the uninsured and underinsured are less likely to seek needed medical care.[1] They may not follow instructions for care because they cannot afford to do so. For example, uninsured and underinsured individuals may not fill an expensive prescription, or they may skip their physical therapy appointments because they are unable to make the co-payment that is due at the time service is rendered. This non-adherence to instructions has detrimental effects by hindering the progress of what would be a minor, manageable health problem into a more serious and expensive chronic problem. An option for the uninsured and underinsured may be to seek care at a federally qualified health center (see Web Resources). More information about types, funding, and services can be found at Department of Health and Human Services, Medicare and Medicaid Outreach and Education services (see Web Resources). See Activity 4.3.

ACTIVITY 4.3
NO INSURANCE COVERAGE

Yvonne Mendoza is the manager of an outpatient clinic with the following policy and procedure:

POLICY: *Physical therapy services may not be provided to patients who are uninsured or unable to make co-payments at the time of service.*
PROCEDURE: *The office manager is to advise each patient of this policy. Visits for physical therapy may not be initiated unless there is documented evidence of insurance coverage and the patient signs an agreement to make co-payments and/or meet deductibles at the time of each visit. Patients with no insurance coverage for physical therapy must pay the total fee for each visit at the time of visit. All fees due must be paid before another visit may be scheduled.*

The following three patients have been referred to Yvonne's clinic. The receptionist/office manager asks Yvonne what she should tell Abigail, Barry, and Carl's nurse. What action should Yvonne take? What are the financial implications of these decisions?

● Abigail is a young woman who was recently laid off from her job as a waitress so she is temporarily unemployed and uninsured. She fell while running across the street and fractured her right distal tibia and fibula. A cast was applied in the emergency room at the time of the accident. It was removed today, 6 weeks later. In addition to the expected limited range of motion (ROM) and atrophy, she appears to have complex regional pain syndrome. The doctor who removed her cast in the emergency room told her she needs physical therapy and gave her a prescription, which she brings to Yvonne's

clinic, the closest one to her home. She is very eager to find a new job.

● Barry is employed as a waiter. He has health insurance and is pleased that it covered so much of the cost of his recent hospitalization when he needed an appendectomy a few months ago. Several weeks later, he hurt his back as he was moving furniture to his new apartment. He has been off work as a result, and his sick days have run out. He is able to move well enough to begin outpatient physical therapy. His doctor gave him a prescription for "PT evaluate and treat 3×/week for 3 weeks for severe lumbar strain" and told him to go to Yvonne's PT clinic that is in the same office complex. Barry is surprised when he is told by the clinic that his insurance does not cover outpatient physical therapy. He wants to get back to work and wants to know his alternatives.

● Carl is a former headwaiter in an exclusive restaurant. However, major reversals in his life resulted in very negative circumstances, leaving him to live on the streets and in various homeless shelters for more than 6 months. He contracted a community-associated methicillin-resistant *Staphylococcus aureus* (CA-MRSA) infection that went untreated, resulting in major surgery to débride his left foot and lower leg. He is also diabetic and relies on services at a clinic for the homeless. The nurse there has called Yvonne to request that she provide physical therapy services to Carl to improve his ability to walk and promote healing of the surgical incision. The clinic is willing to pay a small stipend for a few visits.

The Future

The Patient Protection and Affordable Care Act (ACA) of 2010 (upheld by the Supreme Court's decision in 2012) is expected to affect every aspect of U.S. health care by the time of its full implementation in 2014 and beyond. It may be considered landmark legislation comparable to the passage of the Social Security Act in the 1930s and Medicare and Medicaid in the 1960s.

The major resources for the following review of the 10 titles (sections) of the ACA were *The Affordable Care Act Section by Section* (see Web Resources) and *The Patient Protection and Affordable Care Act: Detailed Summary* (see Web Resources). The U.S. Department of Health and Human Services provides information on the ACA organized by special interests and locations (see Web Resources). See Activity 4.4.

Title I. Quality, Affordable Healthcare for All Americans

This act reduces premium costs for millions of working families and small businesses by providing tax relief for health insurance, and provides reforms in the insurance market, including public justification of any rate increase of 10% or more. It caps out-of-pocket expenses and requires no-cost preventive care. Uninsured people may choose insurance coverage that works for them in new open, competitive insurance exchanges that pool buying power and force insurers to compete on cost and quality. Small business owners may also use the exchanges to receive a new tax credit to help offset the cost of health insurance they offer to their employees. The act reins in insurance abuses such as denying coverage because of pre-existing conditions. The ACA sets the 80/20 rule (Medical Loss Ratio) for insurance companies, which means they must spend at least 80 cents of every premium dollar on healthcare services or improvements to care. It provides people a new power to appeal insurance company decisions.

Title II. The Role of Public Programs

The ACA expands the eligibility of Medicaid beneficiaries and preserves CHIP while treating all states equally. The enrollment process for individuals and families is simplified. It enhances community-based care for Americans with disabilities and provides states with opportunities to expand home-care services to people with long-term-care needs. The act encourages the adoption of innovative strategies to improve care and the coordination of services for Medicare and Medicaid beneficiaries.

Title III. Improving the Quality and Efficiency of Healthcare

The act protects and preserves Medicare. The prescription drug gap in coverage closes to save beneficiaries thousands of dollars. The ACA establishes financial incentives for doctors, nurses, and hospitals to improve the quality of care on common, high-cost conditions and for the reduction of unnecessary errors that harm patients. The act penalizes hospitals for the preventable readmission of patients. Further, it enhances access to healthcare services in underserved areas and controls overpayment to insurers. Finally, the ACA charges a group of doctors and healthcare experts (rather than members of Congress) with the improvement of quality and reduction of costs for Medicare beneficiaries. It implements incentive programs for accountable care organizations (ACOs) and patient-centered medical homes (PCMHs) and revises payments for home health services.

Title IV. Prevention of Chronic Disease and Improving Public Health

The act funds an impetus and infrastructure to re-orient healthcare to prevention, wellness (e.g., no co-payments for Medicare recipients for prevention and screening) and enhances public health (e.g., state immunization programs directed by the Centers for Disease Control and Prevention [CDC]). It creates a national prevention and

---

ACTIVITY 4.4
ANALYZING AS YOU ARE READING

As you read the titles of the ACA and refer to the links provided above for details, put each section in the context of patients, employers, employees, providers, and insurers. Who is the most important stakeholder in each title? What healthcare problems (costs, access, quality) are addressed in each title?

health promotion strategy to improve health status and reduce the incidence of preventable illness and disability (e.g., statewide Medicaid awareness programs, school-based health clinics, oral health education). It includes providing people with tools to find the best science-based nutrition information (e.g., restaurant postings of serving calories) and funds an Institute of Medicine Conference on Pain Care. The act requires all federal health programs to collect and report data by race, ethnicity, primary language, and any other indicator of disparity.

Title V. Healthcare Workforce

The act funds scholarships and loan repayment programs to increase the number of primary care physicians, nurses, physician assistants, mental health providers, and dentists in underserved areas. States and local governments receive resources for health workforce development. The focus is on retention and educational opportunities to combat the critical nursing shortage, and the number of public health professionals prepared to deal with health emergencies (e.g., creation of the Ready Reserve Corps as part of the National Health Service Corps). The act includes funding for expansion of community health centers across the country.

Title VI. Transparency and Program Integrity

The act provides patients more control through information and doctors more access to medical research so that they may make more effective decisions together. Information on nursing homes becomes more transparent. The act requires nursing home staff training to continuously improve the quality of care, which includes the self-correction of errors, background checks on direct care providers, and programs to prevent elder abuse. The act reins in waste, fraud, and abuse by new disclosure requirements to identify high-risk providers who have defrauded the government. It empowers states to prevent providers penalized in one state from moving to another. States have flexibility to propose and test tort reforms that address reduction of healthcare errors, enhance patient safety, encourage dispute resolution, and improve access to liability insurance.

Title VII. Improving Access to Innovative Medical Therapies

The act promotes innovation and reduces costs through the extension of drug discounts to hospitals and communities that serve low-income patients while offering incentives for developing generic versions of biological drugs for lower cost alternatives.

Title VIII. Community Living Assistance Services and Supports Act (CLASS Act)

The act provides for a new self-funded, voluntary long-term-care insurance choice that will cover a wide range of healthcare services based on functional limitations. Medicaid spending decreases as people are able to continue working or they continue living in their homes rather than nursing homes. The act uses no taxpayer funds to pay benefits, and safeguards ensure that premiums cover benefits.

Title IX. Revenue Provisions

The act makes healthcare more affordable for families and small business owners by providing the largest middle-class tax cuts to reduce their premium cost for the purchase of health insurance and increases taxes and penalties for others.

Title X. Strengthening Quality, Affordable Care

This act makes improvements and clarifications in the first nine titles and also adds new content, such as choice vouchers for employees to use in health insurance exchanges, incentives for states to support Medicaid beneficiaries in the community rather than in nursing homes, improvements in Medicare processes for patients and providers, grants for the study of cures and treatments of diseases, and centers of excellence for depressive disorders.

Essential Health Benefits

Another important component of the ACA has been the identification of the essential health benefits that are required of any health insurance plan included in the health insurance exchanges approved by the federal government. These essential health benefits are:

1. Ambulatory patient services
2. Emergency services
3. Hospitalization
4. Maternity and newborn care
5. Mental health and substance use disorder services
6. Prescription drugs
7. Rehabilitation and habilitation services and devices
8. Laboratory services
9. Preventive and wellness services and chronic disease management
10. Pediatric services including oral and vision care

The specifics appear to be negotiable at this time and dependent on action by Congress for fine-tuning, as is expected in all major legislation. Managers and leaders *must* regularly check the implementation and revision of these essential benefits as well as the rest of the important legislation found in the ACA. The Health Care Blog of the Secretary of the U.S. Department of Health and Human Services and the Web pages of the American Physical Therapy Association are important resources for current, new policy developments in practice and patient care, payment, and advocacy (see Web Resources).

Because implementation of the components of the ACA is just beginning, it is premature to predict the impact of this legislation on individuals, healthcare providers, insurers, and other stakeholders. Whether the act will reduce, decelerate, or increase healthcare spending remains a controversial topic. The outcomes of access and quality initiatives in the act that have already been implemented are yet to be determined. Efforts to balance the profits of insurers with the public's need to maintain the health of the population and provide quality care to the sick and injured are expected to continue to evolve. See Activity 4.5.

ACTIVITY 4.5
A HEALTHCARE CASE STUDY

Jerome Kingston is the rehab manager at County Healthcare System. Susan Rosen is one of his neighbors who often asks him for informal advice. What should Jerome tell her when she shares the following information and concerns about her extended family's health insurance issues?

PART I. Susan Rosen has worked for a large manufacturing company in Alabama, ABC Widgets, for 25 years. Her husband, Sam Rosen, is a self-employed electrical contractor with eight contingency employees. He does not have health insurance benefits for himself or his employees. The Rosens have one son who is a 19-year-old college student and two daughters who are 12 and 14 years old.

The Rosens have always been insured by the family coverage plan of the health insurance policy that Susan has had through her employer over the years. ABC Widgets has always contributed 80% of the monthly premium for a health insurance policy for its employees, and Mrs. Rosen has paid the remaining 20% through deductions from her pay. Although the amount of her payroll deduction has been increasing, she is satisfied with the policy and healthcare so she has not taken the opportunities presented by her employer every year to change either the type of health insurance plan she has or her insurance company.

The Rosens have been very fortunate. Except for the usual childhood immunizations and minor injuries, short-term illnesses from viruses and other infections, the birth of her children, and Mr. Rosen's short hospitalization because of a gastrointestinal problem, they have not required healthcare services and have not given their healthcare much thought until now. However, Susan has just been laid off from her job at ABC Widgets.

PART II. Mr. and Mrs. Waterson, Susan's parents, are both 78 years old. They are enrolled in Medicare Parts A and B. In addition, Mr. and Mrs. Waterson continue to receive other health insurance benefits because Mr. Waterson is a retiree of ABC Widgets. He also is a veteran who was wounded in the Korean War; he is eligible for VA benefits and the nearest VA clinic is 20 miles from his home. Mr. Waterson takes medication to control his hypertension and diabetes. He sees his doctor monthly. Mrs. Waterson was

ACTIVITY 4.5
A HEALTHCARE CASE STUDY—cont'd

recently hospitalized for a mild stroke and is receiving outpatient physical, occupational, and speech therapy services. They are confused by the numerous ads they hear on television and receive in the mail almost daily about different Medicare plans and options. Explanation of benefits reports they receive from Medicare and their other insurers are a mystery to them. They pay every bill they receive promptly and without question. They spend part of every winter in Florida and part of every summer in North Carolina in addition to receiving health care at home in Massachusetts.

PART III. Susan's brother and his wife, James and Jane Waterson, have two preschool-aged children. James is the sole wage earner for the family. As an independent computer software contract worker, he makes high hourly wages but has no benefits package. He likes the freedom of selecting jobs that pay the most for the type of work he prefers. They have been uninsured since they have been married, but they are able to afford healthcare expenses,

such as the birth of their children, without difficulty because of their deliberate efforts to maintain a large pool of savings and are able to use payment plans at the hospital in their Colorado community.

Unfortunately, work opportunities for James have been diminishing this year. Although his income has decreased, it is not low enough for the family to qualify for Medicaid to cover their potential healthcare costs. They are dipping into their savings much more than they would like for healthcare because they just learned that their oldest child, who is ready to begin kindergarten, is asthmatic, the baby has been diagnosed as developmentally delayed, and James has developed an unrelenting back problem, which also has contributed to his reduced work effort. They rarely go to a physician and treat the usual run of childhood problems on their own with over-the-counter medications and home remedies. Jane is considering taking a part-time job if she will be eligible for health insurance and can afford the payroll deductions for coverage.

Conclusions

In 2011, according to the Office of the Actuary at CMS, 73% of the $2.7 trillion spent on U.S. healthcare came from health insurance (see Web Resources). That 73% is divided between the 33% that came from private insurance and the remaining 40% that came from all forms of the government insurance discussed in this chapter. The remaining 27% of the $2.7 trillion came from out-of-pocket payments, other health insurance programs such as workers' comp, investments, and public health activities.

This total $2.7 trillion was distributed as payments to providers and others in the following proportions: 31% to hospitals; 20% to physicians and clinics; 10% to pay for prescription drugs; and 14% to pay for other medical products, public health activities, home health care, and other residential care. The remaining 26% was divided almost evenly among dental and other services, government administration, investment in structures and equipment, and nursing care facilities.

The effect of the ACA on revenue and expenses on U.S. healthcare dollars and distribution of payments is yet to be determined. Patients, employers, employees, insurers, and providers have a vested interest in the ongoing implementation of the ACA. The complexity of decisions about U.S. healthcare might be summarized by the efforts of some of these stakeholders seeking to influence liberals, who value collective responsibility and public good, while other stakeholders seek to influence conservatives, who value individual responsibility and choice. Leaders and managers in healthcare organizations will continue to face the challenges of compliance with new and revised regulations of the ACA while political decisions continue to form healthcare policies.

REFERENCE

1. Hadley, J. Insurance coverage, medical care use, and short-term health changes following an unintentional injury or the onset of a chronic condition. *JAMA.* 2007;297(10): 1073-1084.

WEB RESOURCES

2010 Gallup poll. http://www.gallup.com/poll/141785/gov-employment-ranges-ohio.aspx. Accessed July 23, 2013.

The Affordable Care Act Section by Section. http://www.healthcare.gov/law/full/. Accessed July 23, 2013.

America's Health Insurance Plans (AHIP). http://www.ahip.org/. Accessed July 23, 2013.

American Physical Therapy Association. http://www.apta.org/. Accessed July 23, 2013. and clinics. http://www.va.gov/health/default.asp. Accessed July 23, 2013.

Centers for Medicare & Medicaid Services (CMS). http://www.cms.gov/. Accessed July 23, 2013.

Centers for Medicare & Medicaid Services (CMS). Glossary of healthcare terminology. http://www.cms.gov/apps/glossary/default.asp?Letter=P&Language=English. Accessed July 23, 2013.

Department of Health and Human Services, Centers for Medicaid & Medicare. Federally qualified health center information. http://www.cms.gov/Outreach-and-Education/Medicare-Learning-Network-MLN/MLNProducts/downloads/fqhcfactsheet.pdf.

Federal Bureau of Prisons, an agency of the U.S. Department of Justice. http://www.bop.gov/about/co/health_services.jsp. Accessed July 23, 2013.

The Federal Coordinated Health Care Office (Medicare-Medicaid Coordination Office). http://www.cms.gov/Medicare-Medicaid-Coordination/Medicare-and-Medicaid-Coordination/Medicare-Medicaid-Coordination-Office/index.html. Accessed July 23, 2013.

Federal Employees Health Benefits Program (FEHB). Civilian employees of the federal government receive health insurance through FEHB. http://www.opm.gov/healthcare-insurance/healthcare/. Accessed July 23, 2013.

The Federal Health Program for American Indians and Alaska Natives. http://www.ihs.gov/aboutihs/. Accessed July 23, 2013.

Federally Qualified Health Centers (FQHCs). http://www.hrsa.gov/healthit/toolbox/RuralHealthITtoolbox/Introduction/qualified.html. Accessed July 23, 2013.

The Health Insurance Blog of the Secretary of the U.S. Department of Health and Human Services. http://www.healthcare.gov/blog/. Accessed July 23, 2013.

Individual With Disabilities Education Act (IDEA). http://www.ideapartnership.org/. Accessed July 23, 2013.

Medicaid Children's Health Insurance Program (CHIP). http://www.medicaid.gov/Medicaid-CHIP-Program-Information/By-Topics/By-Topic.html http://www.insurekidsnow.gov/. Accessed July 23, 2013.

The National Association of Insurance Commissioners (NAIC). http://www.naic.org/index_about.htm. Accessed July 23, 2013.

National Patient Advocate Association (NPAF). Medical debt, medical bankruptcy and the impact on patients (September 2012). http://www.npaf.org/files/Medical%20Debt%20White%20Paper%20Final_0.pdf. Accessed July 23, 2013.

Office of the Actuary at Centers for Medicare and Medicaid. National Health Dollars, Calendar year 2010. http://www.cms.gov/Research-Statistics-Data-and-Systems/Statistics-Trends-and-Reports/NationalHealthExpendData/downloads/PieChartSourcesExpenditures2010.pdf. Accessed July 23, 2013.

The Patient Protection and Affordable Care Act: Detailed Summary. http://dpc.senate.gov/healthreformbill/healthbill52.pdf. Accessed July 23, 2013.

U.S. Department of Defense's Military Health System, TRICARE. http://www.tricare.mil/Welcome/AboutUs.aspx. Accessed July 23, 2013.

U.S. Department of Health and Human Services. Affordable Care Act state by state. http://www.healthcare.gov/law/information-for-you/index.html. Accessed July 23, 2013.

U.S. Department of Labor, Office of Workers' Compensation Programs. http://www.dol.gov/owcp/. Accessed July 23, 2013.

U.S. Department of Labor's Division of Federal Employees' Compensation. Links for resources and workers' compensation information in each state. Available at http://www.dol.gov/owcp/dfec/regs/compliance/wc.htm. Accessed July 23, 2013.

U.S. Department of Veterans Affairs. Veterans Health Administration's (VA) system of hospitals and clinics. Available at http://www.va.gov/health/default.asp. Accessed July 23, 2013.

U.S. Public Health Service Commissioned Corps. http://www.usphs.gov/aboutus/agencies/. Accessed July 23, 2013.

RESPONSIBILITIES OF THE HEALTHCARE MANAGER

Each chapter in this section addresses one of the major responsibilities of healthcare managers. In the following list, the core managerial responsibilities are shown in bold. In Figure S2.1, they fall under the broad umbrella of responsibility for vision, mission, and goals, resting on a foundation of legal and ethical, risk management, and communication responsibilities.

- Vision, mission, goals (Chapter 5)
- **Policies and procedures (Chapter 6)**
- **Marketing (Chapter 7)**
- **Staffing (Chapter 8)**
- **Patient care (Chapter 9)**
- **Fiscal (Chapter 10)**
- Risk management, legal, and ethical (Chapter 11)
- Communication (Chapter 12)

Strategic Planning

An organization's strategic planning process drives the responsibilities of managers. The classic view of strategic planning is (1) identifying where an organization is now, (2) determining where it wants to be in the future, (3) assessing what it has to work with, and (4) deciding how it will get to where it wants to be. Although the responsibilities of managers overlap and come into play throughout this planning process, it may be helpful to relate the responsibilities of managers to the four general components of strategic planning in this manner:

- Mission: Where are we now?
- Vision, Goals, Legal, and Ethical: Where do we want to be?
- **Staffing, Fiscal, Marketing,** Communication: What do we have to work with?
- **Policies and Procedures, Patient Care, Risk Management:** How will be get there?

The strategic planning process may be applied to reaching the broadest goals of healthcare systems, or it may be used for day-to-day problem-solving—both professional and personal. *All* accomplishments require plans. Like the studies of organizations, management, and leadership, a wide range of disciplines have viewed strategic planning from a wide range

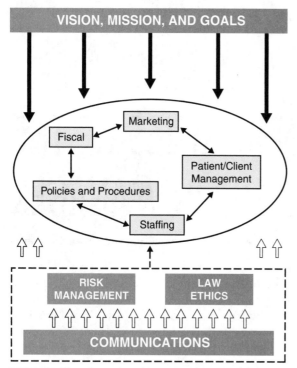

FIGURE S2.1 The relationship of managerial responsibilities.

of perspectives and numerous models and variations.[1,2] For the purposes of this section, the steps of strategic planning are to:

1. Determine where you are (strengths and weaknesses) through honest external and internal reviews.
2. Determine where you want to be in the long term (mission and vision) and set priorities to be addressed.
3. Clearly define the objectives that must be met to address each priority.
4. Determine who is accountable for meeting the objectives (allocation of time, human capital, and finances).
5. Conduct frequent formal reviews of the process to determine progress toward goals.

Although it appears systematic and sensible, the process is actually a series of ups and downs rather than a straight line from where an organization or person is and where he or she wants to be. Strategic planning demands ongoing modifications in response to external forces and internal changes, and not all components of strategic planning are always critical.

One model of strategic planning offers a tool for setting priorities that encourages data analysis of the needs of organizations (need = gap between current status and goal). Answers to the following questions assist managers who must decide which needs are important enough for the organization to invest the resources required to meet them:[3]

● Can the need be easily eliminated or ignored?
● What will it cost to ignore the need?
● What is the effect of meeting the need? On society? On external stakeholders? On internal stakeholders?
● How much will meeting the need cost?
● How high a priority is the need?

Each need that becomes a priority then becomes a problem (challenge) for managers. They are then held accountable for meeting the challenge through the work of others and the resources of the organization. The activities in this section's chapters introduce physical therapists to these challenges.

Program Proposals, Feasibility Studies, and Business Plans

Program proposals, feasibility studies, and business plans are formal written documents used to convey strategic planning processes to others. The documents are also a reference for planners as they adjust components of a plan, and "putting it in writing" is a demonstration of commitment to a project. The differences among them are generally seen as:

Program proposal: Managers may be assigned or take the initiative to prepare a proposal for a patient service or reorganization model (e.g., satellite outpatient physical therapy center or lymphedema management service) that has *already received tentative approval* from upper-level managers. The proposal *fills in details for final decisions* on implementation.

Feasibility study: The purpose is to *determine the viability of an idea.* Will it work? Should we proceed? Managers might conduct feasibility studies *before* presenting an innovative idea to upper-level managers for approval. For entrepreneurs considering independent physical therapy practices, feasibility studies are tools used in preparing business plans.

Business plan: External financial stakeholders such as investors or lenders are the target audience for business plans. Built on feasibility studies, business plans include the details for achieving the goals of new business ventures or new directions for an established business. The focus of a business plan is a detailed description of *how a new business is to achieve its financial goals.*

The outlines for preparing these documents are similar and appear in Appendix 2 (see page 284.).

Chapter activities in this section may be used to guide students in the development of a program plan, feasibility study, or business plan using these outlines. The development of these documents depends on the integration of the responsibilities of managers presented in this section.

REFERENCES

1. Nag R, Hambrick DC, Chen M-J. What is strategic management, really? Inductive derivation of a consensus definition of the field. *Strategic Management Journal.* 2007;28:935-955.
2. Jasper M. What is strategic management? *Journal of Nursing Management.* 2012;20:838-846.
3. Kaufman R. *Strategic Planning for Success: Aligning People, Performance, and Payoffs.* San Francisco, CA: John Wiley; 2003.

CHAPTER 5

Responsibilities for Vision, Mission, and Goal Setting

LEARNING OBJECTIVES

- Distinguish the differences between organizational visions, missions, values, and goals.
- Determine the roles of the statement of a vision, a mission, the values, and the goals in the management of physical therapy practices in healthcare.
- Critique vision and mission statements.
- Relate vision, mission, and values to organizational culture.
- Determine the potential influence of mission statements on individuals in organizations.
- Determine the appropriate relationship between vision, mission, values, and goals of the American Physical Therapy Association and those of healthcare organizations.
- Analyze various levels of goals for the management of physical therapy practices and healthcare services.
- Prepare a vision mission statement and horizon goals.

Overview

The importance of visions and mission statements in the initial start-up and the ongoing development of healthcare businesses cannot be overestimated. The caveat is that they need to be derived from a thoughtful process that includes the input of all stakeholders to identify organizational values and how to accomplish goals. Including key stakeholders in the preparation of visions and missions accomplishes two things: (1) it increases the chance that they will truly reflect the organization at all levels, and (2) it increases the chance of buy-in when it is time for everyone to "walk the talk."

After they are created, the power of visions and mission statements lies in the role they play in the culture of the organization as they guide the expectations and decisions of all stakeholders. This power is dependent on managers effectively communicating and sharing the organization's vision and mission statement to develop a sense of unity and security. A shared common purpose results if

an organization and its members consistently emulate its vision and mission. If, however, the stakeholders perceive the organization's vision and mission as empty expressions that are forced on them, the result is more likely to be disillusionment and low morale.

Because of the importance of the vision and mission, establishing them is a critical beginning step in strategic planning for new organizations or organizations that are changing direction because of external influences or internal disturbances. The physical therapist managing a small independent practice, the healthcare manager leading a multidisciplinary staff, and the chief executive officer guiding a large healthcare system must each establish visions and missions.

Clarifying the difference between vision and mission statements is important, and the question of whether the vision or mission comes first in strategic planning probably is essentially a matter of choice. Typically, however, beginning something new starts with a look to the future and establishes the premise for the business—its vision. It then focuses on what it needs to get there—its mission. A vision is what the business seeks to become and is a source of inspiration for stakeholders. A mission statement reflects what the business is about—its purpose—now. It is a declaration of its values and beliefs and defines customers, processes, and performance expectations.

Often organizations declare their values and beliefs as value statements that are separate from their mission statements. Organizations may choose to separate the two statements when they perceive that the values that drive their decisions are unwavering and their mission statements are evolving. What they believe is separated from what they do— the mission. A value statement clearly presents the guiding principles for expected behaviors of employees and for the strategic plans of the organization. These values drive the establishment of goals that clarify the work of employees in order for an organization to accomplish its mission and realize its vision through strategic planning. See Figure 5.1 and Sidebar 5.1.

SIDEBAR 5.1	
Definitions	
VISION	The future Where you want to be The basic premise of what you stand for Sets the direction
MISSION	Current state Where you are What you are doing What you need Strengths, uniqueness *(Values and beliefs)*
VALUE STATEMENT	Values and beliefs Guiding principles Clarifies behavior expectations
GOALS	Clarify specific work to be done Establish accountability

STRATEGIC PLANNING	
	1. Determine where you are
VISION • Where an organization wants to be • A look to the future • The basic premise of what an organization seeks to become • A source of inspiration	2. Determine where you want to be and set priorities
MISSION • Where it is now • The purpose of the organization • Focus on what it takes to achieve the vision • Definition of customers, processes, performance *(Values and beliefs)*	Review the processes and progress toward goals
VALUES STATEMENT • Values and beliefs • Enduring guiding principles • Organization culture	
GOAL SETTING • Specifics for getting the work done • Steps to be accomplished	3. Clearly define goals for each priority 4. Determine who is accountable for each goal

FIGURE 5.1 Sorting it out.

Visions

Managers cannot dismiss the vision of an organization as unimportant or approach its development casually. Identifying this broad, overriding goal is critical to setting the direction of an organization through a realistic picture of the future. Stakeholders need to be included as important questions about the organization are decided. What should it stand for? What should it become? The resulting visions should challenge the performance and ideas of stakeholders. A vision leads employees and entrepreneurs to:[1]

- Commit to the organization because the vision energizes them.
- Develop a sense of the meaning of their work as part of a bigger whole.
- Strive to achieve a standard of excellence that stimulates improvement.

For instance, compare these vision statements:

ABC Health System Post-Surgical Hip Rehabilitation Program
To provide an efficient and effective multidisciplinary continuum of care within the ABC Health System for patients after hip surgery.

McHale and Associates Physical Therapy
To be the physical therapy provider of choice in Jones City, Alabama.

New Jersey Pediatric Rehabilitation Services
To serve all children with special needs in New Jersey.

The ABC Health System vision suggests a program that is to be implemented in various units of a large system. The McHale vision suggests a small independent business whose future lies in being good at what it does, growing with its community through active engagement. The New Jersey Pediatric Rehabilitation Services vision suggests an expanding organization to meet the needs of a particular population throughout an entire state.

In all three examples, without a vision and overriding goals to strive for, it would be difficult for these organizations to accomplish their business goals. Many entrepreneurs and programs may have a vision but they fail to write it down or share it. The problem with not sharing the vision is that it will be difficult to get others to follow if they do not know where they are headed. The managerial decisions made without a shared vision will have no context. Employees and other stakeholders may then erroneously interpret, or ignore, what appear to be empty decisions.

An unshared vision is problematic, but no vision at all may prove disastrous to an organization. Although a cliché, it is true that it is hard to get anywhere if you do not know where you want to go. It is equally difficult for people to follow or contribute if they do not see the vision. For example, a person who is very good at making pies receives encouragement to sell them. Without a vision, the pie maker may approach her pie-selling business in a hit-or-miss, casual manner by selling pies made on request or by participating in local bake sales. With a vision, she is ready to take steps for her pies to become the pies of choice for all restaurants and catering companies in her community. Another vision may guide her company to become the leading global supplier of frozen specialty pies.

To emphasize the importance of that first vision-setting step, consider the ramifications of hiring a charter group of new employees for a new venture without a vision. For example, physical therapists who take positions with a new physical therapy practice with no vision have no choice but to make assumptions about the organization's direction and may experience dissonance as a result. Developing and then sharing the vision also helps planners of new practices determine which potential employees will be the best match. Finally, with visions as a reference for budget decisions, unnecessary expenses or misdistributions of limited funds are averted.

A vision may not include a target date for realizing the vision, but an estimated date is necessary during its formulation. Beginning the vision with "by 2020" or "in 5 years," whether a date appears in the final written version or not, helps to make the vision concrete rather than an abstract dream. A deadline also provokes discussion about whether or not the vision is realistic and achievable.

For instance, how long should it take ABC Health System to provide integrated services efficiently and effectively or for McHale and Associates Physical Therapy to become the provider of choice in Jones City? How long will it be before New Jersey Pediatric Rehabilitation Services realizes its vision? The level of organizational complexity, resources already available, resources needed, and prior business experience are factors that influence the target date for realizing a vision. A good vision time line for new practices is 3 to 5 years, but new programs within organizations may take only weeks or months. See Sidebar 5.2 and Activity 5.1.

SIDEBAR 5.2

The Vision Statement Checklist

- Clear, vivid picture of the future of the organization
- Challenging
- Hopeful
- Memorable
- Realistic
- Achievable
- Guides long-term decisions

ACTIVITY 5.1
CRITIQUE OF VISIONS

1. Using the characteristics in Sidebar 5.2, improve on the vision statements of ABC Health System Post-Surgical Hip Rehabilitation Program, McHale and Associates Physical Therapy, and New Jersey Pediatric Rehabilitation Services:
   ABC Health System: "To provide an efficient and effective multidisciplinary continuum of care within the ABC Health System for patients after hip surgery."
   McHale: "To be the physical therapy provider of choice in Jones City, Alabama."
   New Jersey: "To serve all children with special needs in New Jersey."
2. Compare the organizational cultures that might be expected in these practices. What would it be like to be employed in each one?
3. Find the vision of a physical therapy practice or other healthcare organization you would like to know more about. What does its vision statement tell you about the organization? Does it meet the characteristics expected of a vision? Does the vision meet your professional expectations for a potential employer?

Mission Statements

A mission statement provides a current path to realize the future that is presented in the vision of an organization. Mission statements may have a direct bearing on the bottom line and success of the organization because, like the organization's vision, they are dependent on the degree of commitment by stakeholders. Like its vision, an organization's mission statement also becomes a source of power for an organization because it enables its sense of purpose. The mission statement clarifies its legal role, expectations of its stakeholders, and, perhaps most important, its moral duty—*what it ought to be doing.* Unless its mission is socially desirable and justifiable, an organization may fail to create the enthusiasm and excitement among its stakeholders to "walk the talk."[2]

A mission statement reflects the principles under which an organization acts and the standards by which it will be judged. It boosts morale and strengthens its reputation when the organization lives up to it. Conversely, it may damage morale and reputation if it is perceived to be weak, hypocritical, or not trustworthy.[3] If the vision for an organization has already been determined, a beginning point for establishing its mission is to ask why the vision exists. What is the purpose of the vision? Other questions to be addressed during development are:

- What does the organization wish to be remembered for?
- What are its unique strengths and weaknesses?
- How is it distinguished from its competitors?

The mission statement is an emotional call to action that is easily transferable to the actions of employees and other stakeholders. It helps an organization focus its energies and drives the organizational culture if it is used consistently in decision-making.[4] For example, McHale and Associates Physical Therapy might ask why Jones City needs its practice to be the provider of choice as it develops its mission statement. The answer may lead to a mission statement such as the following:

McHale and Associates' Mission Statement
McHale and Associates is a group of board-certified physical therapists who provide the highest quality

care to prevent and rehabilitate movement disorders in people of all ages in Jones City. Our individualized, hands-on approach to improving the quality of life of our patients is available at times most convenient for them in our modern, state-of-the-art facility. We believe our patients are at the center of our efforts and the reason we consult with other healthcare professionals to coordinate a comprehensive plan for their health.

A mission statement written with input from an organization's stakeholders assures the inclusion of the values and beliefs of all constituents. Without this input, using a mission statement to make decisions, identify and resolve differences, and clarify expectations of employees becomes more difficult for managers. For instance, when reading McHale and Associates' vision and mission, physical therapists considering employment there may expect that they should hold a board-certified specialization, they will need to be flexible in their work hours, and they will need to be comfortable with one-on-one contemporary patient care in Jones City. Patients who read this mission will have expectations about the qualifications of their therapists and the therapists' collaboration with their physicians and other healthcare providers. Should their experiences fall short of these expectations, the reputation of McHale and Associates may be at risk. See Sidebar 5.3 and Activity 5.2.

ACTIVITY 5.2
MISSION STATEMENTS

1. Using the characteristics in Sidebar 5.3, improve on the mission of McHale and Associates. Review the revised vision created for McHale and Associates in Activity 5.1. Is the new vision aligned with the final mission statement?

2. Given the visions of ABC Health System Post-Surgical Hip Program and New Jersey Pediatric Rehabilitation Services from Activity 5.1, write mission statements for each that meet all of the criteria in Sidebar 5.3.

3. Find the mission statement of a physical therapy practice or other healthcare organization you would like to know more about. What does its mission statement tell you about the organization? Does it meet the characteristics expected of a mission statement using the components in Sidebar 5.3? Does this mission statement meet your professional expectations of an employer?

Broader Healthcare Mission Statements

Because of their importance in the management of healthcare organizations, there is an urgent need for mission statements that capture their unique and enduring purpose, practices, and values. Economic pressures and the service mandate of healthcare often are in conflict. Powerful mission statements motivate individuals and organizations to reconcile these competing interests.[5]

In a thematic analysis of Canadian hospital mission statements, the consistent, outstanding theme was the importance of exemplary patient care. Other than this commitment to patients, the researchers found wide variation in the mission statements they studied. They had expected otherwise because the Canada Health Act recommends specific healthcare values. The mission statements were far from standard boilerplates. They did find common themes among the mission statements that may be expected in the mission

---

SIDEBAR 5.3

The Mission Statement Checklist

- Presents a clear statement of purpose and priorities
- Reflects values or beliefs (culture) of the organization
- Presents the unique attributes of the organization
- Infers the roles of stakeholders in the organization
- Generates commitment to and pride in the organization
- Is consistent with legal and corporate requirements (if applicable) of the organization

statements of physical therapy practices as well.[5] Identified themes included:

- Values
- Identity (image)
- Services provided (geographical area served)
- Employees and staff
- Resources

The analyzed mission statements were considered laudable, and if internalized by the employees, they provided moral guidance that could be translated into behavior. The study reinforced the importance of understanding that behavior is a manifestation of what people truly value and believe. Therefore, for mission statements to translate into action, they must address values. They recommended the following management initiatives to improve commitment to healthcare mission statements:[5]

1. Consider the perspectives of all stakeholders to promote ownership and authenticity of the mission.
2. Make the mission and value statements the central pillars of ethics awareness programs.
3. Increase the relevancy of the mission and value statements by making them part of decision-making and policy-development processes.
4. Provide incentives for mission/value adherence and explicit consequences for non-adherence.
5. Actively promote the mission/values in all relevant internal and external communication.
6. Express and reinforce management's commitment to the mission and values.

In another study, the value of mission statements to organizations was explored through extensive review of the literature and analysis of mission statements. The researchers concluded that mission statements evolving from a broad consensus process do have value to an organization if they are communicated effectively. The effectiveness of mission statements as management tools rather than irrelevant pieces of paper is enhanced by three important factors:[6]

1. Selection of creative, appropriate communication channels (e.g., word of mouth and posters/plaques rather than publication in annual reports) and their frequency positively influence performance outcomes of organizations.
2. Middle- and lower-level managers who transform mission statements into effective management tools by translating the knowledge of missions into action of employees positively influence performance outcomes of organizations.
3. Alignment of every dimension of the organization with tangible and visible evidence of its mission (e.g., organizational structure, rewards, job descriptions) positively influences performance outcomes of organizations.

Value Statements

Recently, some organizations have chosen to separate the values component of the typical mission statement into a separate statement. Value statements often begin with "we believe . . .," or "we are committed to . . .," or simply "we value . . .". This approach results in mission statements that are more direct, typically shorter, and limited to a clear definition of what they do. An accompanying value statement supplies the reasons of the mission and offers support for the vision. See Activity 5.3.

All organizations have values that drive their culture. Although not always explicit, the values of an organization determine the qualities that command respect. They generate the principles that guide the actions of the employees and other stakeholders as they judge themselves and are judged by others.[3] The value statement typically identifies the four to six most important values, or things that are valued, which are presented in rank order with the most important value listed first. A physical therapy practice's value statement may address (in alphabetical order):

- Access
- Accountability

ACTIVITY 5.3
WALK THE TALK

Select the vision and mission statement from an actual healthcare organization. Does it include a value statement? What might you expect to see or actually see if you visited an organization with these values?

- Diversity
- Education
- Financial success
- Honesty
- Innovation
- Productivity
- Quality care
- Respect
- Teamwork
- Work/home balance

See Activities 5.4 and 5.5.

Goal Setting

The goals, or results desired, for the organization are equally powerful and important in strategically planning and implementing a new practice or new program in an organization. Organizational goals are also a means for controlling, coordinating, and evaluating work performance. In large organizations, conflict commonly arises because the many goals established to carry out a mission and achieve a vision may seem to contradict one another. The focus of an organization's goals also may change at different times as factors influencing the business of healthcare force a change in the priority rank of goals. Some general rules for goal setting are in bold in this list using holiday shopping as an example:[7]

1. Goals must be **phrased in terms of outcomes** (accomplishments), not processes. Example of an unacceptable goal as process: Go shopping.

   Example of an acceptable goal as outcome: Purchase all gifts for family members by end of the day on December 15th.

2. Goals must be **measurable:**

   Example: Purchase five stocking stuffers for under $10 each by the end of the day on December 10th.

3. Goals must be **challenging but realistic:**

   Example: Make all gift purchases at the Midway Mall.

4. Goals must be **communicated:**

   Example: Use text messages, emails, phone calls, or a family meeting to get the point across.

The following example combines all of these goal criteria:

In a phone message to Sam from Susie:

"We will meet at Midway Mall at 9 a.m. on Saturday, December 15, to complete our entire holiday gift shopping by 5 p.m. The gift list includes five stocking stuffers for less than $10 each for the neighborhood children and 10 total gifts for our parents, your three sisters, my brother, and our bosses, limiting our spending to less than $50/person."

Another common approach to goal writing is SMART,[7] an acronym for:

- **S**pecific
- **M**easurable
- **A**ction-oriented
- **R**ealistic
- **T**imebound

SMART may appear as SMARTER or SMARTERS (in which E stands for *Evaluate*, R for *Reevaluate*, and S for *Satisfactory*). To compare the

---

ACTIVITY 5.4
VALUES STATEMENT

Take this opportunity to brainstorm 10 additional values or beliefs that might support physical therapy practices or multidisciplinary programs that include physical therapy services. Define these values in terms of the actions of employees.

ACTIVITY 5.5
VALUES AND THE AMERICAN PHYSICAL THERAPY ASSOCIATION

1. What are the vision and mission of the American Physical Therapy Association? Do they meet the criteria for a vision and a mission statement provided in Sidebars 5.2 and 5.3? How do you think they might be improved?
2. Why did the American Physical Therapy Association separate its core values from its vision and mission statement?
3. What should be the relationship between the vision, mission, and core values of the profession and those of individual physical therapy practices?

general guidelines for goal setting with SMART, in the shopping example, SMART criteria are met as:

"We'll meet at Midway Mall at 9 a.m. on Saturday, December 15 (A), to complete (A) our entire (S and R) holiday gift shopping by 5 p.m. (T and R). The gift list includes five (M) stocking stuffers for less than $10 (M) each for the neighborhood children and 10 total (M) gifts for our parents, your three sisters, my brother, and our bosses, limiting (A) our spending to less than $50/person (M)."

Three types of goals are included in any strategic planning. They all demand deadlines and evaluation feedback to determine whether they have been met:[8]

- **Horizon goals**—broad and less specific goals that are to be met over the course of the overall planning time span, typically years.
- **Near-term goals**—also called short-term goals, with results or accomplishments expected in the next operating cycle, typically 1 year. They serve as progress points toward horizon goals.
- **Target goals**—very short-term and specific to time and measurement. They generate action that can be accomplished in days or weeks. Target goals need to be checked regularly to determine whether they remain consistent with near-term and horizon goals.

Target goals require action plans that include the identification of barriers to reaching the targets. Barriers can be insurmountable, in which case the target is abandoned and an alternate goal is set. Other barriers are temporary if the target can be set aside for a short time so that the barrier can be overcome or resolved.[7] For example, a near-term goal may be that all staff earns transitional doctor of physical therapy (t-DPT) degrees by the end of the year. A barrier may be that one of the contracts with a third-party payer was not renewed and revenue did not meet projections. As a result, funds to support the tuition of staff in transitional programs were not available so their studies were postponed.

Because there is no practice too small for strategic planning, the following fictitious solo practitioner's private practice is used to demonstrate the target goal-setting component (goals) of strategic planning.

Michael Somski's vision and mission for his Chronic Pain Relief practice are the following:

VISION: To practice physical therapy exclusively to resolve complex chronic pain conditions of people who have previous failed attempts for relief of their pain.

MISSION: To provide focused, one-on-one care to people with chronic pain through an efficient, effective multifaceted approach provided by a board-certified physical therapist who is a fellow of the International Pain Society that results in the clients' ability to participate in meaningful work and leisure activities.

This vision and mission statement may lead to the following horizon goals for Chronic Pain Relief:

By 2017:

- 100% of patients receiving care at Chronic Pain Relief will be referred or seek care on their own initiative because of its reputation for success in resolving complex pain problems.
- Chronic Pain Relief's start-up debt will be paid in full.
- 100% of the patient load will be patients with chronic pain.
- Patient volume will be consistently six patient visits/day.
- 85% of patients who receive care at Chronic Pain Relief will report either a return to work or normal daily activities if not employed.

Near-term goals for Chronic Pain Relief may include the following:

In 1 year:

- Twenty-five physicians will refer at least one patient/month to Chronic Pain Relief.
- The practice's treatment area, reception room, and office will be completely furnished.
- The Chronic Pain Relief webpage will be recognized by ABC Website Review for excellence.
- Contracts with 20 health insurance companies will be fully negotiated and in place.

Typically, target goals are presented in a chart like the one in Table 5.1 for a given week. See Activities 5.6 and 5.7 for more attention to goals.

A Manager's Responsibility

Healthcare managers have responsibility for the development, implementation, and ongoing review of visions, mission statements, and goals as a major component of strategic planning for a new

TABLE 5.1   Chronic Pain Relief practice

TARGET	BARRIERS	ACTION	DEADLINE
Hire receptionist/ office manager.	Timely posting of ad for position Time for interviews during patient care	Have ad in Sunday paper. Select applicants and schedule three interviews after 5 p.m.	Wed. noon By the end of the next week Start date for receptionist first of month
Market-call three physicians.	Arranging appointments with physicians	Call to confirm office appointment. Make reservations for lunch. Pick up muffin basket for office staff.	By end of week
Finalize and implement billing system.	Limited computer skills	Arrange 8-hour session with computer consultant.	Saturday
Average three appointments/ day next week.	Limited referrals	Follow-up calls to 10 physicians to ask for referrals.	In next 2 days

---

ACTIVITY 5.6
CRITIQUE OF GOALS

1. Critique the goals established for Chronic Pain Relief using SMART or the general rules for goals. Revise as necessary.
2. Determine how attainment of the goals will be evaluated.

ACTIVITY 5.7
ESTABLISHING GOALS

Write goals for ABC Health System Post-Surgical Hip Program, McHale and Associates, and New Jersey Pediatric Rehabilitation Services based on the final versions of their visions and mission statements.

---

organization or program. Managers must persuade and empower people to achieve the vision and live the mission to accomplish the goals of an organization.

Independent (private) practitioners cannot afford any less investment of time and thought in establishing these tools for a new practice. Particularly in the early developmental stages of a new business, all decisions about a new practice depend on understanding where the organization is headed and how it intends to get there. These processes also assist new entrepreneurs in clarifying answers to the tough questions posed by investors or lenders as they determine how well thought through a business plan is. Managers in established organizations may devote more time to looking for gaps between a current vision, mission, and goals and one that will best prepare them for the future. See Activity 5.8.

REFERENCES

1. Lansdell S. *The Vision Thing* (ExpressExec Strategy; 03.04) (eBook). Oxford, England: Capstone Publishing Ltd; 2002.

ACTIVITY 5.8
TIME-OUT FOR WRITING

All three strategic planning documents described in the Introduction to Section 2—program proposal, feasibility study, business plan—require a vision, mission statement, and goals. If you have been assigned the preparation of one of these documents, the conclusion of this chapter is a good time to prepare its vision, mission, and goals. Refer to Appendix 2.

2. Bryson J. *Strategic Planning for Public and Nonprofit Organizations: A Guide to Strengthening and Sustaining Organizational Achievement.* San Francisco, CA: Jossey-Bass; 1995.

3. Talbot M. *Make Your Mission Statement Work: Identify Your Organisation's Values and Live Them Every Day.* Oxford, England: How to Books Ltd; 2003.

4. Luke RD, Walston SL, Plummer PM. *Healthcare Strategy: In Pursuit of Competitive Advantage.* Chicago, IL: Health Administration Press; 2004.

5. Williams J, Smythe W, Hadjistravropoulos T, et al. A study of thematic content in hospital mission statements: a question of values. *Health Care Management Review.* 2005;30: 304-314.

6. Desmidt S, Prinzie AA. The organization's mission statement: give up hope or resuscitate? A search for evidence-based recommendations. In: Wolf JA, Hanson H, Moir MJ, Friedman L, Savage GT, eds. *Organization Development in Healthcare: Conversations on Research and Strategies.* Bingley, England: Emerald Group Publishing Ltd; 2011:25-41. *Advances in Health Care Management;* vol 10.

7. Doran GT. *How to Be a Better Manager in 10 Easy Steps.* New York, NY: Monarch Press; 1983.

8. Fry FL, Stoner CR, Weinzimmer LG. *Strategic Planning for New and Emerging Businesses: A Consulting Approach.* Chicago, IL: Dearborn; 1999.

CHAPTER 6

Responsibilities for Policies and Procedures

LEARNING OBJECTIVES

- Determine the purpose of policies and procedures.
- Distinguish between policies and procedures.
- Identify some expectations of The Joint Commission for policies and procedures.
- Identify managerial actions that increase the value of policies and procedures.
- Compare policies and procedures with other documents used by healthcare organizations.
- Critique given policies.
- Prepare a policy and procedure using a given guideline.
- Discuss the responsibilities of managers for policies and procedures.

Overview

In large healthcare organizations, the development, review, and implementation of policies and procedures are driven by The Joint Commission (formerly The Joint Commission on Accreditation of Healthcare Organizations) and other accreditation and licensure requirements. One intent of these requirements is to ensure that policies and procedures are multidisciplinary in order to reduce confusion and inconsistencies about patient care that may occur among various units and disciplines.[1]

Because of this requirement, and the complexity of large healthcare organizations, responsibility for policies and procedures often falls to a systemwide standing committee devoted to the ongoing development and review of its policies and procedures manual.

Usefulness of Policies and Procedures

Although it will be less complex, a policies and procedures manual is important to even the simplest

organization—an independent physical therapy practitioner. Regardless of size, there are several good reasons to develop and implement policies and procedures:

- To avoid the potential trap of relying on memory to assure consistency in conducting business over a period of time.
- To demonstrate thoughtful, thorough attention to business details for all stakeholders.
- To serve as evidence during legal proceedings. NOTE: Wording that suggests absolutes such as *always* should be avoided; use *typically* or *usually* instead.
- To meet the requirements of licensing or other agencies that may demand them.
- To reflect the compliance of an organization's commitment to state and federal laws.

Policies and procedures cover the gamut of operations and reflect an organization's vision and mission. A sampling of the range of topics that might be found in the table of contents of any healthcare organization's policies and procedures include:

- Charges for Patient Cancellations and No-Shows

- Recognition and Reporting of Abuse
- Use of Patient Restraints
- Interpreter and Translation Services
- Medical Device Safety
- Patient and Family Education
- Universal Precautions
- Verbal and Telephone Orders

Basic Principles of Policies and Procedures

A policies and procedures manual has value only if it is used. Access to the manual is the first important criterion. A cumbersome manual that serves only as a space-taker on a manager's bookshelf will be of no value if it is opened only when a compulsory review of it must be done. An online version of a manual in which employees may search for terms increases its usability and implementation. It also reinforces the use of standardized formats as they are developed. To be more functional, the policies and procedures manual for any healthcare organization must:[1]

- Be current and relevant to contemporary work.
- *Exclude* clinical guidelines and protocols.
- *Exclude* entries that are simply information sharing.
- Be consistent in format (e.g., worded as do's rather than do not's).
- Emphasize expectations rather than what is unacceptable.
- Be accessible and easily retrievable.
- Include a complete history of changes made to the document.
- Include guidelines for writing, revising, and reviewing the manual.

Deleting outdated policies and procedures is probably as important as writing new ones, particularly for healthcare organizations that struggle to keep up with ongoing changes in technology, employees, and organizational structures. Not only do managers want everyone to be on the *same* page, but also it is critical that the page they are on is the *right* page. Acceptance of a policy and procedure to manage policies and procedures is the critical first step. Fortunately, computer software programs

and other resources have made the development, review, revision, and tracking of changes in policies and procedures manuals easier and timelier.

Preparing Policies and Procedures

Policies and procedures are more likely to be effective if they accurately describe an activity using consistent terminology to make results more uniform. They must be logical, detailed, free of spelling and grammatical errors, and understandable. There should be no gaps in the steps to ensure adherence and the desired outcome. A template or standard format for policies and procedures is valuable for improving their effectiveness. Although the layout of a policy and procedure may vary, they typically include the following sections:

- Title and tracking number
- Effective date
- Review/revision date
- Policy
- Purpose
- Persons affected
- Scope
- Background
- Definitions
- Procedures
- Responsibilities
- Approval signatures

This format reflects a system that combines policies and procedures in one document. Some organizations may choose to separate policies and procedures into two manuals that are cross-referenced. There is a risk that people are less likely to look up the information they need in two sources because it is more cumbersome for readers, and because procedures are revised more frequently than policies, some organizations find it easier to maintain procedures separate from policies.

Policies

A policy is a broad statement of an expectation that guides decisions regarding actions to be taken. The general rules that govern organizational procedures are found in policies. A policy also addresses the who, what, when, and where about some component of an organization. Some examples of policies in fictional healthcare organizations are:

- **KEYS AND LOCKS.** The Chief of Physical Plant Services is responsible for responding to all requests for replacement or issuance of new keys or keycards, duplication of existing keys, keying changes, installation, or repair of locks (rooms, desks, file cabinets, deadbolts, etc.) throughout the ABC Health System. Reproduction of keys is prohibited by anyone other than the locksmith designated by the Chief of Physical Plant Services. It is a misdemeanor crime to possess, use, duplicate, or cause to duplicate any keys to buildings or other secured spaces without proper authorization of the Assistant Vice President of Operations.

- **PATIENT SCHEDULING.** Each new patient is scheduled for an initial appointment within 48 hours of receiving a request for an outpatient physical therapy appointment. Inpatients must be seen on the same day when a referral is received before noon.

- **INTERVIEW EXPENSES.** ABC Health System reimburses certain travel expenses of applicants who are invited for an interview but not offered a position or if the applicant accepts the position offered. However, reimbursement for travel expenses will not be granted if the applicant is offered a position with ABC Health System but declines the offer.

- **REIMBURSEMENT TRAINING.** All physical therapy staff receives effective and timely education on federal and state statutes, regulations and guidelines, and corporate policies that are related to the billing of patient services.

- **PERFORMANCE EVALUATION.** Adherence to and promotion of the Code of Conduct is a required element in performance evaluations of all employees. All employees are to be held accountable for behaviors displayed relative to the values articulated in the mission and values statements. Managers and supervisors are held accountable for setting an example and being a role model to ensure that those on their team have sufficient information to comply with laws, regulations, and policies as well as the resources to resolve ethical dilemmas.

- **EMPLOYEE BACKGROUND CHECKS.** Such checks provide a standard requirement and process for obtaining and evaluating background information on candidates for employment, students, volunteers, and staffing agency and contracted staff/employees. This policy articulates notice of investigation and documentation requirements.

- **GIFTS POLICY.** Establishes parameters for the extension of gifts to and the receipt of gifts from individuals or organizations that have a business relationship with ABC Health System but who are not referral sources.

See Activity 6.1.

Procedures

A procedure describes a particular way of accomplishing an action. It is a series of steps to provide details to reach an end or to describe how to carry out a policy. Unlike policies, which tend to be more enduring, the wording of procedures generally allows some variation in actions that are acceptable as long as the intent and outcome of the procedure are reached. They tend to evolve more over time because of the impact of new technology and processes on tasks completed and responsibilities met. For example, a policy on reimbursement of interview expenses is not likely to change, but the procedures for an applicant to receive reimbursement may change.

Despite this flexibility and modification, procedures are the established methods for conducting the business of an organization so that it may reach its goals. Therefore, it is important that they be thoroughly and thoughtfully prepared if they are to be

---

ACTIVITY 6.1
POLICIES REVIEW

Discuss your impressions of these sample policies:

- Do they need to be improved?
- Are the who, what, when, and where addressed?
- What do these policies tell you about the culture of ABC Health System?
- What can be done to improve them?

of value. Procedures must be presented in a way that is easy to follow including accurate, step-by-step tasks with user options whenever possible. See Activity 6.2 and Activity 6.3.

ACTIVITY 6.2
WRITING PROCEDURES

For a Nonsmoking Health Campus Policy, a procedure may be:

The Chief of Physical Plant Services posts and maintains placement of nonsmoking signs at all entrances and other appropriate locations. The steps are:

1. *Designates two outdoor smoking-permitted areas and posts smoking-permitted signs.*
2. *Places appropriate receptacles in each designated smoking-permitted area.*
3. *Checks on the condition of the signs and smoking areas biweekly.*
4. *Replaces or repairs signage or areas as necessary within 24 hours.*
5. *Receives reports of incidents of smoking in violation of the policy from employees and guests.*
6. *Reports incidents of smoking violation to the Assistant Vice President of Operations within 24 hours.*

Prepare an accompanying procedure(s) for a selected policy reviewed in Activity 6.1. Include a *draft* of the steps necessary to carry out the policy.

ACTIVITY 6.3
YOUR CHOICE

Select a current policy in your school of physical therapy such as the policy on classroom absences. Begin with a strategic plan: (1) What is the school or PT department's policy now? (2) What do you want it to be? (3) What do you or the school have to work with? (4) How will you or the school get it to where it wants to be? With the answers to these questions, prepare a new or revised policy and procedure. NOTE: A policy from a healthcare organization may be selected instead, for example, Assignment of Staff to Weekend Coverage.

Other Organizational Documents

In addition to policies and procedures, managers may also need to become familiar with other important documents (see Activity 6.4). For example, discussions with executives may include references to the organization's bylaws. They might also refer to specific clinical guidelines and protocols as managers monitor the care of a particular patient or groups of patients. Policies and procedures should be distinguished from the bylaws of a healthcare organization, clinical guidelines, and protocols:

- *Bylaws* are the essential legal framework of a corporation that typically addresses procedures for holding meetings, electing officers, and defining the duties and powers of the corporation. Shareholders or boards of directors adopt *bylaws* to provide detailed implementation of the articles of incorporation of their organizations.
- *Clinical practice guidelines* (pathways) are systematically developed statements based on established standards to assist in the decision-making of practitioners and patients about appropriate healthcare for specific clinical conditions.
- *Protocols* are specific, detailed plans for treatment regimens (or a scientific study). Protocols are about doing and clinical practice guidelines are about deciding. See Web Resources for bylaw, guideline, and protocol sources.

A Manager's Responsibility

Policies and procedures are about accountability for decisions at all levels of an organization and the

---

ACTIVITY 6.4
OTHER DOCUMENTS

Use online resources to find examples of an organization's bylaws, a clinical guideline, and a protocol that are of interest to you. Compare their formats. Discuss how each of these documents is different from policies and procedures. See Web Resources for suggested types of online resources for this activity.

processes that are required to accomplish its goals. Managers are responsible for preparing them from the reader's viewpoint to assure their implementation. It is unreasonable to expect people simply to know what to do. They may bring assumptions from prior work experiences that are no longer applicable, or they may be expected to perform duties that are new to them. Even experienced employees may need to be reoriented to their work as changes in the organization or technology result in new ways of doing things or new responsibilities.

Managers need to be policies and procedures experts. Questions often arise because of the difficulty in identifying every possible step and possibility in a procedure. They arise because the actual performance of a procedural addition or change occurs faster than it can be written or revised. Questions about why a policy even exists also demand answers and action from managers. Managers must see to it that any policies and procedures in question are revised. Writing policies and procedures earlier rather than later saves time and diminishes the chances for potential errors or inconsistencies in performance.

Encouraging those affected by policies and procedures to participate in their review and to make recommendations for improvement is likely to be an important institutional policy that increases commitment to the manual. Managers who assign new employees to read and then sign off on a policies and procedures manual during the orientation process may discover this is a meaningless exercise. An alternative approach may be to introduce questions or problems during orientation sessions or meetings and ask employees to find the relevant policy and procedure to address them. This approach also presents the ongoing opportunity to update or revise policies as questions are raised in these sessions.

Particularly important are policies and procedures related to the legal rights and responsibilities of employees. Because employees may rely on a policies and procedures manual when they seek legal solutions to problems with their employers, or patients may seek answers in the manuals when they question the care they have received, managers also must consider the manual a potential risk management and quality assurance tool.

If confronted with a manual during legal proceedings, a manager would not want to be caught in the awkward position of reporting that it is outdated, or that it is *not really* the way procedures are implemented, or that it has not been applied consistently across all employees. When forced to choose, courts often will interpret actions by organizational personnel as representative of the organization's preferred course of action over related, documented policies that may not be consistent with those actions. See Activity 6.5 and Activity 6.6.

ACTIVITY 6.5
POLICY AND PROCEDURE REVIEW

Currently, staff at ABC Health System has not been involved in the review of policies and procedures. Now that they are more easily accessible online by all employees, Greg Ovinio, the CEO, has asked Marsha Morris, the rehabilitation manager, to come up with a plan to assure that all of her 23 staff members review the policies and procedures pertinent to them and make their recommendations to her for changes and additions during the next 3 months. Using a strategic planning process, how would Marsha meet this need? HINT: (1) Where is the staff now? (2) Where will they be in 3 months? (3) What is there to work with? (4) How will she get the staff there?

ACTIVITY 6.6
TIME-OUT FOR WRITING

A completed policies and procedures manual is typically not included in program proposals, feasibility studies, or business plans. However, some people may choose to include a table of contents for policies and procedures as evidence of the detailed approach taken in the preparation of one of these documents. At the very least, particularly in strategic plans for new businesses, budgeting for a packaged plan or software to develop policies and procedures is indicated.

REFERENCE

1. Paige JB. Solve the policy and procedure puzzle. *Nursing Management.* 2003;34(3):45-48. http://www.nursingmanagement.com. Accessed January 12, 2008.

WEB RESOURCES

Agency for Healthcare Research and Quality National Guideline Clearinghouse. http://www.guideline.gov/content.aspx?id=36828. Accessed July 23, 2013.

American Physical Therapy Association bylaws. http://www.apta.org/uploadedFiles/APTAorg/About_Us/Policies/General/Bylaws.pdf. Accessed July 23, 2013.

By-laws of North Florida Regional Medical Center. http://nfrmc.com/professionals/physicians/bylaws.dot. Accessed July 23, 2013.

World Confederation of Physical Therapy clinical guidelines. http://www.wcpt.org/node/29657#australian. Accessed July 23, 2013.

Post-operative rehabilitation surgical protocols of the Orthopedic Specialists of North Carolina. http://www.orthonc.com/physical-therapy/physical-therapy-postoperative-rehabilitation-protocols. Accessed July 23, 2013.

Rehabilitation protocols of Massachusetts General Hospital. http://www.massgeneral.org/ortho/services/sports/rehab.aspx. Accessed July 23, 2013.

CHAPTER 7

Marketing Responsibilities

LEARNING OBJECTIVES

- Discuss the reasons for modification of the traditional Four Ps of Marketing in healthcare.
- Compare the characteristics and purposes of inbound and outbound marketing.
- Distinguish among advertising, publicity, promotion, and public relations.
- Compare traditional and social marketing strategies.
- Compare the cost and effectiveness of branding and other marketing tools.
- Discuss the need to consult with marketing professionals.

Overview

Despite the long history of marketing, its role as a management tool is relatively new to healthcare organizations. Marketers seek to define new relationships with healthcare stakeholders and to face the challenges of evolving healthcare policy. Patients are more likely to take the initiative in finding the healthcare information they need and to ask providers more questions about their personal healthcare. More than ever, people seek healthcare relationships that are based on an exchange of information and direct participation in decisions made. Along with these system changes, new hospital executives have brought trusted business tools, including marketing plans, with them from other industries. As a result, marketing is now enmeshed in the responsibilities of managers at all levels of all healthcare organizations.

According to the American Marketing Association, "marketing is the activity, set of institutions, and processes for creating, communicating, delivering, and exchanging offerings that have value for customers, clients, partners, and society at large."[1] Some examples in healthcare of the *exchange of something of value* include the following: a physical therapist treats a patient in exchange for money from the patient and/or from a third-party payer, a physician receives staff privileges at a hospital in exchange for admitting patients there, or an employer pays insurance premiums in exchange for healthcare coverage for its employees. Marketing is the process for these exchanges and relationships that is considered successful when the goals of both parties are met.[2]

Many marketing professionals have modified or abandoned traditional marketing approaches for healthcare because of the uniqueness of its business. For example, a classic approach to marketing is control of the Four Ps of marketing—product, price, place, and promotion—which may be applied in healthcare as follows:

- **PRODUCT**: the goods, services, and ideas offered by an organization. A lasting, loyal relationship is often considered the product of healthcare for marketing purposes.

- **PRICE**: the charge for the product including professional fees, insurance premiums, deductibles, and co-payments. *Effort costs* are often included in healthcare marketing. In addition to money, patients and clients must relate costs to long-term benefits of care, including lifestyle changes that demand a great deal of effort on their part.

- **PLACE:** the manner in which goods and services are distributed to consumers. Place often enhances the perceptions of quality in healthcare. Place includes communications that are not face-to-face such as online information, 24-hour nursing consultations, and the ability to share medical records electronically.

- **PROMOTION:** any means used to inform a market that an answer to its need is available to facilitate an exchange. It is often a mix of advertising, direct sales, sales promotions, and publicity.

The application of the Four Ps to healthcare has not been easily accomplished. Customer satisfaction became patient satisfaction, and new ways to measure satisfaction have been developed. Unlike other customers, though, patients are rarely the ultimate decision makers about "buying" healthcare services, and they usually do not have a choice when they need a service. Patients do not know the price of a healthcare service so they do not base selecting a service on price, even when they have a choice. Patients require the referral of professionals to services that they often know little about, making it difficult for them to judge the quality of those services.[2] Consider the differences in the buying processes when a person needs a new television and when a person needs a total joint arthroplasty, for example.

One View of Marketing

For the purposes of this chapter, marketing is a managerial process that includes a wide range of activities to assure that an organization meets its goals by meeting the needs of its customers. In one model marketing is viewed as processes that are both inbound to the organization and outbound from the organization:[2]

- **Inbound marketing** includes marketing research to identify potential customers and their needs, the means to meet those needs, analysis of the competition, and positioning and pricing a new service (finding a niche).
- **Outbound marketing** is the promotion of a product or service through advertising, public relations, and sales strategies.

Marketing typically focuses on one particular service or product at a time because the activities used to be successful may be very different from one another. Success depends on attention to *both* inbound and outbound marketing processes. Until recently, healthcare focused primarily on outbound marketing, typically without much attention to or analysis of its effect. Physicians were often the only focus of hospital marketing efforts. Patients, employers, third-party payers, and many others also have become important customers of healthcare organizations. Today, healthcare systems often have vice presidents of marketing or marketing consultants who guide plans that managers implement at all levels of an organization. Even solo practitioners must assume responsibility for marketing to reach the goals of their smaller organizations.

Inbound Marketing

The perspective of managers with primary responsibility for marketing is taken to introduce several important components of inbound marketing in this section. In large organizations, mid-level managers who are developing new programs may work in collaboration with marketing professionals who are accountable for a broader, systemwide marketing plan.

Target Markets

The first inbound marketing responsibility is to identify the potential groups of patients or clients with specific needs to be met or to survey a broad group of people in a community to identify opportunities for new programs that may need development. This development is particularly important in healthcare in which increasing the patient base is very important to increasing revenue and profits when costs and reimbursement are so tightly controlled. Managers identify target markets that can be described by age, sex, income/educational levels, profession/career, type of residence, and ZIP code. Technology for data collection and analysis has made these processes easier (see Web Resources).

Marketing success is dependent on knowing customer likes, dislikes, goals, and expectations, in other words, answering the question: What will satisfy these particular, specific customers? In addition to databases, more direct data collection techniques include having employees report what patients and other customers ask for or complain about, directly asking them in person about their needs (focus groups), or having patients submit comment cards or complete electronic or paper surveys. See Activity 7.1 and Activity 7.2.

Product Demand and Clarification

Because of this inbound process, managers should be able to describe clearly the product or service from the perspective of the target market group. Emphasizing special features that have been designed to anticipate their particular needs builds satisfaction and loyalty. Determining how a product or service is packaged and priced is the next step. Finally, the demand for a product or service in healthcare needs to be identified as specifically as is possible. Understanding the demand can be challenging because of the complexity of access to services, variable payment for those services, the unpredictable nature of injuries and diseases, and frequent changes in reimbursement policies. The U.S. Census Bureau (see Web Resources) provides demographic data that may be added to economic development information from the local chamber of commerce as resources to answer questions such as:

- Is this a seasonal community?
- Who are the major employers?
- What percentage of the population is over 65? Over 85? Under age 5?
- What percentage of the population is uninsured?
- Do existing practices have waiting lists for appointments for physical therapy?
- What is the impact of physician-based services in the community?
- How far do people currently travel to receive physical therapy? How long does it take them to travel for services?
- Who are the potential referral sources?

Managers and entrepreneurs become sleuths or spies in gathering some of this information, yet cannot be shy about asking questions of any potential source of information while determining how important it is to keep these inquiries confidential. Networking at professional meetings and other business gatherings is a way of discovering potential sources of information. Talking to people who have received

---

ACTIVITY 7.1
A STUDENT FOCUS GROUP

Roberta Robinson is the manager of rehabilitation services in a large, multi-site healthcare system. There are between 20 and 30 students from all of the rehabilitation disciplines assigned to the center at any point in time. One of her goals for this year is to develop a centralized, rehabilitation-services clinical education program for all centers of the system that is more consistent with the mission of this church-affiliated organization:

Extending the healing ministry focused on healing the whole person—mind, body, and spirit.

She is considering conducting a focus group of selected students. She has gathered some information on focus groups in preparation that includes the following:

- Focus groups are used to assess services and test new ideas.

- For about an hour, discussion leaders interview 6 to 10 people with similar characteristics, who do not know each other, in a group.
- Five or six questions are prepared that focus on a clearly defined objective for addressing the issue at hand.
- Ground rules typically include an opportunity for everyone to be heard, staying on task, and achieving closure on the questions posed.
- The meeting is recorded so that content may be analyzed later.
- Facilitating discussion, summarizing what is heard, and assuring participation are important skills in conducting focus groups.

With these guidelines, plan the focus group composed of current students assigned to rehabilitation services.

services in the competition's practices may reveal additional factors important to potential target markets. Being open and honest about plans for a new business may cause others to put up a defense, making it harder to get information, or, conversely, it may encourage people to be helpful. Determining the loyalty of the target market to existing healthcare organizations may be as important as determining other facts and figures.

Competition

Managers also need to direct their attention to the competition. If a product or service is new or unique, there may be no direct competition. More often, in healthcare there may be a great deal of competition. Managers need to determine their attitudes about their competition as the first step. Competitors may be ignored so that all energy is focused on other aspects of the business. At other times, managers may obsessively track the strategies of competitors to outdo them, or they may imitate them. In any case, managers need to establish the uniqueness of their products and identify a name, or brand, to reflect that image to set them apart from the competition.

The starting point of this process is competitor analysis that helps to determine the advantages an organization has over another. It helps in forecasting returns on possible future investments in the organization. One way to analyze the competition is for managers to ask some key questions:

- Who are all of the competitors for meeting specific customer needs or preferences?
- What is the competition's profile? Location? Vision, mission, and goals? Organizational structure? Market segments served? Capacity? Numbers and types of employees?
- What strategies do they use to meet their objectives?
- How do competitors' products and services differ from one another and your organization?
- What are the strengths, weaknesses, and threats of the competitors?
- How satisfied are the competition's customers?
- Who are the competition's partners and supporters?
- What are possible actions to beat the competition? Can they be done?
- How will the competition react to the projected changes if they are made?
- Who are potential new competitors?

Gathering data to answer these questions requires putting together information from a variety of sources such as published reports and brochures and asking suppliers, customers, and former employees. Simple, disciplined, direct observation of advertising, press releases, trade-show presentations, and other social contacts also provides information. Tracking changes in the competition's advertising may reveal new directions, products, and services or a change in the focus of their strategies.

Benchmarking

Benchmarking is a tool for comparing competitors. Using ideal standards for best practices, organizations are compared across a variety of key success factors. Comparative scores are expressed as ratios. The Association for Benchmarking Health Care provides more information on benchmarking processes and results (see Web Resources). Managers may use benchmarks to identify necessary initiatives to improve their competitive position. The challenge is the accurate analysis of benchmarking data and then developing a plan to meet or exceed the competition. This may mean doing the same things better or developing an entirely different approach. Other challenges for physical therapy include improving the internal validity of clinical data that are used in benchmarking.[3]

The SWOT Strategy

SWOT is another classic marketing analysis strategy.[4] SWOT identifies the **S**trengths and **W**eaknesses of an organization (i.e., internal factors, such as resources and capabilities) and the possible **O**pportunities and **T**hreats (i.e., external factors, such as competition, reimbursement, and governmental policies). SWOT is generated through an environmental scan, which is a systematic surveillance of the internal and external events and conditions that affect the organization. SWOT allows managers to summarize and filter key points about their organizations. See Activity 7.3.

Outbound Marketing

Outbound marketing has shifted somewhat from image advertising to specific, targeted promotions that include more informational content for specific products and services. Advertising and promotions are supplemented with sales and public (or media) relations that focus on an organization as a whole. They are complemented by customer service and satisfaction efforts. If inbound marketing efforts have been effective, outbound marketing should easily fall into place. If inbound marketing is skipped or ineffective, no amount of outbound marketing may lead to the desired level of use of a product or service. The standard practice of developing a product or service and then convincing people they want it seems to be over.

Branding

Healthcare faces the challenge of marketing intangible concepts such as quality, caring, and professionalism to develop a perception of an organization. This requires establishing a mindset of the image of the organization and its services. Healthcare services are often difficult to quantify and evaluate because they are personal, subjective experiences that are not open to the same types of quality controls as are tangible products. They reflect the persons who are providing them and really cannot be owned or transferred. The solution to this dilemma is a brand—some name, symbol, or other feature that distinguishes an organization from other similar organizations or services. Branding is less common in healthcare, but because brands incorporate intangible values, images, and benefits into some visual feature that stimulates demand, branding may become a more important healthcare marketing tool. See Activity 7.4.

Selecting Outbound Marketing Tools

Managers have to decide the comparative value of efforts expended, funds available, and costs associated with a wide range of outbound marketing possibilities. Particular attention must be given to which target market(s) to appeal to and what message is to be communicated. The most preferred and effective means for delivering the message is balanced against what is affordable and practical. Some selected tools are the following:

- Sponsorships of sport teams, charities, and the arts
- Memberships in professional associations and community and civic organizations
- Community outreach, such as participation in health fairs and other educational programs

---

ACTIVITY 7.3
DETERMINING A MARKET

Sid Williams is a physical therapy manager of his own practice. He learns of a rehabilitation program that targets people with chronic gastrointestinal disorders. He thinks he would like to develop a similar program in his practice. It might be good for business and the community. How could Sid use SWOT to decide whether this would be a good business decision?

ACTIVITY 7.4
HEALTHCARE BRANDS

Sid Williams is a physical therapy manager of his own practice. He feels he needs a brand to help his business. Sid is aware of the American Physical Therapy Association brand campaign to "move forward." He is not certain it will help his practice stand out. What do you think? What advice do you have for Sid?

HINT: Explore the APTA's marketing webpages available at www.apta.org/PRMarketing.

- Logos on stationery supplies, apparel, and signage
- Publication of newsletters and brochures
- Hard-copy advertising in newspapers, community directories, entertainment programs, billboards, and banners
- Radio and television ads or public service announcements

The measurement of the consumer response to these tools is limited so it is difficult to determine their effectiveness in meeting an organization's goals. A shift to more consumer-driven tools such as interactive websites with webpages that include message boards and links for clients and potential clients to use to request more information, podcasts, stealth ads, blogs, social networks, and word-of-mouth referrals are often more cost-effective, and the rate of usage and consumer responses are more measurable and more quickly available.[5]

The increased availability of healthcare outcome data has allowed them to become a resource for savvy consumers and a potential outbound marketing tool. Examples of consumer resources are found in the Web Resources. Sidebar 7.1 clarifies some marketing terminology. See Activity 7.5.

Marketing Physicians and Others

Physicians and other health professionals who may refer patients remain a target market of particular concern to all independent practitioners as well as to large healthcare systems. Not only must managers establish referral relationships and identify and meet the needs of the people who refer, but they must also be able to sustain a consistent commitment from the physicians and others for referrals. Establishing and sustaining relationships with case managers, vocational rehabilitation counselors, employers, and attorneys to increase referrals are equally important in many practices. As physical therapy practices compete with one another for a limited number of contracts with third-party payers, strategies to meet the needs of decision makers in insurance companies also become critical. See Activity 7.6.

ACTIVITY 7.5
CONSUMER-DRIVEN MARKETING

1. Identify healthcare organizations with webpages that include message boards or links for more information, customized interactive websites, networking, podcasts, stealth ads, blogs, or social networks.
   - What is your impression of them?
   - Who is the target market for these marketing efforts?
2. Give an example of how word of mouth has affected a decision you made.

SIDEBAR 7.1

Advertising, Publicity, Promotion, and Public Relations

Advertising is publicity and non-media efforts that are paid for and controlled by an organization. EXAMPLE: A flyer on bulletin boards in local restaurants reads—Fourth St. Physical Therapy Center. Hours 7 a.m. to 7 p.m. Mon.–Sat.

Publicity is appearing in the media. Organizations do not control the message that is developed by media reporters and writers. EXAMPLE: An expert on peripheral vascular disease gives a 1-hour presentation on Open House Night at Fourth St. Physical Therapy and is interviewed by a reporter for the health section of the newspaper.

Promotion is ongoing advertising and publicity that keep the product or service in the mind of the customer and help stimulate demand. EXAMPLE: One-hour presentation on a different diagnosis the first Friday of every month during Fourth St. Physical Therapy Open House Night.

Public relations ensures that an organization has a strong public image and helps the public understand the organization. Advertising and publicity contribute to this image either negatively or positively, so the message conveyed is very important. EXAMPLE: Fourth St. Physical Therapy receives an award for outstanding physical therapy practice in the state.

Social Marketing

The discussion so far has focused on commercial marketing to bring about voluntary exchanges that result in an organization meeting its goals and patients, meeting their needs. Social marketing is the application of commercial marketing techniques to services that are designed to influence the *voluntary* behavior of target groups to improve their personal welfare and that of society. Examples include smoking cessation, safe sex practices, breast cancer screening, family planning, and seat-belt use programs. The key concepts in social marketing include the following:[6]

- A patient/customer-centered orientation
- Segmentation of target markets
- Accounting for real and perceived barriers that prevent people from adopting a new behavior
- Demonstrating the benefits of the desired change for people in the target markets
- Using a variety of means to reach target markets
- Pretesting and monitoring marketing interventions as they are implemented
- Forming partnerships that enhance credibility and facilitate access to target markets
- Coordinating with other approaches to social change

- Making a long-term commitment to the social marketing strategy

Managers must distinguish between traditional marketing efforts directed at meeting the needs of customers and social marketing efforts directed at changing the behaviors of a group of people. For example, physical therapists may be involved with a program created by a healthcare system to increase the number of at-risk women who are screened for breast and ovarian cancers each year. Social marketing strategies may include asking female patients for the date of their last mammogram as part of the physical therapy admission screening process, reminding them of the importance of screening during therapy sessions, or providing general information pamphlets in the waiting room on the importance of breast cancer screening. Social marketing shifts the emphasis of marketing from what is good for the organization to what is good for the broader society.

A Manager's Responsibility

There are many complex aspects of inbound and outbound marketing. Managers in healthcare organizations and private practitioners typically rely on marketing experts to assist in their decision-making, particularly as implementation of the Affordable Care Act presents new challenges in all aspects of healthcare. Efforts to increase efficiency and a focus on outcomes of quality care may require organizations to focus on a different set of marketing tools. To meet these new demands, an organization may outsource its entire marketing function to a full-service marketing firm that plans, implements, and monitors all marketing activities. Larger organizations may have in-house marketing staff who coordinate with a contracted agency for specific components of marketing such as direct-mail campaigns or media purchases. Smaller organizations may rely on a marketing agency intermittently as needs arise, for example, graphic art for a logo or website building. In any case, familiarity and comfort with the unique features of healthcare organizations are important factors in the selection of a marketing professional partner.[7] The webpages of the American Physical Therapy Association provide profession-specific tools that may be of value to independent practices as well as to larger organizations that seek to increase the visibility of physical therapy services. See Web Resources.

Even the best efforts at inbound and outbound marketing may fail. Managers need to be comfortable that they made the best effort to arrive at the best decision, particularly as it relates to the needs of people who are often in crisis when they require healthcare services. Managers also need to consider the ethical implications of both commercial and social marketing plans—considering whether actions are persuasive or coercive, for example. How the organization addresses these issues so that the target markets are respected and treated fairly is somewhat enhanced by the shift from straight advertising to promotions that emphasize education.

Evaluating the effectiveness of marketing efforts is another challenge because direct relationships between efforts and results may not be obvious or even measurable. For instance, increased profit margins, satisfaction of staff and patients, increased demands for services, or the number of new patients may or may not be associated with advertising and public relations. It may indicate that inbound processes were effective or ineffective. Managers must be prepared to contribute to both establishing and evaluating marketing efforts. See Activity 7.7.

ACTIVITY 7.7
TIME-OUT FOR WRITING

Use the following more robust strategic planning process and the resources and questions raised in this chapter to address the inbound and outbound marketing required for your program proposal, feasibility study, or business plan. Follow this strategic planning process:

1. Determine where you are through honest external and internal reviews (SWOT).
2. Determine (review) where you want to be in the long term (mission and vision) and set priorities to be addressed.
3. Clearly define the objectives that must be met to address each priority.
4. Determine who is accountable for meeting the objectives (allocation of time, human capital, and finances).
5. Conduct frequent formal reviews of the process to determine progress toward goals.

REFERENCES

1. American Marketing Association. Definition of marketing. http://www.marketingpower.com/AboutAMA/Pages/DefinitionofMarketing.aspx. Accessed April 13, 2013.
2. Thomas RK. *Marketing Health Services.* Arlington, VA: Health Administration Press; 2005.
3. Resnik L, Liu D, Hart DL, Mor V. Benchmarking physical therapy clinic performance: statistical methods to enhance internal validity when using observational data. *Physical Therapy.* 2008;88(9):1078-1087.
4. Humphrey AS. SWOT analysis for management consulting. *SRI International Alumni Association* [Newsletter]. December 2005:7. http://www.sri.com/sites/default/files/brochures/dec-05.pdf. Accessed April 15, 2013.
5. Rooney K. Consumer-driven healthcare marketing: using the web to get up close and personal. *Journal of Healthcare Management.* 2009;54(4):241-251.
6. Longest BB. *Health Policymaking in the United States.* 4th ed. Chicago, IL: American College of Healthcare Executives; 2006.
7. Thomas RK. *Marketing Health Services.* 2nd ed. Arlington, VA: Health Administration Press; 2010.

WEB RESOURCES

American Physical Therapy Association. Public relations and marketing. http://www.apta.org/prmarketing/. Accessed November 21, 2013.

American Statistics Index (ASI). Comprehensive guide and index to the statistical publications of the U. S. government. http://library.truman.edu/microforms/american_statistics_index.asp. Accessed November 21, 2013.

Association for Benchmarking Health Care. http://www.abhc.org/. Accessed November 21, 2013.

Centers for Medicare & Medicaid Services (CMS). Interactive tool: Hospital compare with links for nursing home compare, dialysis compare, physician compare, and Medicare plan finder. www.hospitalcompare.hhs.gov. Accessed November 21, 2013.

Dartmouth Atlas of Healthcare. www.dartmouthatlas.org/. Accessed November 21, 2013.

U.S. Department of Commerce. U.S. Census Bureau. http://www.commerce.gov. Accessed November 21, 2013.

U.S. Department of Health and Human Services. Agency for Healthcare Research and Quality's HCUPnet for consumer access to data on utilization and quality. hcupnet.ahrq.gov/. Accessed November 21, 2013.

CHAPTER 8

Staffing Responsibilities in Healthcare

LEARNING OBJECTIVES

- Identify compensation and benefits costs.
- Compare the types of employees.
- Prepare a job description for a physical therapist.
- Analyze staff mix and productivity decisions based on job analysis.
- Critique tools for recruitment and for retention of staff.
- Review hints for interviews.
- Address the challenges of performance evaluation.
- Set performance goals for a given person using observable behaviors.
- Investigate approaches to staff development.
- Discuss the management of employee grievances.

Overview

Healthcare managers devote a great deal of time and effort to staffing responsibilities. Having employees who consistently cooperate and collaborate to provide the expected level of quality of care is essential to achieve an organization's goals. Numerous factors influence staffing in contemporary healthcare organizations, for example, recruitment of healthcare professionals who are in short supply, ongoing education and training needs, reduction of services provided, increased technology to support work, reorganization of work flow, increases in ancillary or support staff, and the resulting adjustments of the healthcare skill base.[1]

Managers are held accountable for the use of overtime, on-call, and per diem expenses; staff vacancies; turnover rates; understaffing; and on-the-job injuries. They must attend to the motivation and satisfaction of employees for patients to be satisfied. Patient satisfaction may depend on *how* clinicians and others do their work as much as on the actual outcomes of the work they do. For most patients, their interactions with staff members are their only impressions of an organization.

Because of its dependence on employees for achieving patient outcomes and overall organizational goals, a healthcare system's most powerful asset is its staff. Protecting and sustaining staff to provide 24/7 healthcare services is a major focus of managers. Although opportunities may be limited for some people, employment is generally a matter of voluntary free choice. To be the employer of choice reduces staff turnover and recruitment costs while increasing an organization's reputation. This chapter introduces several of the key staffing responsibilities of managers in contemporary healthcare.

Staff Mix

Managers of physical therapy practices may not have a great deal of flexibility in determining the mix of physical therapists, physical therapist assistants, and non-licensed personnel on staff because of legal constraints, reimbursement issues, the availability of potential employees, and related costs. In some jurisdictions, the ratio of physical therapists to physical therapist assistants is regulated. Most third-party payers and many jurisdictions recognize that only services provided by physical therapists or physical therapist assistants under their direction or supervision can be billed as physical therapy.

As a result of reimbursement constraints, the duties of any other support personnel (aides or techs, for example) typically do not include direct patient care. In many states, practice acts include precise regulations about support personnel. Generally, however, the expectation is that supportive personnel are trained to perform only very specific tasks that are related to the general operations of the physical therapy practice. If aides or techs are engaged in direct patient care, they typically must perform their duties under the direct, continuous, personal supervision of a physical therapist or a physical therapist assistant who is physically and immediately available.

The same staff mix issues apply to all rehabilitation professions. To make effective decisions, the managers of interdisciplinary teams must be aware of the staff mix within a professional group before deciding on a staff mix that includes several professions.

Job Analysis

Staff mix decisions are never easy. Managers cannot afford to have higher-paid employees occupied with duties that can be performed by other levels of workers. They cannot risk the safety of patients and quality of outcomes by assigning tasks to workers who are not qualified to perform them. Managers determine what combination of clinical staff can do the most for the least cost. This serious attention to job analysis requires managers to observe actual work performance to ask the following questions:

- What tasks are currently performed by each level of worker?

- What tasks are performed by each type of worker within a level of work?
- What tasks can each level of worker legally perform?
- What tasks can be eliminated?
- Who is the least expensive worker who can perform each task safely, legally, and effectively?
- What tasks are more easily completed personally by the physical therapist or other professional than they would be by someone who requires the time and attention of the physical therapist for direction and supervision?
- When is work time unproductive?

Any shift in duties and responsibilities resulting from this analysis must be confirmed by the people who actually do the work. A regular re-examination of job descriptions and the number of positions required may lead to surprising conclusions. For instance, it may not always be the best clinical decision to hire an aide if it means that physical therapists' salaries will be frozen to accommodate that new position, or it may be better to hire a physical therapist assistant rather than a physical therapist if the number of new patients per week is low and patient cancellations are high. Hiring physical therapist assistants when physical therapists prefer a one-on-one, hands-on approach in a specialized practice may result in reduced productivity for the assistants because their patient care assignments will be limited.

These decisions are further complicated by the fact that not all employees in the same category of work are equally effective. Managers must be fair in expecting the same performance and amount of work from everyone with the same job description. Strong employees become resentful if they feel that managers tend to reward their outstanding performance with more work while mediocre performers receive fewer assignments. See Activity 8.1.

Types of Employees

Another staff-mix issue is the ratio of full-time employees to all other types of workers who are not full-time. This "other" group includes permanent part-time employees and contingent workers who do not have an implicit or explicit contract for ongoing employment. Contingent (alternative

---

ACTIVITY 8.1
AN AIDE FOR THE SUMMER

Kim Bartholomew's younger brother, 4-year-old Ken, has been receiving intermittent outpatient physical, occupational, and speech therapy at Smith and Associates Pediatric Rehabilitation for most of his life. Kim has approached Anita Smith about a summer job in the practice. She wants to be a physical therapist and feels that a job will not only help her pay for college but will also give her work experience.

Anita is shorthanded and almost said yes immediately, but she asked Kim to give her a chance to think about it. She employs therapists only and has no assistants on staff.

What does the physical therapy practice act in your state say about supportive personnel in this situation? What duties might Anita assign to Kim? Consider: Where is Anita's staffing now? Where does she want it to be? What does she have to work with? How will she get there?

---

or flexible) employment arrangements involve persons employed as independent contractors who work per diem (day by day) at will, on-call workers, temporary help agency workers, and workers provided by contract agencies. Managers must consider the potential higher staffing costs in these arrangements weighed against the costs of paying employees with benefits.

Contingent workers may be long-term substitutes for staff on extended leave or vacation or for positions that remain unfilled for extended periods. They may also be assigned short-term assignments that occur very intermittently as unexpected staffing needs arise or they may be assigned consistent intermittent assignments such as weekend coverage only. Many large organizations may have an in-house pool of contingent workers who are available on call to fill in as needed.

The U.S. Department of Labor Web pages provide information related to these work issues as well as explanations of the Fair Labor Standards Act (FLSA) that must be applied in categorizing employees:[2]

Wage-based employees (non-exempt status). FLSA requires that employees be paid at least the federal minimum wage for all hours worked and overtime pay at time and one-half the regular rate of pay for all hours worked more than 40 hours in a work week. These hourly workers typically log in and out to determine actual time worked. FLSA does not set the number of hours that define full-time or part-time employee status. This determination is at the discretion of the employer. However, the Patient Portability and Affordable Care Act (ACA) currently requires employers to provide full-time employees health insurance coverage. It defines working at least an average of 30 hours/week as a full-time employee during a given measurement period (e.g., 1 year).[3]

Salary-based employees (exempt status). Currently, executive, administrative, professional, computer, and outside sales employees are exempt from FLSA if they are paid a salary of at least $455/week rather than an hourly wage. Specific job duties and salary rather than job title determine exempt status. The test of a professional is met if the employees make at least $455/week and their primary duty is work requiring advanced knowledge in science or learning that is intellectual and requires consistent exercise of discretion and judgment. The advanced knowledge is acquired through a prolonged course of specialized study.

Exempt employees receive a predetermined amount of compensation each pay period (salary) that is not reduced because of variations in their work, and they receive full salary regardless of the number of days or hours worked. As long as they are ready, willing, and able to work, exempt employees are paid even if no work is available. Although not stated in the law, employers expect exempted employees to work as long as it takes to get their work done and to meet all of their responsibilities.

Fee-based employees (may be exempt status). Employees paid an agreed sum (fee) for a single, unique job (rather than a series of jobs repeated a number of times for the same payment each time) are another category of worker. If the fee is at a rate that would amount to $455/week, the employee is exempt from FLSA. Example: A project that takes 20 hours to complete for a fee of $250 would be equivalent to $500 in a 40-hour week.

Contract staff may be defined as professionals according to FLSA but are paid as non-exempt employees by staffing agencies. Independent contractors may fall into any FLSA designation. Managers often seek legal advice or consultation with human resource experts as contracts with registries, staffing agencies, and independent contractors are negotiated. See Activity 8.2.

Job Descriptions

Job descriptions are useful for evaluation of work performance only if they are well written and provide detailed guidance. They need to be updated often to reflect a rapidly changing healthcare environment so that they do not limit the scope of work but do remain in compliance with legal requirements. Job descriptions must be general enough for a broad category of workers but not so vague that they provide little guidance for the specific duties of workers in a category. Jobs need to be structured to allow for a greater variety of duties, more autonomy in decision-making, and increased control of individual work schedules (flex time). They also need to reflect the tasks of individuals who are part of work groups.[1] Prior to recruitment and hiring, each position in an organization must have an accompanying job description that serves several purposes:

- To establish qualifications and other criteria to recruit the right person for the position
- To classify a position into a pay scale by comparing it with all other job descriptions
- To provide details of duties and responsibilities, physical demands, and other performance expectations
- To serve as the basis for evaluation of work performance

The creation of new positions and job descriptions is serious because of the financial implications of expanding an organization's workforce or expanding job responsibilities with increased salaries. Managers often face a series of approvals to justify that the creation of a new position is aligned with the strategic plans and goals of the organization. Demonstrating how and why a new position is different from those in place is part of this process. Determining whether the job description for a contingent worker is different from that for comparable full-time employees is another important consideration that will influence staff mix decisions. If performance expectations are different, two job descriptions are necessary.

Preparation of Job Descriptions

Job descriptions typically include a heading section that includes the job title, grade or level, a unique job code, FLSA status, and implementation date. The body of the job description usually includes a brief overview of the job, essential and nonessential functions, requirements, and other desirable skills

---

ACTIVITY 8.2
FULL-TIME VERSUS CONTRACT

Candace Peterson has been a full-time staff physical therapist at Wilson County Health Care for 8 years and she is now the only employee there. She is increasingly unhappy; it seems that her new manager prefers to contract with outside companies for temporary placement of physical therapists because he has not attempted to fill the three open full-time positions. Because of the continual employee turnover (every 13 weeks or so) of contracted physical therapists, Candace is often called on to assist temporary employees with a wide range of daily patient care problems. She falls behind in her own work and struggles to meet productivity goals. In addition, she has become resentful because the

"temps" seem to choose the new referrals that are considered the easier patients.

She has asked to meet with her manager, Larry Edwards, to discuss her frustrations. She is apprehensive because she cannot risk the potential loss of income if she converts to contract status should the work available decrease. She also needs the health insurance she receives as a full-time employee. Put yourself in Candace's situation and use strategic planning to prepare what she might say to Larry. Consider: Where is Candace now? Where does she want to be? What does she have to work with? How will she get there?

or abilities. A statement that the job description may not be all-inclusive and other duties may be assigned is always included. See Activity 8.3.

Compensation and Benefits Costs

Another important staffing responsibility for managers is establishing the compensation for each position, the total cost for the compensation and benefits of all employees, and fees for contingent staff. It may be risky for an organization to deliberately, or unknowingly, deviate from the going rates for wages and salaries offered by the competition. Underpayment may lead to the inability to fill vacant positions, and overpayment may dip into funds needed for other expenses. For large organizations and independent practitioners, software programs are often used to manage all aspects of compensation and payroll benefits that may include:

- Direct wages and salaries
- Mandatory benefits: payroll taxes including Social Security and Medicare Part A, unemployment compensation, workers' compensation, health insurance under the Affordable Care Act
- Voluntary benefits: vacation and sick leave; family and medical leave; uniform allowances;

tuition; other insurance; child care; other perks such as cell phones, club memberships, expense accounts, home offices, stock options, bonuses and incentives, severance packages, retirement plans

Managers must keep an eye on all compensation and benefits expenditures in relationship to the accomplishment of the organization's goals. Realizing that the value of a given benefit is a major concern of the employee, and because not all employees value the same benefits, many employers have moved to cafeteria benefit plans that allow employees to select those benefits of most value to them. For example, a single worker in his 40s may find retirement options important while a younger married man may find subsidized child care more important. As long as they are administered fairly and equitably, cafeteria benefit plans may be an important deciding factor for potential employees. Having flexibility in changing benefits as personal needs demand may also be a powerful employee retention tool.

Most of these details fall to centralized human resources experts in healthcare organizations. They interact with managers of units and programs who are responsible for verifying work hours for non-exempt employees and salaries to be paid to exempt employees. These experts provide data to managers for analysis of total personnel costs and per-patient personnel costs. They also work together to determine pay scales, ongoing review of wages, and salaries for adjustments to remain a competitive employer.

Salary adjustments for cost-of-living increases, meritorious performance, seniority, or performance-based incentives are typically codetermined, too. They are often negotiated by managers because controlling the costs associated with human resources is a shared organizational goal. Independent practice physical therapists may be at an advantage in recruiting employees because they have more flexibility in offering salaries and wages, but they may not be as competitive in terms of the cafeteria benefit plans they are able to offer.

Staff Recruitment

Recruitment requires creativity and the use of a variety of outbound marketing strategies that go beyond newspaper advertisements and professional

---

ACTIVITY 8.3
WRITING JOB DESCRIPTIONS

As a result of his meeting with Candace (Activity 8.2), Larry realizes that the physical therapist job description has not been reviewed since Candace was hired. How might Larry begin to address modification of the outdated job description? What are the key components of the job description he needs to focus on? Consider: What is the current job description? What does it need to be? What do we have to work with? How will we get there?

HINT: The extensive resources of the Occupational Information Network (O*NET at http://www.onetonline.org/link/summary/29-1123.00), which is a component of the U.S. Department of Labor, may provide a foundation for preparing job descriptions.

publications to include social networking and other online resources. The websites of healthcare organizations are frequently the first place potential applicants look for employment opportunities. Other online job boards (including those of professional associations) may be effective for many healthcare employers who can post vacancies for a fee. In conjunction with these tools, employers may use applicant tracking systems and recruitment software.

Other recruitment strategies may include promoting the organization's brand to new graduates by attending college job fairs, developing clinical education relationships with schools, and promoting a classroom presence through staff who provide guest lectures. Staff members may think that there is some prestige associated with these assignments, and students may be more likely to work in practices that have provided positive clinical and classroom learning experiences.

Managers need to weigh these supplementary efforts of staff against a potential negative effect on their productivity. Recognition or reward for these activities that may not be included in a job description (or appear as other assigned duties) may be indicated. Offering new graduates sign-on bonuses or student loan forgiveness programs and establishing referral bonus programs to reward current employees with referral bonuses when their efforts lead to a new hire are other recruiting tools.

Recruitment efforts should lead to hiring people who are the best match with the organization and who also have the greatest potential to do the work in the positions they were hired to fill. Determining this ability to contribute requires the identification and nurturing of employees' important skills, knowledge, and talents that are necessary for patients to have superior healthcare experiences. Reviewing credentials and gathering information during employment interviews are the typical means for making these determinations about job applicants. Conversely, becoming the employer of choice requires serious attention from a variety of perspectives. Recruitment needs to begin with a manager having clear answers to these questions:[4]

- Why does the job exist?
- What does the jobholder need to achieve for the organization?
- How can responsibilities be shifted for the best employer/employee match?

- What changes in the organization could affect the available job?
- What skills are needed to make transition into a new organization easier?

See Activity 8.4.

Hiring

With a clear description of the job to be filled and a pool of qualified applicants available, the next management challenge is selection of the best person for the position and the organization. After an initial screening and ranking of applicants based on job description criteria for the position, managers need to develop a plan for interviewing selected candidates. The interview cannot be left to chance, be conducted ad lib, or be inconsistent among applicants for the same position. It is a subjective process so the development of a scoring rubric for assessing desirable qualities becomes important for comparison of applicants and for the comparison of impressions of several interviewers. For example, in addition to the necessary technical skills or competencies, strong interpersonal and communication skills, willingness to learn, and problem-solving abilities might be assessed.

ACTIVITY 8.4
RECRUITMENT TEAM

Mercy Hospital has created a recruitment committee that includes the Director of Human Resources and the managers of each of the hospital's units. Their charge is to develop a new recruitment plan to fill four positions in rehabilitation services, 12 positions in nursing, and six positions in other units. The usual extensive advertising campaigns and contracts with professional recruitment companies have not been successful. Mercy is a good place to work. The other hospital in the city is having similar problems filling vacant positions. The Vice President of Clinical Services wants the committee to address the following questions: Where are we now? Where do we want to be? What do we have to work with? How will we get there?

The manager's goal in interviewing is to confirm the applicants' credentials and the compatibility of their values with those of the organization. Identifying those people with that little something extra that improves patient care and the work environment can be wonderful, too. This is much easier said than done, particularly when managers must pay strict attention to the legal requirements of interviewing during limited interactions to assess someone's values and behaviors. Posing open-ended questions facilitates this information gathering. Some examples are:

- Tell me about _____.
- How important is _____?
- What do you think the problem is with _____?
- What will _____ do for you?
- What prevents you from _____?
- What would you change about _____?
- What have you learned about _____?
- What are your views on _____?
- Give me your impressions of _____.
- Please expand on _____.
- What is involved in _____?
- What achievements are you proudest of?
- What is your assessment (opinion) of _____?

The Interview

A plan for the format, length, and proposed outline of discussion points requires thoughtful consideration so that a good employee/employer match results. The interview may be held one-one-one, in pairs, or with a panel of three or four interviewers.[4] The panel interview allows more time for depth of discussion without sacrificing the input of several people for comparison of impressions. It also provides the applicant an opportunity to witness the group dynamics of current employees. Each member of the panel may be assigned particular questions or topics to avoid duplication of effort while using a standardized evaluation form to rate candidates more objectively. A form also serves to keep interviewers focused. Characteristics expected should be identified ahead of time and then confirmed through discussion of past experiences that may be used to predict future behaviors.

Interviews should begin with an understanding that the goal is to learn about one another and a potential match with the organization. Interviewers should only ask questions that pertain to the person's ability to perform the job with a focus on selected aspects of résumés and reference letters for further exploration or confirmation of facts. To be fair, all applicants for one position should be asked similar questions. Some other considerations for the interview include the following:[4]

- Present a balanced view of the organization so applicants gain a full understanding.
- Be truthful.
- Share the purpose and objectives of the position, state the job title, describe the context and scope of the job.
- Supplement the interview with a tour of facilities and assess spontaneous reactions.
- Allow 45 to 60 minutes for face-to-face meeting time.
- Provide applicants questions ahead of time so they may prepare for the interview.
- Set the tone, eliminate distractions, minimize personal items, create a comfortable setting and a welcoming mood, and pronounce the applicant's name correctly.
- Videoconferencing may be used to involve more people in the interviewing.
- Know the precise desired competencies and ask questions to get insight into them: How have you handled _____? Tell me about a time you _____.
- Verify credentials: How long were you _____? Could you elaborate on _____?
- Identify potentially important cultural considerations: association memberships, corporate dress, dietary needs, availability of religious facilities, gestures, eye contact.
- Seek advice on potentially illegal, discriminatory questions. Examples: Not—Where are you from? Rather—Do you have a legal right to work in the United States? What languages can you speak? Not—What is your religion? Rather—Can you work all days of the week?
- Avoid personal discussions and initiating or accepting inappropriate overtures.
- Observe non-verbal behavior: fidgeting, crossing arms, eye rolling, drumming fingers, shaking foot, twisting hair.
- Provide an opportunity to add more information, cover any missed topics, and ask questions.

- Advise the applicant of any required aptitude or personality assessments and the next steps.

A few questions that are generally considered important in interviewing are:[5,6]

- Why are you interested in this position?
- Why are you looking to leave your current position?
- What is important to you in a work environment?
- Why should we hire you?
- What makes you the best candidate?
- Tell me about a specific situation in which you failed.
- Tell me about a past accomplishment you are especially proud of.
- Tell me how you handle conflict at work.

The Hire

Managers should avoid quick employment decisions, allowing time for impressions to form. If the impression is that goals and values are aligned and the credentials have been confirmed, an applicant may be offered a position. The offer typically includes salary, benefits, work hours, and start date. Before finalizing employment, required background checks, drug screens, and other legal documentation must be collected, all credentials verified, and any other negotiations closed. Candidates who are not offered a position should receive a formal letter of rejection that also includes something positive and encouraging.

At the other end of employment, exit interviews require that managers engage in the same preparation for the interview and offer plenty of opportunities for the employee to talk, focusing on the strengths and weaknesses of the organization's vision, mission, and goals. Interviewing employees who have chosen to terminate employment may provide insights that would not otherwise be shared. A supervisor or manager who is not directly involved with the employee should conduct an exit interview.

Orientation

Preparing the new hire for the position is dependent on a strong orientation to highlight responsibilities and expectations with an emphasis on safety and communication channels. Managers should not assume the level of assistance a new employee may need to transition to a new organization. The needs of someone starting his or her first full-time job are very different from the needs of someone who brings other work experience to a position. Managers may make themselves available, particularly during the first few months, to serve as a mentor or appoint someone to mentor a new employee. A mentor may facilitate the important socialization in the new organization and reduce the amount of nonproductive time that accompanies all new work. Providing training to serve as a mentor, including mentoring in a job description, and rewarding those efforts may relieve concerns about these responsibilities to encourage more participation.

Employee Retention

Some turnover is expected and desired for an organization to remain fresh with new ideas and enthusiasm and to have new people question the status quo. However, except when employee retirement or expansion of the organization requires it, retention is always preferred because of the time and expense of recruiting to fill open positions. Employees are most likely to remain loyal to organizations that meet their unique needs while also meeting the general needs of all employees who want to take pride in a safe, fair, and interesting workplace.

Retention is difficult because turnover is dependent on market demands that make competitive compensation a key factor. Jobs need to be appealing and satisfying and performed under excellent managers. Identifying and finding the resources to meet these needs is a primary management responsibility. Some examples of services to meet the needs of employees include counseling, employee financial assistance, child care, educational opportunities, social events, and discounts on goods and services; these all suggest that the organization values its employees and supports them in the achievement of their personal and professional goals.

Incentives and rewards that supplement basic compensation also may lead to personal job satisfaction and recognition of the importance of work efforts of individuals and groups. Incentives are typically related to contributions to the accomplishment of financial goals but may apply to quality improvement goals as well. Managers contribute less tangible rewards in their daily interactions with the people they supervise by encouraging, recognizing, and reinforcing actions that contribute to the success of the organization. Some suggestions for rewards that promote a positive, supportive work environment are:

- Sincerely praising accomplishments and efforts
- Presenting tokens of appreciation in celebration of significant actions or performance
- Practicing "do as I do" rather than "do as I say" by role modeling expected behaviors
- Admonishing in private and praising in public
- Relating actions to the vision, mission, and goals of the organization
- Encouraging growth and development
- LISTENING, LISTENING, LISTENING

Perhaps the most important aspect of work, and therefore the most important retention tool, is providing the opportunity for employees to be heard. People quit their supervisors, not their jobs.[5] If employees are not satisfied, the cause must be identified and fixed. See Activity 8.5.

ACTIVITY 8.5
RETENTION

The hospital's Vice President of Clinical Services, Chief Executive Officer, Jack Belfonte, has become concerned about rehabilitation services. Exit interviews conducted by the human resources staff have led to the conclusion that the problem lies with Betty Montrose, the Director of Rehabilitation Services. The rate of staff turnover under her leadership has doubled. When Jack meets with Betty, she expresses surprise that she is the source of dissatisfaction. She is proud to share her accomplishments in improving staff productivity and overall efficiency of their work. She states that she has been consistently reducing the department's budget while maintaining patient quality outcomes. What should Jack's strategy be with Betty? Consider: Where is rehabilitation services now? Where does he want it to be? What does he have to work with? How will he get there?

Productivity

Successful efforts to recruit and retain the right staff reduce the need for managers to monitor the day-to-day work performed by professionals, which includes work productivity. Some managers feel that productivity goals and outcome measurements are difficult to determine because of the nature of the work in healthcare services. Unpredictable patient cancellations, no-shows, variations in patient acuity level, along with the style and skills of physical therapists and physical therapist assistants all influence a manager's efforts to reach target goals for number of patients treated or units billed for the services provided in any setting. Because of these intervening variables, managers have to be careful that setting productivity or outcome goals is neither punitive nor threatening.

Managers need to start somewhere and may rely on the history of productivity in their organizations, or they may compare their productivity numbers against the numbers of other similar organizations. Employees need to understand work expectations so productivity goals expressed in number of patient visits or some other measure are important in all practice settings. Employees may self-assess their own performance by comparing their productivity numbers with the efforts of coworkers. The danger for managers is focusing *only* on numbers without putting them in the context of the work practices and processes. Asking how much time physical therapists spend working must be followed with a question about what specific tasks are performed.

It is not enough to know the ratio of productive hours compared with total hours worked. The more productive hours there are per day may sound like a good idea, but this could actually mean fatigued, disgruntled staff and dissatisfied patients. Scheduled breaks should be encouraged even for salaried employees and mandatory for nonexempt employees. At the other extreme, managers cannot afford too much unscheduled non-work time among staff members. Distracters, such as personal phone calls, text messaging, private conversations, and poor patient scheduling among departments, should be minimized so they do not interfere with the delivery of efficient, effective patient care.

Although not common in healthcare organizations, professionals with exempt-FLSA status may choose collective bargaining to resolve their employment concerns. Physical therapist assistants and other staff in a rehabilitation department who are nonexempt employees are more likely to be represented by a union that has negotiated productivity, pay scales, and other issues for them. Having employees who belong to a union may lead to adversarial rather than cooperative interactions. However, a commitment to compliance with negotiated agreements by both sides eliminates the need for managers to negotiate with each individual about assignments, productivity, time off, and the like. In those organizations with collective bargaining units, managers should expect that the organization provides them education to function effectively in their interactions with both staff who are members of a bargaining unit and those who are not. See Activity 8.6.

Evaluation of Staff Performance

Typically in any organization, a designated probationary period (usually 90 days) gives both the employee and employer an opportunity to evaluate their new relationship. It ends with a formal review at the end of the probation period and the opportunity for everyone to decide about continuation

---

ACTIVITY 8.6
PRODUCTIVITY

At a recent staff meeting, as usual, Janek Breznov, the rehabilitation manager, reported productivity statistics for the department as a whole. Hearing mumbling, Janek discovered that his staff is very unhappy about these reports and feels that they just cannot win. Every time they reach a goal, Janek raises the bar. He says he cannot just eliminate measuring the performance and work of the department because he is held accountable for justifying the costs of their salaries. The attitude of upper management is that higher salaries mean people need to work harder to generate revenue. The staff says something has to be done about this. Janek is out of ideas and arranges a meeting devoted to resolving this dilemma. What ideas do you have? Consider: Where are they now? Where do they want to be? What do they have to work with? How will they get there?

---

in the position as a permanent employee. Should either party decide during probation that the relationship is not as expected, employment is ended without prejudice on either side.

Employment that continues beyond the probationary period includes formal, regularly scheduled performance appraisals that must be fair, objective, and related to set standards or established performance goals and plans. Face-to-face evaluation meetings with the immediate supervisor are conducted on a timetable established by accrediting or licensing bodies, or managers themselves. The meeting is documented with a standard form that aligns with job descriptions and becomes part of permanent employment records. The report may also serve as the basis for merit salary increases. A compilation of all actions to praise work or take corrective action since the previous evaluation is included in the report. This process provides employees with the opportunity to praise or express their concerns, issues, and suggestions for the organization.

Ongoing Feedback

Between these formal evaluation meetings, managers are responsible for addressing any employee deficiencies or problems (critical incidents) by setting performance goals and documenting plans for improving performance that may deter formal disciplinary procedures. Goals also may be set for professional development or upward mobility in the organization. Assisting employees to adopt a process for setting objective, measurable work goals for themselves rather than setting goals for them allows managers the opportunity to provide employees with a powerful tool in all aspects of their lives. Managers also have the responsibility to follow up to determine whether actions toward established goals have been implemented and to assist in implementing them if necessary.

Whether formal or informal, performance evaluations increasingly need to address team efforts, which are best determined by multi-rater (360-degree) appraisals that include input from members of the immediate work team, self-assessment, and the supervisor. The collected feedback becomes the foundation for improvement plans for individual behaviors and work results. This multi-rater process may be very important to managers of multidisciplinary staff. Reliance on professional peers for assessment of clinical performance that are not within a manager's skill set may be necessary. See Activity 8.7.

Performance evaluations should include interpersonal relationships, problem-solving skills, and patient care responsibilities that are related to the mission and values of the organization. Managers may need to find the courage to address impressions that specific behaviors are not consistent with these values so that employees have the opportunity to improve. Particularly when team performance depends on people who bring a wide diversity of generational and cultural views to their work, managers need to direct the focus of employee behavior on its influence on the organization to decrease concerns of favoritism or bias.

For example, asking an employee to be less rude may not result in a change in behavior. What the manager thinks is rudeness, the employee may not. The employee may be even puzzled by the comment. Instead, identifying the behaviors that portray rudeness may lead to goals to be achieved. For example, to reduce rudeness, suggested behaviors may include to allow others to finish their thoughts without interruption, address people by their proper names, or respond to people without prompting when they ask questions. See Activity 8.8.

Staff Development

Organizations are expected to demonstrate their commitment to meeting specific goals and the importance of employees in these endeavors through

---

ACTIVITY 8.8
SPECIFYING WORK BEHAVIORS

Using the example of rudeness behaviors mentioned in the text, complete the following table by identifying two or three *behaviors* that reflect the vague goals listed:

INSTEAD OF SAYING: **SAY:**

Be less shy
Improve your attitude
Work harder
Take more initiative
Be respectful of coworkers
Work faster
Be more friendly
Be more creative
Care more
Stop bullying

---

solid staff development programs. These efforts may take several forms:

- In-house sessions on topics related to guest relations, safety, and so on
- Support for continuing education courses that support professional *and* organizational goals
- Formal degree programs in preparation for career advancement

In exchange for financial support of an external degree program, an employer may require an employee to commit to continued employment for a specified time. Financial support for travel and tuition to attend continuing education programs or professional conferences that may include paid release time is often provided with no return obligation expected. It is not unreasonable for managers to ask employees to apply for this type of financial support by justifying the request in terms of the goals of the organization. It is also reasonable for managers to expect employees to present a report on the application of new knowledge attained through the educational experience to an assigned program or task.

In-service programs require an investment of managers to plan, prepare, and schedule them. The urge to offer in-services on a regular basis just for the sake of offering them may lead to more frustration than learning. Unless it is viewed as important and relevant, employees will tune out as they go through

---

ACTIVITY 8.7
GOAL SETTING

Frances Newsome wants to help Carol Bradford set some performance goals to improve her ability to complete tasks, particularly patient documentation, on time by answering: Where is Carol now? Where do we want her to be? What do we have to work with? How will we get there? What are two or three goals, using the SMART approach (Specific, Measurable, Action-oriented, Realistic, Timebound; see Chapter 5), that Frances and Carol might come up with to improve Carol's performance?

the motions of attending required in-services. Conversely, employees may appreciate the convenience and opportunity to improve their performance when the programs are well prepared and relevant to their work. In-services also are used to update and inform employees of policy changes and new developments in the organization.

Employment Law and Related Issues

Managers in large organizations rely on human resource experts to deal with employment-related legal responsibilities. Smaller physical therapy practices may be legally exempt from some of these employer requirements, but everyone has a duty to protect the public and to treat employees fairly. Federal and state statutes, their accompanying administrative laws, and judicial decisions have been passed or ruled on to protect employees and their relationships with employers. Links to a few laws of most interest in healthcare organizations are listed in the Web Resources.

These federal statutes are supplemented with state laws that address important issues such as employment-at-will, dismissal for cause, collective bargaining, the right to due process, unemployment benefits, and workers' compensation.

Grievances

Employers must meet the legal requirements for grievance or complaint processes to address each of these laws because of the serious implications of violations that include discrimination. These requirements include mechanisms for appealing decisions if employees are not satisfied with responses to a major complaint they receive in the regular chain of command.

Managers may do well to have a simpler process of resolution for employees' less serious concerns. The process may simply involve holding meetings in which employees trust that a manager patiently hears a disagreement among coworkers, negotiates a vacation schedule fairly, resolves patient assignments, or gives sound advice about clinical decisions. Managers normally spend a great deal more time addressing these complaints about the daily routine than they do more serious grievances about the rights of employees.

Assuring employees that they are able to present concerns and problems to a manager who will respond fairly and consistently may relieve a great deal of job-related emotional stress. Managers help employees realize that they may perform their duties effectively although not all coworkers may be people whom they admire or choose to socialize with outside the organization. Employees are relieved when they can trust their managers to follow through on promised actions, which often reduces staff turnover.

Coworker relationships that evolve into more serious relationships also may require the attention of managers. Finding a work-home balance is challenging for all employees, but new, evolving relationships that begin in the workplace may become disruptive and even legally risky if the parties involved are different levels of workers (e.g., supervisor and physical therapist assistant). Managers may need to remind employees of policies related to romantic relationships while understanding that the workplace is likely to be where many people meet their significant others.

Background Checks and Other Credentials

Managers also must attend to the verification of credentials (academic records, professional credentials, right to work documents) and criminal background checks and public records of potential employees. The requirements must be the same for each applicant. These responsibilities are directly connected to the protection of the public and serve to protect patients from caregivers with potential harmful behaviors that place patients and others at risk. For instance, the practice acts governing professions may include measures to be taken when alcohol or drug abuse, mental or physical impairment, felony convictions, failure to meet continuing education requirements, or providing false information to a state occur. Managers are responsible for identifying these high-risk behaviors, beginning with the application for employment so that they take all appropriate action to protect patients. See Activity 8.9.

Managerial Responsibilities

Achievement of the organization's goals depends heavily on the selection and retention of people

---

ACTIVITY 8.9
STAFF DEVELOPMENT

Vincent Vasquez receives a phone call from Tricia Conrad, a professional colleague whom he trusts. Tricia wants to put in a good word for a former employee of hers, Mark Haskins. Mark is applying for a staff position that Vincent has had open for more than a year. Tricia wants Vincent to know that Mark was an excellent clinician who ran into some trouble and dropped out of the profession for a couple of years. His physical therapist license has been reinstated and he is eager to get back to patient care. Should Vincent decide to hire Mark, what action might he consider? Consider: What is Mark's current status? Where does Vincent want him to be? What does Vincent have to work with? How will he get there?

ACTIVITY 8.10
TIME-OUT FOR WRITING

The staffing section is a critical component of program proposals, feasibility studies, and business plans. Decision makers want to know the details of the staff mix, your job analysis, types of employees, compensation and benefits costs, recruitment plans and costs, retention plans and costs, productivity, plans for the evaluation of work performance, and costs of staff development.

---

who fit best with its vision and mission. This selection is particularly important for mid-level managers who have a powerful influence on their staffs. With the support of either human resource experts or consultants, healthcare managers bring all responsibilities along with the most important one, assisting people to perform their highest quality of work. Because of the complexity of the legal and interpersonal aspects of these staffing responsibilities, ongoing development is required of managers who must balance the needs of their staffs with the needs of their organizations.

Managers must seriously reflect on their perceptions of people and their ideas about work to define an approach to their staffing responsibilities that includes patience and fairness. Managers who believe people are eager to learn and do their best approach their staffing responsibilities differently from managers who believe most people need to be persuaded and monitored to work to their fullest potential. Responsibility for staffing is fulfilling, rewarding work for most managers. It is also the most complex and challenging aspect of their work and becomes more so as multidisciplinary staffs become more common. See Activity 8.10.

REFERENCES

1. Fottler MD. Job analysis and job design. In: Fried BJ, Fottler, MD, eds. *Human Resources in Healthcare: Managing for Success.* 3rd ed. Chicago, IL: Health Administration Press; 2008.
2. United States Department of Labor, Wage and Hour Division. http://www.dol.gov/whd/flsa/. Accessed July 28, 2013.
3. Workforce. IRS notice gives employers clarity on definition of "full time." http://www.workforce.com/article/20120924/NEWS01/120929979/irs-notice-gives-employers-clarity-on-definition-of-full-time. Accessed April 18, 2013.
4. DK Essential Managers. *Interviewing People.* London, England: Dorling Kindersley Ltd; 2008.
5. Tuckerton R. *Hiring Manager Secrets: 7 Interview Questions You Must Get Right.* Published December 19, 2010. http://www.interview-aid.com/. Accessed November 21, 2013.
6. Fried BJ, Gates M. Recruitment, selection, and retention. In: Fried BJ, Fottler MD, eds. *Human Resources in Healthcare: Managing for Success.* 3rd ed. Chicago, IL: Health Administration Press; 2008.

WEB RESOURCES

Americans With Disabilities Act of 1990. http://www.ada.gov/. Accessed November 21, 2013.

Consolidated Omnibus Budget Reconciliation Act (COBRA) 1974. http://www.dol.gov/dol/topic/health-plans/cobra.htm. Accessed November 21, 2013.

Consumer Credit Protection Act (Title III). http://www.dol.gov/compliance/guide/garnish.htm. Accessed November 21, 2013.

Drug-Free Workplace Act of 1988. http://www.dol.gov/elaws/asp/drugfree/screenr.htm. Accessed November 21, 2013.

Employee Retirement Income Security Act of 1974 (ERISA). http://www.dol.gov/compliance/laws/comp-erisa.htm. Accessed November 21, 2013.

Equal Pay Act of 1963. http://www.eeoc.gov/laws/statutes/epa.cfm. Accessed November 21, 2013.

Executive Order 11246 amended. http://www.dol.gov/ofccp/regs/statutes/eo11246.htm. Accessed November 21, 2013.

Family and Medical Leave Act (FMLA) of 1993. http://www.dol.gov/whd/fmla/. Accessed November 21, 2013.

Immigration Reform and Control Act of 1986. https://secure.ssa.gov/poms.nsf/lnx/0500501440. Accessed November 21, 2013.

Occupational Safety and Health Administration (OSHA). http://www.osha.gov/. Accessed November 21, 2013.

Rehabilitation Act of 1973. http://www.hhs.gov/ocr/civil-rights/resources/factsheets/504.pdf. Accessed November 21, 2013.

Uniformed Services Employment and Reemployment Rights Act (USERRA) of 1994. http://www.dol.gov/vets/programs/userra/. Accessed November 21, 2013.

Worker Adjustment and Retraining Notification Act (WARN). http://www.dol.gov/compliance/laws/comp-warn.htm. Accessed November 21, 2013.

CHAPTER 9

Responsibilities for Patient Care

LEARNING OBJECTIVES

- Discuss the management needs of professional employees.
- Distinguish between utilization management and case management.
- Discuss the role of managers in utilization management and case management.
- Determine the status of quality care and outcomes in contemporary healthcare.
- Analyze physical therapy practice for quality dimensions and defects.
- Analyze quality measures and models.
- Analyze factors contributing to patient satisfaction.
- Discuss managers' roles in protecting patient rights and identifying patient responsibilities.

Overview

The amount of direct patient care that a manager engages in varies widely. Solo physical therapy practitioners may spend at least half of their time in patient care while middle-level managers in large organizations may be one or two steps removed from direct patient care. Others may fall somewhere in between. In all instances, managers have indirect responsibility for all of the patient care provided by their subordinates. They must have a plan for monitoring the processes and outcomes of that care and patients' responses. This chapter addresses patient care responsibilities of managers that are not included in other chapters: managing professionals, utilization management, case management, quality care, patient satisfaction, and patient rights.

Managing Professionals

Healthcare managers do not have direct responsibility for individual patient–therapist interactions. Instead, direct patient care responsibility belongs to *each* physical therapist and extends to other staff

members that the therapist directs and supervises. The *Guide to Physical Therapist Practice* reinforces the importance of the supervisory relationship.[1] The guide states that all physical therapists of record remain responsible for *all* aspects of a plan of care although they may direct physical therapist assistants to perform components of that care. Their deciding if and when to utilize the physical therapist assistant should be based on ensuring safe, effective, and efficient care at each treatment session. They must provide oversight of documentation for all services delivered by support personnel as well.

In all settings, physical therapists currently have a great deal of freedom in day-to-day patient care. They are individually accountable for the care of the patients and the ongoing collaboration and consultation with other health professionals involved in the care of a patient to coordinate a patient's goals and the plans to meet them.

Needs of Professionals

It should be no surprise that professionals who assume such a high level of responsibility for the care of others do not really require much management to fulfill their clinical responsibilities. They control their own work to a high degree after assignments have been made and may even have a great deal of control in selecting the patients they will care for in some settings. This autonomy in clinical decision-making is confirmed by the recent trend for rehabilitation managers from one discipline to manage professionals from others. The shift to business rather than clinical roles of healthcare managers reflects the level of professionalization of individual rehabilitation specialists who neither turn to supervisors for directions, nor rely on specific physician's orders to make clinical decisions. Instead, professionals with strong technical skills, good problem-solving ability, sound judgment, and sense of responsibility may need managers only to empower their actions; assist with nonclinical problems; provide performance feedback; and reaffirm the vision, mission, and goals of their organizations.

Work Stress

Managers also play a role in reducing the sources of work stress including heavy workloads, interprofessional role conflicts or ambiguity, scarce resources, understaffing, physical strain, emotional labor (maintaining and juggling emotions to present a socially acceptable presence at all times), work/home conflicts, and limited input into organizational decision-making. These stressors affect the physical and emotional health of employees, which then affects the patient care. Poor employee health is costly to organizations in terms of absenteeism, staff turnover, or poor work performance that may lead to clinical errors. Managers may help employees deal with these stressors through several means such as encouraging coworker support as a coping mechanism, arranging flexible work schedules, rewarding positive efforts to provide quality care, and encouraging high levels of control over their work.[2,3,4]

The Big Picture

Rather than micromanaging patient care, therapists want managers to focus on interpreting the big picture of healthcare policy, reimbursement, and organizational goals so that they may care for patients safely, efficiently, and effectively. Therapists may not want to be told what to do with patients, but they do want to know why the organization

functions as it does. Managers who provide this overall perspective and clearly delineate the roles and responsibilities of all members of the rehabilitation service are appreciated.

Monitoring provider–provider and provider–patient communication is essential to achieve coordination of care, which includes a coherent, harmonizing team with shared responsibility for patient outcomes and healthcare results.[5] That does not mean that managers have little to do with patient care. On the contrary, everything managers do rests on the provision of quality patient care that is safe, legal, and ethical. See Activity 9.1.

Utilization Management and Case Management

Utilization Management

Another important component of a manager's responsibility for patient care is responding to the efforts of third-party payers to manage their costs and the quality of the care that they pay for. Controlling the utilization of services is now an expected

---

ACTIVITY 9.1
CLINICAL EXPERTISE

Rachel Gibson is the regional manager for six outpatient rehabilitation centers in the northeast region of All-Sports Rehabilitation. Each center is staffed with one physical therapist, one physical therapist assistant, a per diem occupational therapist, and a per diem speech-language pathologist. A recurrent issue has been troubling her. Although she has more years of clinical experience than the current staff combined, she has been a full-time manager for 5 years. She is uncomfortable when staff members ask her to help with clinical questions because she feels her knowledge has become outdated, and she is often not readily available when they need answers. What might she do to provide the means for her staff to collaborate more effectively? Consider: Where is All-Sports Rehab now? Where does it need to be? What does it have to work with? How will it get to where it wants to be?

component of healthcare. Third-party payers may conduct utilization management directly or outsource it to independent review organizations.

Their reviews of patient care are based on written standards, which are drawn from historical data and typically approved or developed by physician panels in health insurance companies. Those conditions that are the most costly, most utilized, or result in questionable outcomes receive the greatest scrutiny, but any patient's care may be managed for effective utilization.

In any case, the purpose of these reviews is to determine whether patient care is efficient, effective, medically necessary, and appropriate. As a consequence, determining that quality standards have been met precedes payments to providers in essentially all inpatient and outpatient centers.

Each payer addresses the quantity of services, timetable for delivery, and appropriate sources of evaluation and treatment. The decisions of reviewers (typically nurses) about certification or authorization of care are driven by these standards through reviews of medical records and direct communications with providers and billing staff. They are essentially asking if patients received a level of care that was efficient, effective, and consistent with their individual needs and the needs of previous patients with similar conditions.

Utilization review becomes territory that lies between the patient care and fiscal responsibilities of managers. They must be familiar with utilization reviews that occur at various points in an episode of patient care. The standards may vary from setting to setting and payer to payer. The types of utilization review are:

- *Precertification reviews.* This process certifies the medical necessity of care *before* a patient can be admitted for inpatient or outpatient care, and that the anticipated care is provided in the most appropriate setting (e.g., inpatient or outpatient elective surgery). Emergency admissions are reviewed within 48 hours and are based on the same standard guidelines. Managers are involved in the processes necessary for providing required information to reviewers. The purpose of this form of review is to control costs *before* admission.
- *Admission reviews.* These are reviews conducted after a patient has been admitted for care to determine medical necessity and the

appropriateness of inpatient care within 1 working day. Standard guidelines are followed to confirm precertification information, review additional information that has been discovered during admission and to assess documentation that the planned course of treatment has been implemented to determine the expected costs associated with an episode of care. This review is often conducted on-site in large hospital systems.

- *Continued stay (concurrent) reviews.* These scheduled reviews apply to all admissions and are conducted periodically until a patient is discharged. Objective patient data are collected and compared with the standard guidelines or criteria for each patient's diagnosis or diagnoses. The intent of this review is to approve the continuation of care for only as long as necessary to reach the expected outcomes. Identifying options for alternative, less expensive continued care settings is part of this process as a means of controlling costs. The need for intensive case management services for catastrophic conditions and discharge planning are components of this type of review. Typically, these concurrent reviews do not directly involve the patient as decisions are made about lengths of inpatient stays or the duration of outpatient care.
- *Discharge planning.* This is the process of facilitating the transfer of a patient to an alternative, most appropriate setting when the goals of care have been reached. It begins when the provider or setting is notified of the certification of a patient's care. Discharge planning includes arranging for any continued care that is needed in advance to avoid transfer delays, which can be costly to all involved parties. Discharge planning was a component of patient care for physical therapists long before utilization management was implemented. Including patients in the process has always been important. Managers typically are not involved in this professional decision-making unless conflicts arise among the care team engaged in this process.
- *Retrospective review.* This review occurs post-discharge and the same utilization standards used in other reviews continue to be applied. The obvious disadvantage of this type of

utilization review is that involved parties do not know until after the fact whether or not the care provided was deemed medically necessary and appropriate. This type of review, which was originally referred to as a utilization review, has evolved into the broader prospective of utilization management.

Managers may represent their staffs during any of these utilization management stages as important decisions are made from pre-admission to discharge of patients. Managers must ensure that staff involved in direct patient care are prepared for the high-level clinical decision-making involved in continued stay reviews and discharge plans in all settings. Rehabilitation staff are expected to be immediately available to provide data when called on to do so by physicians or utilization review staff. Physical therapists are called on to determine their patients' ability to walk and function safely and independently, their level of endurance for activity, and their response to exercise. Because of their knowledge of function and movement, they provide important recommendations for less costly, alternative healthcare settings.

Case Management

A parallel process common in contemporary healthcare is case management. Case management is another cost-control process of hospitals, insurance companies, and employers primarily directed to patients with high-cost medical conditions. It is a collaborative process that includes assessment, planning, facilitation, and advocacy to meet a person's needs through available resources to achieve cost-effective outcomes. Patients may or may not have the option to use case management services. Depending on the setting, the duties of case managers may include:

- Screening to identify appropriate patients for case management services (e.g., patients with high-risk pregnancy, multiple trauma, or renal disease)
- Planning and coordinating the delivery of care by the healthcare team
- Making discharge arrangements and following up with patients
- Evaluating the outcomes of care for each patient

- Checking benefits available and coordinating with other benefits (e.g., a patient has both Medicare and workers' compensation benefits)
- Recommending insurance policy coverage exceptions where appropriate
- Coordinating referrals to specialists and arranging for other special services (e.g., durable medical equipment)
- Coordinating care with community services
- Verifying medical reasons for employee absences
- Educating workers with chronic conditions

Physical therapists and their managers have a long history of professional collaboration with case managers because of their involvement with patients who have work-related injuries and other complex, chronic conditions requiring rehabilitation.[6]

In hospitals, daily collaboration with case managers takes place for discharge planning decisions. Managers may need to intervene to help clarify the roles of case managers and the policies of particular third-party payers because not all insurance companies follow the same standards in their utilization and case management decisions. Managers need to keep abreast of policy decisions and establish strong communication channels with utilization managers and case managers so that they are prepared to address concerns of staff should conflicts arise in these decision processes. In some instances, managers may represent all of the physical therapists as they serve as "go-betweens" with case managers. See Activity 9.2.

Quality Care in Healthcare Organizations

The concept of quality has not transitioned easily to healthcare from other types of businesses. The nature of healthcare is so different from manufacturing and other industries, where the study of quality began, that the concept of healthcare quality continues to develop as an offshoot of these industrial models. See Sidebar 9.1 for a brief historical perspective of the quality movement in non-healthcare businesses.

The recent report *Crossing the Quality Chasm*[7] was an effort to span this difficult gap between healthcare and other types of businesses. The

ACTIVITY 9.2
FRUSTRATION AND CONFUSION

Mindy Hanson appears frustrated after 2 months as a staff physical therapist in St. Anne's Rehabilitation Hospital. Joanna Freedman, her supervisor, asks whether there is anything she can do to help. Mindy says no because she is generally disturbed about patient policies. She just cannot understand how some of her patients were admitted for an intensive rehabilitation program when they are so sick that they can hardly participate in therapy, and others who have the potential to make significant functional gains are discharged quickly. Mindy is also challenged by the expectation that she provide input for patients' discharge plans when she has barely completed their initial evaluations. What should Joanna do? Consider: What are the policies now? What do they need to be? What do they have to work with? How will they get to where they want to be?

report presents a goal-driven definition of healthcare quality with six dimensions of patient care:

1. *Safe:* Care should be as safe for patients in healthcare facilities as in their homes.
2. *Effective:* The science and evidence behind healthcare should be applied and serve as the standard in the delivery of care.
3. *Efficient:* Care and service should be cost-effective, and waste should be removed from the system.
4. *Timely:* Patients should experience no waits or delays in receiving care and service.
5. *Patient-centered:* The system of care should revolve around the patient, respect patient preferences, and put the patient in control.
6. *Equitable:* Unequal treatment should be a fact of the past; disparities in care should be eradicated.

Regardless of the type or size of healthcare organizations, including physical therapy practices, these dimensions may serve well to clarify quality so that the concept may be more easily incorporated

SIDEBAR 9.1

Brief History of Quality Models

- Avedis Donabedian is often considered the father of modern quality assurance that began in the 1980s. He conceived quality as the interaction of structure (characteristics of systems and providers), process (patient/practitioner activities), and outcome (health status of an individual or community). See his article, "The Quality of Care: How Can It Be Assessed?" *JAMA*, 1988;260(12), for a historical perspective.

- Also in the late 1980s and 1990s, Motorola developed the Six-Sigma program for quality improvement that was adopted as General Electric's business strategy. It then received widespread application to a range of industries and businesses. In manufacturing, a six sigma means that 99.999998% of the products and processes are error free.

- Lean is a process developed about the same time (usually associated with Toyota) that

focuses on elimination of waste, which is defined as anything that does not add value to a product or service for the customer. More recently these two models have merged into the Lean-Six Sigma Model. Several texts and articles may be explored for more information on these quality concepts and procedures for people and organizations to be certified in their use.

- Robert Kaplan and David Norton developed the Balanced Score Card framework as a management tool in the 1990s. This tool has become one of the most popular models for determining the balance of financial and non-financial factors that drive an organization's vision and mission. Their text, *The Balanced Scorecard: Translating Strategy Into Action* (Harvard Business Review Press, 1996), provides the foundation for this strategy that continues to evolve.

into their visions, missions, and goals, and serve as a basis for both managerial and clinical decision-making. The report goes on to classify quality defects as:[6]

- *Underuse:* Failure to employ many scientifically sound practices as often as they should be
- *Overuse:* Failure to eliminate diagnostic tests and interventions when they are not indicated
- *Misuse:* Failure to appropriately execute the proper clinical care process

In other words, quality may be defined as the degree to which a healthcare organization increases the likelihood of desired health outcomes, consistent with current evidence about the scientific, interpersonal, and organizational components of healthcare. Quality depends on the integration of all of its levels: (1) what happens to the patient; (2) the care delivered by healthcare provider teams; (3) the organization's management and coordination of all of its units; and (4) the external environment where regulations and policies are made.[8] See Activity 9.3.

Despite efforts to raise awareness and to increase the value of quality in healthcare, attention to quality is often displaced by other urgent priorities, and it is difficult for patients to grasp this concept. However, this has not stopped healthcare organizations from gathering data on hundreds of measures related to the complex, interrelated components of quality. Some data are required by The Joint Commission and the Centers for Medicare & Medicaid Services (CMS), while other data seem to be collected for no clear reason.

Fortunately, software systems are available for analysis of large amounts of data related to key performance indicators. The use of visual representations of data as dials on a dashboard helps to facilitate analysis and decision-making about financial and clinical aspects of healthcare. However, the data collection and analysis tools do not matter much unless managers have clearly decided what they should measure and for what purpose. Measures of clinical quality remain challenging as links between everyday key operations and strategic goals are pursued, analyzed, and shared with stakeholders. See Activity 9.4 and Activity 9.5.

Because quality care is a continually evolving concept that has the attention of licensing and accrediting bodies, its concepts, tools, and terminology seem to change at a rapid rate. Managers must be prepared for modifications in related responsibilities, and develop an approach for keeping abreast of this important aspect of patient care.

Patient Satisfaction

The two key aspects of patient satisfaction may be represented on a continuum anchored with content quality and service-delivery quality. All patient care includes both components of service. But depending on their circumstances, patients may perceive that they receive technical excellence and clinical expertise if these components of care are more important to them. Other patients may perceive their care as humane and culturally appropriate if that is what they value. See the examples in Figure 9.1.[8]

ACTIVITY 9.3
QUALITY PHYSICAL THERAPY

Select any physical therapy practice or rehabilitation unit in a healthcare system. What are your impressions of the practice in terms of the six dimensions of patient care—safe, effective, efficient, timely, patient centered, and equitable? Are there any potential quality defects—underuse, overuse, misuse?

TIME-OUT FOR WRITING: Review your program proposal, feasibility study, or business plan in terms of the quality dimensions and defects. Do the mission and goals reflect a commitment to quality care? Make any necessary revisions.

ACTIVITY 9.4
QUALITY AND OUTCOME MEASURES

1. Go to the U.S. Agency for Healthcare Research and Quality (AHRQ) webpages available at http://www.qualitymeasures.ahrq.gov and http://www.guidelines.gov. Identify content relevant to physical therapy practices and other rehabilitation professions.
2. Go to the American Physical Therapy Association (APTA) webpages for more information on outcomes available at http://www.apta.org/OutcomeMeasures/. How important are these tools to healthcare managers?

ACTIVITY 9.5
IMPROVING QUALITY

Jeremy Hines has identified a few quality defects in his private physical therapy practice. Analyze each problem using the six dimensions of quality. For each scenario, ask, Is Jeremy's practice safe? Is it effective? Is it efficient? Is it timely? Is it patient centered? Is it equitable? What actions should Jeremy take to improve the quality of care in his practice?

- It seems that the physical therapists have fallen into the habit of "rewarding" patients who exercise well with a hot pack or cold pack at the end of each session.
- Patients have complained that they often wait almost 30 minutes in the waiting room before beginning their therapy sessions.
- Patients have complained that they are left unattended during treatment sessions and just exercise on their own.

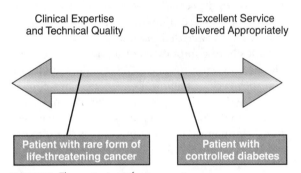

Clinical Expertise and Technical Quality

Excellent Service Delivered Appropriately

Patient with rare form of life-threatening cancer

Patient with controlled diabetes

FIGURE 9.1 The patient satisfaction continuum.

Managers must ensure both aspects of quality are present. Quality content depends on performance evaluations, staff development as new approaches and technology advance evidence-based care, and compliance with evolving guidelines and standards. Patient satisfaction with the service delivery component depends on managers having processes that meet patient expectations for convenience and timeliness. The development of strong interpersonal relationships with their direct caregivers and other nonclinical support staff are equally important in service delivery.

Guest Relations and Patient Satisfaction

Many managers value patient satisfaction as highly as they value clinical outcome indicators such as functional status. Because many healthcare organizations reach common benchmarks for clinical outcomes, patient satisfaction is among those factors that may set one organization apart from the others. It can be argued that certain aspects of healthcare are similar to the hospitality industry. Managers who take a hospitality approach may improve patient satisfaction through attention to personal preferences, physical and emotional comfort, and directly asking patients what is important to them.

Like the hospitality industry, patient satisfaction is dependent on staff committed to excellent service throughout all aspects of a healthcare experience. Hiring competent people who also seek to serve is a good starting point. Simple courtesy matters. Employees who smile and introduce themselves, make eye contact, say please and thank-you, address patients by their names, knock before entering, explain what they are doing, and maintain a clean, neat environment contribute to a positive healthcare experience. Preparation for patient service goals is as important as the development of clinical skills in many organizations.

Assuming that people have come to their work with these service skills may be risky, so formal efforts to address them are necessary. Managers may need to direct their efforts at encouraging employees to care about patients while taking care of them. Empowering employees to eliminate patient disappointments immediately and to anticipate patient needs may lead to a seamless and positive healthcare experience for patients. Although more difficult in complex, busy organizations, making people feel that they matter is an important point in establishing good customer relations. Patients should not feel that making their needs known and having them met constitute an intrusion in the work of their healthcare providers. Employees must move past an "it's not my job" attitude when a patient's immediate needs are not part of their usual duties.

Managers are also responsible for creating a welcoming environment that gives the perception of quality, cleanliness, security, and caring. Attention to sights, sounds, smells, and temperatures can promote a sense of healing and comfort. Overloading the environment with too much information may be threatening and confusing rather than helpful. Over-decorating may make it difficult for people to find their way when knowing where to go and how to get there should be easy. Managers need to scan the environment from the patient's viewpoint rather than their own.[9] Efforts to measure patient satisfaction in outpatient physical therapy practice can be found in Web Resources. See Activity 9.6.

Patients' Rights and Responsibilities

A bill of rights for patients is a list of guarantees while receiving medical care, which may be a voluntary declaration developed by an organization for its own members or goals. If working in a larger healthcare system, managers may be familiar with its patient's bill of rights. Web Resources include other examples.

Generally, these patients' rights include items such as:

- Right to be treated with respect
- Right to make a treatment choice
- Right to refuse treatment
- Right to obtain medical records
- Right to privacy of medical records
- Right to informed consent
- Right to make decisions about end-of-life care

ACTIVITY 9.6
PATIENT SATISFACTION

Amy Allen is pleased in one way and offended in another. She has received a great deal of positive feedback from patients on the care that they receive from her staff, but recently she overheard a patient say to another that the place was such a dump. She works hard to keep it neat and clean but has decided that she may need to do more. What other factors should Amy consider? What kinds of things would give the impression that a professional practice is a dump? Consider: What is the current status? What does Amy want it to be? What does Amy have to work with? How will she get to where she wants to be?

To ensure quality care, patients are also expected to meet certain responsibilities that may include:

- Being respectful to providers
- Being honest with providers
- Complying with treatment plans
- Meeting financial obligations
- Reporting fraud and waste

Patients and their families may be encouraged to assume increased responsibility for their care by:[10]

- Training patients in the skills and knowledge they need
- Providing opportunities to practice skills
- Encouraging patients to monitor employees
- Having patients teach other patients

Handling patients who do not seem to be vested in their own care is another management challenge. In the same vein, despite the best efforts of employees, some patients are rude and perhaps even dangerous to employees. Managers need a plan for serving as a buffer between people in conflict. They may need to take direct action to reassign difficult patients to staff with the most patience or to counsel patients about their inappropriate behavior. Expelling patients or employees from the premises may require the support of security or law enforcement officers.

State Laws

Some states have enacted patients' bills of rights. For example, the link to Florida's Patient's Bill of Rights can be found at Web Resources. Managers should investigate similar legislation in their states to identify their responsibilities. For example, managers might be legally required to ensure therapists seek, receive, and document a patient's consent to care. Managers may need to determine whether a patient simply signing a form during the intake process meets the intent of the legal expectations for consent in their jurisdictions.

Federal Laws

The Health Insurance Portability and Accountability Act of 1996 (HIPAA) protects the privacy of patients' medical records as they are shared among providers and insurers. The Patient Safety and

Quality Improvement Act of 2005 (PSQIA) establishes a voluntary reporting system to enhance the data available to assess and resolve patient safety and healthcare quality issues.[11]

To comply with these laws, managers must investigate their organizations' involvement in PSQIA and determine their roles in quality assurance and risk management programs to reduce medical errors. Managers are more likely involved in HIPAA requirements to assure that healthcare providers do not disclose the personal and medical information that they hold without a patient's permission.

Creating an environment that discourages casual discussions about patients may be difficult, particularly in small organizations in which patient–therapist relationships are often long term, and the practices pride themselves on providing a family atmosphere. It is essential that patients trust their caregivers so that a warm and accepting relationship may develop. However, even if unintentional, when confidentiality is breached in any way, patients may have the right to sue if harm is a result of even inadvertent disclosures. HIPAA also includes policies about securing medical information and the use of electronic equipment to store and transfer records and a process for patients to file complaints. See Activity 9.7.

Patient Portability and Affordable Care Act (ACA) of 2010

Despite numerous congressional attempts to pass legislation over the years until passage of the Affordable Care Act in 2010, there has been no federal patient's bill of rights. The focus of patient rights in the ACA is the rights of people to gain *access* to healthcare. The 10 titles (components) of the act address insurance coverage for adults and children with preexisting conditions, extension of insurance under their parents' plans for young adults until age 26, a choice of doctors, no annual dollar or lifetime insurance limits, an end to arbitrary cancellation of insurance policies, a requirement that insurance premiums collected by insurers be spent primarily on patient care, removal of emergency service barriers, access to preventive care, and the right to appeal payment denials.[12]

A Manager's Responsibility

Generally, patients expect respect and the best efforts of the people who care for them. Although many may be disappointed with the outcomes of their care because their conditions simply do not allow cures or total relief of their problems, few are truly dissatisfied with rehabilitation experiences. The ability to establish strong relationships with professionals during the rehabilitation process may be a key factor. Managers who are able to make these distinctions in patient expectations may discover that resolving conflicts is all that is necessary because of the clinical skills and compassion of the professionals they supervise. It is not surprising that melding utilization management and quality of care to achieve expected patient outcomes and satisfaction is a critical area of a manager's responsibility for patient care within the context of patients' rights and responsibilities. See Activity 9.8.

ACTIVITY 9.7
MUM'S THE WORD

Ramon Latoya owns a small independent practice in a rural community. He overhears two patients in the waiting room discussing a third patient who is not there. He is concerned because they are saying that more than one member of his staff has provided them the personal information on the person they are discussing. What should he do? Consider: What is the current status? Where does Ramon want it to be? What does Ramon have to work with? How will he get to where he wants to be?

ACTIVITY 9.8
TIME-OUT FOR WRITING

Determine whether your program proposal, liability study, or business plan needs to address patient care issues such as outcomes, satisfaction, and rights and responsibilities.

REFERENCES

1. American Physical Therapy Association. *Guide to Physical Therapist Practice* [Ebook]. Vol 81. 2nd ed. Alexandria, VA: American Physical Therapy Assoc; 2001. http://guidetoptpractice.apta.org/. Accessed November 27, 2013.

2. Apker J, Ray EB. Stress and social support in healthcare organizations. In: Thompson TL, ed. *Handbook of Health Communication.* Mahwah, NJ: Lawrence Erlbaum Associates; 2003:347.

3. Barnes CM, Van Dyne L. "I'm tired": differential effect of physical and emotional fatigue on workload management strategies. Human Relations. 2009;62(1):59. http://hum.sagepub.com/content/62/1/59. Accessed May 7, 2013.

4. Campo MA, Weiser S, Koenig K. Job strain in physical therapists. *Physical Therapy.* 2009;89:946-956.

5. Van Servellen G. *Communication Skills for the Healthcare Professional: Concepts, Practice, and Evidence.* 2nd ed. Sudbury, MA: Jones & Bartlett; 2009.

6. Commission for Case Manager Certification. FAQs about case management. http://ccmcertification.org/healthcare-organizations/faqs-about-case-management Accessed July 26, 2013.

7. Committee on Quality of Healthcare in America, ed. *Crossing the Quality Chasm: A New Health System for the 21st Century.* Washington, DC: National Academies Press; 2001.

8. Ransom SB, Joshi M, Nash DB. *The Healthcare Quality Book: Vision, Strategy, and Tools* Washington, DC: Health Administration Press; 2005.

9. Longest BB. *Health Policymaking in the United States.* 4th ed. Chicago, IL: American College of Healthcare Executives; 2006.

10. Fottler MD, Ford RC, Heaton CP. *Achieving Service Excellence: Strategies for Healthcare Management Series.* Chicago, IL: Health Administration Press; 2002.

11. United States Department of Health and Human Services. Health information privacy. http://www.hhs.gov/ocr/privacy/. Accessed July 27, 2013.

12. Centers for Medicare & Medicaid Services. Patient's bill of rights. http://www.cms.gov/CCIIO/Programs-and-Initiatives/Health-Insurance-Market-Reforms/Patients-Bill-of-Rights.html. Accessed July 27, 2013.

WEB RESOURCES

American Hospital Association (AHA). Patient care partnership. http://www.aha.org/advocacy-issues/communicatingpts/pt-care-partnership.shtml

Centers for Medicare & Medicaid Services. Medicare rights & protection. http://www.medicare.gov/Publications/Pubs/pdf/11534.pdf.

The development of an instrument to measure satisfaction with physical therapy. Goldstein MS, Elliott SD, Guccione AA. *Physical Therapist.* 2000;80:853–863. http://physther.org/content/80/9/853.full.pdf. Accessed November 13, 2013.

Florida Agency for Health Care Administration. Patient's bill of rights and responsibilities. http://www.floridahealthfinder.gov/reports-guides/patient-bill-rights.aspx

Italian version of the Physical Therapy Patient Satisfaction Questionnaire: cross-cultural adaptation and psychometric properties. Vanti C, Monticone M, Ceron D, et al. *Physical Therapist.* 2013;93:911-922. http://ptjournal.apta.org/content/93/7/911.full. Accessed November 13, 2013.

Longitudinal continuity of care is associated with high patient satisfaction with physical therapy. Beattie P, Dowda M, Turner C, Michener L, Nelson R. *Physical Therapist.* 2005;85:1046-1052. http://www.physther.net/content/85/10/1046.full.pdf. Accessed November 13, 2013.

Patient satisfaction with musculoskeletal physical therapy care: a systematic review. Hush JM, Cameron K, Mackey M. *Physical Therapist.* 2011;91:25-36. http://ptjournal.apta.org/content/91/1/25.full. Accessed November 13, 2013.

Patient satisfaction with outpatient physical therapy: instrument validation. Beattie PF, Pinto MB, Nelson MK, Nelson R. *Physical Therapist.* 2002;82:557-565. http://www.expertclinicalbenchmarks.com/pages/Patient_Satisfaction_Tool_Development_2002.pdf. Accessed November 13, 2013.

Scale to measure patient satisfaction with physical therapy. Monnin D, Perneger TV. *Physical Therapist.* 2002;82:682-691. http://physther.org/content/82/7/682.full.pdf. Accessed November 13, 2013.

Spanish-language version of the MedRisk instrument for measuring patient satisfaction with physical therapy care (MRPS): preliminary validation. Beattie PF, Nelson RM, Lis A. *Physical Therapist.* 2007;87:793-800. http://ptjournal.apta.org/content/87/6/793.full. Accessed November 13, 2013.

CHAPTER 10

Fiscal Responsibilities

LEARNING OBJECTIVES

- Discuss healthcare managers' typical fiscal responsibilities.
- For a given physical therapy practice assets, analyze property, location, equipment selection factors, costs, and depreciation.
- Identify fixed, variable, direct, and indirect costs and potential sources of waste or excess that increase practice costs.
- Compare different payer mixes to analyze their impact on revenue.
- Discuss other possible sources of revenue.
- Analyze factors that enhance reimbursement from third-party payers (i.e., authorizations, coding, billing, contract negotiation).
- Discuss the use of Current Procedural Terminology (CPT) codes.
- Identify alternative revenue sources.
- Discuss the importance of financial statements and budget reports.

Overview

All aspects of healthcare finances and accounting are scrutinized for compliance with a range of laws, regulations, contracts, and operation systems. Compliance leads to a standardization of many financial systems in any type of healthcare organization. The responsibilities for these systems are either led by professional financial experts in large organizations or managed with the assistance of financial consultants in smaller organizations.

All organizations have two components to their finances. The first component is financial management, which is a factor in strategic planning that includes funding of assets with a focus on profits and losses. The other component is the controller functions for the day-to-day operations of the business. The functions include recording all business transactions; focusing on revenue and expenses; and guarding against theft, waste, or loss of assets and other resources.

To communicate effectively with these experts about finances, upper-level managers should be able to grasp:[1]

- financial statements
- basic principles of accounting and finance
- cost accounting
- capital and operational budgeting
- reporting and control
- reimbursement and capitation
- databases
- information systems' relationship to financial and strategic planning
- basic economics (supply and demand)
- contracts

Healthcare financing has become so complex that organizations are compelled to prepare mid-level managers at varying levels of involvement for many of these financial responsibilities. Large organizations develop ongoing training programs because financing decisions are tightly linked to changes in healthcare policy and reimbursement requirements. Because small private practices face the same challenges, ongoing education of owners and staff is necessary to remain current with changes. The American Physical Therapy Association (APTA) webpages provide the latest information to assist in meeting these needs. Links are available in Web Resources.

This chapter is a basic introduction to the complexities of fiscal responsibilities. Outpatient practice is used as the example in all of the activities to demonstrate the interaction of these factors in a straightforward manner and to guide the development of program proposals, feasibility studies, and business plans. The general concepts, however, may apply to any type of healthcare service with consideration for how it fits into a larger organization, its major source of funding, and whether or not it is a cost center (a center that generates expenses but no direct revenue). Section 3 of the text delves into these unique aspects of each type of physical therapy setting.

Assets, Liabilities, and Net Worth

For large healthcare organizations, assets are property such as goods, equipment, buildings, installations, land, investments, and retained earnings. Business ownership has both financial and psychological implications that may drive professionals into establishing freestanding private practices in which they take pride in both financial and patient care accomplishments. For individuals, assets also include personal cash savings, interest on savings and investments, and other valuable items that are owned outright. For both organizations and individuals, net worth equals assets minus liabilities (debts). Entrepreneurs must be brutally honest about their personal net worth when preparing feasibility studies and business plans for their own businesses.

Current funds available or large-scale loans for expansion or development of new programs may be of little concern for many healthcare organizations with large assets and sound credit ratings. For entrepreneurs, credit sources may be challenging and often include loans from family and friends, banks, and credit unions. It is difficult to borrow money without a strong positive net worth and credit history. The beginning of a new career is a good time to take a financial planning course or consult a financial planner whether intending to be an entrepreneur or not to assure long-term financial success. An accurate accounting of assets is important to determine how many, if any, additional funds are needed to financially support a new business. As an academic exercise, students may assume a net worth of $100,000 for the development of proposals for new businesses or programs.

Real property and equipment assets are the focus of this section. Managers may rely on financial consultants to make decisions about cash, bonds, stocks, and other investments that affect an organization's assets.

Real Property Assets

Particularly for new business owners, owning outright or mortgaging a property (freestanding or condominium) may not be realistic. It is a decision based on the same factors used to decide to rent rather than buy a home. People decide between the investment of ownership and the expense of leasing with attention to the tax implications of those decisions. Determining the square feet of space and how that space is arranged is also important. Patient privacy, employee comfort, and safety must all be considered in relation to space requirements of the government agencies that license healthcare organizations.

Location

Deciding where to place a practice is critical. Location contributes to property value and it also contributes to the value of the practice to its customers. The better the location is, the greater is the value of the asset to a physical therapy practice. The value of the location is just as important for inpatient rehabilitation services within a building and for outpatient satellite centers on the campuses of healthcare systems. Managers have to weigh the pros and cons of possible locations carefully by answering some questions:

1. How important is public transportation to the target markets of patients and employees? If important, where is the location in relationship to transportation system stops?

2. What are local traffic patterns and commuting times to the location for the target market?

3. Is parking convenient, available, and safe?

4. How important are face-to-face interactions with physicians? If this level of interaction is important, what is the travel time or distance to these referral sources?

5. Is the location of the building safe? Is the building secure? Is it freestanding or part of a larger complex?

6. What are the neighboring businesses? How do they impact the appeal of the practice?

7. Is the location of an office within a building safe and secure? Is it a convenient, visible space within the building? Is it important to be on the first floor?

8. Do people with physical disabilities have convenient access to the practice?

See Activity 10.1.

Equipment Assets

For convenience, managers may determine that anything over a particular price is capital equipment, $500 or $1,000, for example. Another approach is to classify equipment that is more permanent (lasts more than 1 year, typically) as an asset from that which is more dispensable, is expendable, or requires frequent upgrading. For

> **ACTIVITY 10.1**
> **LOCATION**
>
> Select an existing physical therapy practice for critique. Begin with identifying the advantages and disadvantages of the location of the selected practice against the list above. Add other factors to be included on the list of questions about location. What does the location say about the vision, mission, and goals of the practice?
>
> *TIME-OUT FOR WRITING: Analyze the location and space needs for your program proposal, feasibility study, or business plan. What is the cost of the space? If you are establishing a program in an existing organization, the business office would provide the prorated space cost.*

example, a cold-pack machine is capital equipment and the cold packs that are in it are expendable, frequently replaced, and noncapital items. The need for different request and approval processes for capital and noncapital equipment and supplies partially drives these classifications. Managers want employees to identify and request capital equipment needs supported by rationale and the potential to generate revenue, but they do not want to be overwhelmed with paperwork to replace expendable supplies and less expensive equipment. More important, the classification of equipment has tax implications.

Depreciation

Equipment classification decisions may require the advice of a tax consultant because of the financial and legal implications of depreciation of any asset. Depreciation is an income tax deduction that allows the taxpayer to recover the costs of owned property or other assets placed in service over time that have a determinable useful life. For example, if a physical therapy practice purchases an exercise system for $80,000 and expects the equipment to last for 10 years, the expense would be recorded as $8,000 per year for 10 years. Depreciation preserves revenue and increases profits by reducing tax payments. Because expenses are deducted from revenue when they occur, converting as much property and equipment as possible into assets defers these losses to taxes. Increasing assets for tax purposes is weighed against the costs of either borrowing the funds or depleting funds to obtain them. Another fiscal strategy is reinvesting profits back into the organization to reduce income taxes. To repeat, these are complex decisions that may demand consultation with tax or other financial experts.

Equipment Choices

As real property, equipment and other furniture may be purchased or leased. Similar to the decision of buying or leasing a car, managers also need to consider the pros and cons of these choices:

1. Will there be frequently updated models of the equipment?
2. Is the technology associated with the equipment rapidly changing?
3. Are there classic or traditional pieces of equipment that must be included?
4. Is there a minimal set of equipment required to meet external licensing requirements?
5. What furniture is needed in the staff and/or business offices? Are there special ergonomic needs?
6. What computers, phones, and other means of communication are needed?
7. What furniture and other décor are needed in the reception and waiting areas?
8. What scientific evidence supports the purchase of equipment for particular patient populations?

See Activity 10.2.

Costs

A top priority for managers is determining the cost of doing business, which is usually expressed as the cost per patient visit. Without knowing how much it costs to deliver services, managers are unable to determine how much to charge for services to end up with a profit. Negotiating with insurance companies for contracts to provide services may be disastrous if a manager does not know whether the reimbursement rate offered will cover the costs of the treatment sessions to care for patients.

ACTIVITY 10.2
EQUIPMENT

Select an existing physical therapy practice for critique. Determine the pros and cons of purchase or lease of each piece of equipment beginning with the list above. Add other factors to be included on the list. What is the estimated value of the equipment? What does the equipment say about the vision, mission, and goals of the practice?

TIME-OUT FOR WRITING: Analyze the major equipment needs for your program proposal, feasibility study, or business plan, and prepare a draft list for your budget. Will you borrow money to buy it? Will you lease all or some of it? Include these costs as start-up and operational expenses (discussed later). Does the equipment fit into the space needed that you identified in Activity 10.1? You may choose not to depreciate the equipment for the purposes of this exercise.

Kinds of Costs

The two major categories of costs are:

- Direct costs: Expenses for delivering services, which include salaries, equipment (loans or leases), and clinical supplies. NOTE: Inventory control is important in controlling direct costs related to clinical and office supplies so that sufficient quantities are available when needed while avoiding the expense of stockpiling excess supplies for extended periods of time.
- Indirect (overhead) costs: Rent or mortgage payments, utilities, janitorial services, equipment maintenance, office supplies, and so on that underlie the direct delivery of services. Overhead costs are those items necessary regardless of the number of patients there are in a practice or service. For example, even if there is only one patient, the practice needs electricity, temperature control, software packages, telephone and Internet services, medical records, and the like.

Costs are also classified as:

- Fixed: The same cost regardless of the number of patients who are treated (e.g., rent, loan payments)

- Variable: The cost increases as the number of patients increases (e.g., laundry services)
- Semifixed: A fixed cost, such as wages and salaries that may vary because of need for overtime or when work hours are decreased as patient census fluctuates

Direct Labor Costs

Managers may use some historical data to begin to determine an estimated amount for direct costs. The total labor costs of all employees (i.e., salaries, wages, benefits, and payroll taxes) divided by the average number of treatment sessions in a unit of time gives an average labor cost per treatment session. Labor costs are the major expense of any business. For example:

Total labor costs per month = $50,000

Average number of treatment sessions per month = 1,000

Formula: $50,000 ÷ 1,000 = $50 (average labor cost per treatment session)

Total direct costs per month = Labor costs ($50,000) + equipment loan payment ($2,000) + clinical supplies ($250) = $52,250

Average number of treatment sessions per month = 1,000

Formula: $52,250 ÷ 1,000 = $52.25 (average total direct cost per treatment session)

Labor costs include other payroll expenses (i.e., workers' compensation, contributions to taxes), which may be estimated to be about 2% of the total labor cost, and the salaries that owners pay themselves. The salaries of managers and other non-patient care staff in large institutions may be prorated among several departments according to some given formula. Determination of the most appropriate staff mix to control these labor costs is an important management consideration. For example, the fixed labor costs of salaried, exempt employees may be weighed against the potentially variable labor costs of more expensive hourly contingent workers.

Managers strive to fill as much work time with treatment sessions as possible and reasonable, typically applying a productivity expectation. Revenue cannot be generated unless patients are being treated. A commonly used standard is that 80% of the time a professional employee should be engaged in direct patient care that is billable. That means an employee working 40 hours per week for 52 weeks a year (2,080 hours) would be generating revenue 1,664 hours per year. The rest of the time is paid time off, meetings, breaks, documentation of care, submitting charges, and so on.

Scheduling

Other factors influencing the number of treatment sessions (billable time) are patient cancellations and no-shows, which may result from weather conditions or personal choice. One solution to avoid empty treatment sessions is to double-book (assign two patients to one therapist at the same time) or overlap patient appointments. However, reducing non-billable time through scheduling patients concurrently may lead to reduced reimbursement. Medicare and some other insurers who define skilled service as one-on-one professional care reduce the reimbursement per patient when treatment time is shared by more than one patient.

Even with the best attempts to schedule treatment sessions consistently, not all staff members work at the same pace so treatment times may vary to achieve the same patient results. The complexity of patients with the same condition also varies, and each patient's condition varies in acuity and complexity over time. This provider and patient variation makes establishing a standard workday difficult for managers. Rushed and harried therapists and unhappy patients must be avoided while also keeping non-productive time and unexpected employee absences to a minimum. Deciding whether or not one non-clinical person is assigned the duties of scheduling and reminder calls to patients or whether therapists make their own appointments with patients is an important management decision that partially depends on the ability of therapists and a scheduler to work well together. Managers weigh the labor cost of a scheduling position against the increased non-productive time when therapists do their own scheduling. Therapists creating their own schedules may increase productivity because they are able to consider factors unknown to schedulers such as patient conditions and equipment availability. See Activity 10.3.

ACTIVITY 10.3
FILLING IN

The issue of "filling in" has become a contentious one for the staff in Rosemont Physical Therapy. Mark Potter has called a staff meeting to brainstorm some ideas to solve the problem of what to do when a therapist or assistant is unexpectedly out sick or on planned leave. In the past, the staff simply met briefly to review the schedule and divided the work of the absent therapist among themselves. However, because the volume of patients has increased for each therapist, it is almost impossible to take on more work. Use the strategic planning process to develop a plan for coverage of patient care during unexpected absences. Consider: What is the current situation? What should it be? What do they have to work with? How will they get to where they want to be?

TIME-OUT FOR WRITING: Determine the labor and other direct costs for the budget in your program proposal, feasibility study, or business plan. Consider the fixed and variable labor costs per average treatment session depending on your staff mix (contingent, contract, employees).

Prorate costs if staff are assigned to more than one unit in a large organization.

ACTIVITY 10.4
CUTTING COSTS

Mark Potter feels that the staff is working as hard as they can and efficiency has significantly improved, but he feels that he still needs to reduce his costs. Other than salaries, wages, and benefits, what other direct and indirect costs might he be able to reduce (i.e., linen, electric, janitorial services)? Consider: What is the current situation? What should it be? What does he have to work with? How will he get to where he wants to be?

TIME-OUT FOR WRITING: Estimate the indirect (overhead) costs per average treatment session for the budget in your program proposal, feasibility study, or business plan. Prorate these costs if they are spread across units in a large organization based on some given formula.

Other Cost Determinations

This section includes some other considerations in determining costs. Beginning with capital equipment, managers need to be careful to avoid impulse buying by considering the impact of a large purchase on profits and on the generation of revenue. For example, an unused expensive piece of gym equipment can be a costly expense to the organization. Managers need to ask whether the equipment is worth the cost of a long-term loan and whether it adds to the value of patient care. Finally, is there evidence to support positive changes in the expected outcomes of patient care because of the new equipment? A typical formula for predicting the costs of expensive equipment is:

Total capital clinical equipment cost ÷ years that the equipment will last × 1.00 + the interest rate = annual cost
Example: Borrow $100,000 at 6% interest to buy equipment expected to last for 10 years
Formula: $100,000 ÷ 10 years × 1.06 = $10,600 annual cost ÷ 12 = $883.33 monthly cost for 10 years

Managers also need to consider the cost of space that is calculated as cost per square foot per month whether it is leased or purchased. How much space is needed for effective patient care

Indirect Costs

The average indirect costs per treatment session are determined by adding all of the indirect costs and dividing by the estimated total number of treatment sessions per month. Although some expenses (e.g., education, bonuses) may be expended only if surplus funds are available others expenses are embedded in the business. As a simple example with a partial list of indirect costs:

Per month costs: Lease = $6,000 + phone/Internet services = $500 + electricity = $700
Average number of treatment sessions per month = 1,000
Formula: $7,200 ÷ 1,000 = $7.20 (average indirect cost per treatment session)

See Activity 10.4.

becomes an important question to control this cost. Some industry minimal standards that may be used for academic exercises are:

Each clinical staff = 500 sq. ft

Each clerical staff = 60 sq. ft

Waiting room/reception area each = 100 sq. ft

Medical records = 100 sq. ft

Example: A practice includes four therapists (4 × 500 = 2,000 sq. ft), two clerical staff (2 × 60 = 120 sq. ft), reception and medical records (100 + 100 = 200 sq. ft) for total space of 2,320 sq. ft. The lease is $20 per sq. ft.

Formula: 2,320 sq. ft × $20 = $46,400 per year ÷ 12 = $3,866.66 per month

Equipment size and arrangement, patient and employee safety, patient privacy, and healthcare or business licensure requirements may affect these general guidelines.

Revenue (Income)

Revenue, or income, is the total of all monies received for services provided or goods sold during a given period. Managers, perhaps obviously, need to know where the money will be coming from.

Payer Mix

Physical therapists and other healthcare professionals are paid in different reimbursement models depending on type of setting and the insurer. See Table 10.1. The payer mix (the percentage of a target population insured in each model) becomes very important. For instance, if the average cost of treating the mix of patients in Table 10.1 is $50 per visit and each of the 4,000 patients in the payer mix averages 12 visits (48,000 total visits per year), it would cost $2,400,000 to treat the patients. The average revenue per treatment session must be greater than $50 to make a profit (revenue – costs). A manager may receive reimbursement in one model for more than $50 per visit, and in other models for less than $50 per visit, but the average revenue from all reimbursement contracts must be $50.

For another example of the impact of payer mix on potential income, see Table 10.2. The facts and figures in this table demonstrate what would happen if a physical therapy practice were to have 4,000 patients in only one type of the reimbursement model. The last column suggests the management implications of each single-payment model if the average cost of each visit to the physical therapy center remains at $50.

Insurance companies' preferences, obviously, are for models that reduce the amount of reimbursement they are likely to pay per patient that

TABLE 10.1   Examples of reimbursement models on an annual basis with 1,000 patients in each mode

FORM OF REIMBURSEMENT	DEFINITION	EXAMPLE	TOTAL REVENUE/ YEAR
Fee schedule based on price/ Unit of care	No. of patients per year × No. of visits per patient × No. of units per visit × payment per unit	1,000 patients × 12 visits/patient × 3 units/visit × $25/unit	$900,000
Per diem or Per visit	No. of patients per year × No. of visits per patient × Payment per diem or per visit	1,000 patients × 12 visits/patient × $50 flat fee	$600,000
Per case	No. of patients × Payment per patient for 1 year	1,000 patients × $500/patient/year regardless of number of visits	$500,000
Capitation	No. of covered people × Premium per patient per month × 12 months/year	1,000 patients × $25/patient/month × 12 months regardless of number of patients who receive services	$300,000
TOTALS		4,000 patients	$2,300,000

TABLE 10.2 Revenue of each reimbursement model on an annual basis where all patients have the same insurance model with managerial considerations

FORM OF REIMBURSEMENT	TOTAL REVENUE/YEAR FOR 4,000 PATIENTS	MANAGEMENT TOOL BASED ON COST/PATIENT VISIT OF $50
Fee schedule based on price/unit of care	With average revenue of $900 per patient = $3,600,000	4,000 patients × average of 12 visits × $50 cost per visit = $2,400,000 total cost. $3,600,000 revenue – $2,400,000 costs = $1,200,000 profit. To increase profit margin: ↓ cost/visit, ↑ average revenue/visit.
Per diem or per visit	With fee of $50 per visit and average of 12 visits per patient = $2,400,000	4,000 patients × average of 12 visits × $50 cost per visit = $2,400,000 total cost. $2,400,000 revenue – $2,400,000 = 0 profit For profit: ↓ costs/visit, ↑ number of visits/patient or ↑ number of patients.
Per case	$500 per patient for an episode of care = $2,000,000	Dependent on number of visits per patient. If each person in this group has 12 visits per year, the reimbursement per visit averages $41.66. The cost is $50 visit. $50.00 – $41.66 = $8.34 loss per visit (about $320,000/year). For profit: Must ↓ the cost per visit to less than $41.66, ↓ the average number of visits per patient.
Capitation	$600 per patient each year = $1,200,000 An accountable care organization (ACO) receives $10,000 for each patient with total hip arthroplasty.	4,000 patients × $600/year. At a cost of $50/visit, if each patient receives 12 visits, there are significant losses. However, not each patient may need physical therapy or may not need 12 visits and PT still receives $600/patient. For profit: ↓ the number of people who receive physical therapy, ↓ the number of visits/patient so that average revenue/visit is more than $50.
Bundled services		A physical therapy practice that is part of the ACO negotiates for a flat fee for each patient receiving outpatient services. For profit: The flat fee must exceed an average of $50 in order to exceed the cost/visit.

they insure. Providers prefer models that give the most flexibility in the number of sessions and payment per session they receive to meet the needs of each individual patient. With utilization review methods and models of reimbursement to consider, managers must know organizational income on a daily basis. Attention to contract details in negotiations with insurance companies must be taken very seriously as well.

Co-Payments and Deductibles

The other aspect of payer mix for consideration is the percentage of direct reimbursement in each model of payment. Patient deductibles and co-payments may vary within a model and among models and affect the level of reimbursement,

which is often 80%. For example, for a $100 charge for a physical therapy, the insurer pays $80 and the patient pays the provider a $20 co-payment. Managers would prefer no deductibles or patients who have already met their deductible amounts before beginning physical therapy to reduce the risk of nonpayment of these out-of-pocket expenses by patients. High co-payments may make it difficult for patients to attend 12 scheduled visits. For instance, if the co-payment/visit were $25, a patient would pay $300 out of pocket for his physical therapy care over the course of 3 or 4 weeks. Other patients' policies may limit the total number of visits per year. Knowing the contract limits and levels of reimbursement for each patient is critical information for a manager to relay to staff.

Contract Negotiation

Managers in large organizations developing new programs may be less concerned with insurance contracts that may already be in place for a broad range of healthcare services. Managers may need only to confirm that there are no limitations in those agreements that might negatively influence a proposed new service. For private practices, the details of contracts with insurers drive revenue so that managers need to:

- Identify the types and sources of health insurance for the potential target markets.
- Identify the model(s) of reimbursement for each of those health insurance policies.
- Determine the coverage for physical therapy services in those models.

Negotiating contracts with insurance companies presents risks. Managers or owners need to know their cost per treatment and desired profit per treatment before entering these negotiations. They cannot afford to enter into payment contracts that do not cover their costs per treatment, nor can they accept a fixed rate that places profits at risk if the number of patient visits suddenly increases. Likewise, accepting discounted fees and relying on increased volume to make up the gaps created by accepting a lower rate of payment may be unaffordable without contracts at rates high enough to counterbalance these risky agreements.

To negotiate these contracts, managers may need the assistance of attorneys and financial experts with a broad view of numerous kinds of contracts. Having a checklist of items that need to be addressed in a contract is important for mangers to have on hand. Independent practitioners may join networks of practitioners that provide power in numbers during negotiations with insurance companies. Networks also provide services to their members to help implement and monitor these negotiated contracts.

With the emergence of accountable care organizations (ACOs), private practice physical therapists and rehabilitation corporations have potential opportunities for revenue through bundled payments. Bundling (bundled payment systems, case rates, episode-based payment) is single payment reimbursement for all services related to a treatment or condition, possibly spanning multiple providers in multiple settings. This new payment methodology is in its trial stage of development for the care of people with given diagnoses. It is a way to link the payment to providers with patient outcomes within an episode or continuum of care delivery. Clinicians engaged in bundling models are expected to focus on coordinating patient care to share in the potential savings and financial risk through increased quality and efficiency of all of the care within an episode of care for a patient. For example, the bundled costs of caring for a patient who undergoes a total knee arthroplasty would include pre-surgical diagnostic tests and physician office visits, the surgery and acute care, post-operative rehabilitation, and follow-up physician visits. Determination of the effect of bundling on providers, insurers, and patients is unclear at this time. See Activity 10.5.

Additional Revenue

Managers may decide that they wish to supplement revenue from direct patient care or identify other sources of income as a cushion during times of unpredictable patient visits. Selling medical equipment, developing fee-for-service programs that patients pay for privately because they are not included in health insurance policies, or adding

---

ACTIVITY 10.5
CONTRACTS

Most of the patients at Rosemont Physical Therapy work at a regional distribution center at the edge of town. This year that company offered a cafeteria benefit plan, so employees now have many healthcare benefit choices. The previous single health insurance plan included generous reimbursement for physical therapy. What are the potential financial implications that Mark Potter needs to consider for this change in his target market?

TIME-OUT FOR WRITING: Determine the potential revenue sources and contracts for reimbursement to support your program proposal, feasibility study, or business plan. You may average the revenue/treatment session across multiple insurers for ease of calculations. NOTE: Programs in acute care hospitals may be cost centers that do not generate revenue.

services that complement physical therapy (massage therapy is an example) are possible options. Managers must be sensitive to the ethical and legal issues in establishing these additional services so that patients referred to them do not feel coerced into using them.

As businesses and services become established, managers need to decide whether marketing and increased referrals are really what they want. Increased visits usually mean increased staff and space to maintain the quality of services provided. The amount of growth that a practice can handle without increased personnel costs becomes an important question. Competition for the most desirable patients (such as those who need the least amount of therapy or those who have the ability to pay) becomes a serious consideration. See Activity 10.6.

ACTIVITY 10.6
OPPORTUNITIES

1. Mark Potter is intrigued but unsure about what action to take. The local arts consortium has approached him to exhibit paintings on the walls in his practice. They offered him 10% of any exhibited artwork that is purchased. Neighboring businesses want to place brochures and business cards in the waiting room. A company that sells nutritional supplements wants to set up a display in the Rosemont waiting room and will pay Mark 10% of documented sales. What should Mark do? Accept both offers? Why? What are other possibilities for this type of supplemental income?

2. The space next door to Rosemont Physical Therapy has become available. The leasing office is giving Mark Potter first choice on renting it. Mark does not think there is a market for expanding his physical therapy services, but he thinks this may be an opportunity to develop a related yet separate new business using the profits from his practice. What are the possible alternative business opportunities that might be most appropriate?

TIME-OUT FOR WRITING: Although not necessary, identify and include any additional sources of revenue in your program proposal, feasibility study, or business plan.

Reimbursement Challenges

Strict adherence to the rules of carriers about authorizations for payment is necessary to avoid payment denials and delays. Business staff and therapists must work together closely so that patients begin therapy services with all necessary pre- and continuing authorizations in place. Therapists need to know the number of sessions that have been authorized and the Current Procedural Terminology (CPT) codes they may use in billing for services for each insurance intermediary or carrier. Procedures for justifying and seeking reauthorizations or extension of services to meet patient goals must be in place. The time these processes take away from patient care is a managerial concern. However, providing patient care that is not reimbursable is unsustainable. Guiding staff to make certain that patient needs are reconciled with insurance requirements is a primary consideration in clinical decision-making that cannot be lost in the process. The American Physical Therapy Association webpages on coding and billing are indispensable references for this aspect of management. The link can be found in Web Resources.

In addition to bad debts (e.g., a patient fails to make out-of-pocket payments), pro bono services may reduce profits and claims for payments may be denied for a variety of reasons. Managers must avoid failure to document as necessary to support the medical necessity of care, and technical errors in billing, coding of units or documentation that does not match billing. In some practices, these combined factors may mean that as much as 30% of the expected revenue is lost—or really that the revenue was never had to begin with. As a result, profit margins (income – expenses) vary widely in physical therapy. Profit margins may also vary from year to year as insurance companies and employers negotiate contracts that affect coverage of rehabilitation services in the target market of a practice. Congress continues to cut Medicare costs, and intermediaries and carriers adjust their rules to control their payment of claims for rehabilitation services.

Coding and Billing

After contracts are created based on fee schedules, managers need to assure that all services provided are accurately coded and billed to avoid the potential for fraud and abuse. Accuracy also ensures that practices receive all revenue to which they are entitled. Clinical and business office staffs typically require outside training for coding and billing, ongoing in-services, other communication methods, and audits to determine accuracy and completeness of billing and documentation of care. Many insurers increasingly require the use of computerized billing systems for submission of claims for payment. These systems may be integrated with broader information systems, including documentation and scheduling software. These technological interventions are efforts to increase the accuracy of coding and billing and the documentation to support them. They also reduce the time to complete these administrative tasks and to receive payment, allowing more time for direct patient care—and the generation of more billable units. See Activity 10.7.

CPT Codes

Fee schedules used by insurance companies may be based on more than 8,000 CPT codes. Developed primarily as the basis of payment for services provided to Medicare recipients, the system has been adopted by some workers' compensation and other private insurers as their fee schedules as well. However, managers should not expect absolute adoption because each insurer may use the codes

as they see fit, or may use older versions of the CPT that better suit their purposes.

The CPT codes are established and reviewed each year by a special committee of the American Medical Association that includes other health professionals. This system has provided a uniform language and description for many aspects of medical and other health professional practices, but they are particularly important for reimbursement. For rehabilitation services, about 46 codes in the 97000 set of codes are used most frequently. For example, the code for physical therapy evaluation is 97001, modalities that do not require direct patient contact by the provider are in the 97010 to 97028 range, and therapeutic procedures that are charged by the minute are in the 97110 to 97140 range of codes.

It is important to note two things about CPT codes. First, they are reviewed and modified each year to reflect changes in healthcare practice that are determined by surveys of practitioners. For example, changes in the 2008 version of the CPT codes include the additional new codes for non–face-to-face services, such as telephone or e-mail to manage patient care and a code for attending team conferences. The addition of these codes means that other codes have been eliminated or the value of other codes was reduced because CPT coding is a neutral budget system that contributes to controlling healthcare costs. The establishment and revision of the codes involve a great deal of negotiation and analysis of practice. Managers must be mindful of these changes in codes and their values to avoid denial of claims or appeals to correct coding errors.

Second, just because codes exist does not mean insurers will pay for them. For example, many third-party payers do not reimburse for services that are coded as modalities that do not require direct patient contact by the provider, such as hot packs and cold packs. Many insurers have decided that these passive interventions do not require the skill and knowledge of professionals, and therefore do not pay for them.

Values of CPT Codes

The following constitutes the American Medical Association process for review of CPT Codes:

1. Resource-based relative value scale (RBRVS) is established by the American Medical Association every fall and implemented each January.

ACTIVITY 10.7
DOING BETTER

Although Mark is pleased with the changes implemented as a result of cutting costs (Activity 10.4) and some additional revenue sources (Activity 10.6), Rosemont Physical Therapy's profit margin remains dangerously slim. The only component of the business he has yet to address is coding and billing. What might be a plan for improvement in this area? Consider: What is the current situation? What should it be? What does he have to work with? How will he get to where he wants to be?

TIME-OUT FOR WRITING: Identify and include any expenses related to billing and coding in your program proposal, feasibility study, or business plan.

2. The basic value of each CPT code is set and then modified based on the costs of providing a procedure, test, etc. from one practice to another and from one geographic area to another.

3. The established uniform relative value is modified by a geographic adjustment factor (GAF) and a nationally uniform conversion factor that changes each year.

4. For example, payment for code 97110, Therapeutic Exercise, may be $26.04 for every 15 minutes of exercise in a rural part of the country and $28.79 in a large metropolitan area where the cost of doing business is higher because of GAF modifications on the RBRVS value for CPT 97110.

Payment based on this coding system has presented many challenges to physical therapists. Additional information on specific aspects of current billing and coding can be found at the webpages of the American Physical Therapy Association. Meanwhile, efforts are under way to seek adoption of an alternative payment system that may reduce administrative costs. Use the link in Web Resources for more information. The change in focus from interventions performed to patient outcomes may be one important effect of the suggested alternative. This proposed change is directed at moving from the current fee-for-service payment to a per-session payment. Many existing CPT codes would then be replaced with the alternative payment system. This system has 12 codes—three for evaluation and nine for examination and intervention. The three evaluation codes are differentiated by the level of complexity of decision-making required. A matrix of patient severity and intensity of service is designed to categorize treatment sessions that involve combinations of examination and interventions. Although not adopted at this time, this session-based payment system appears to align with healthcare policy shifts to new pay4performance (P4P) models that link quality outcomes to reduced costs and provider incentives. In this model, the likelihood that claims reviewers and insurers will be the primary decision makers about the specific care provided to accomplish an individual patient's goals will be significantly reduced. Payment of claims would be based on the severity of the patient's condition and the intensity of service required

rather than the current system of assigning CPT codes to a particular diagnosis regardless of individual patient factors.

Other Financial Considerations

Managers must ensure that bills are paid in a timely manner and payroll is met to avoid the embarrassment of debt collectors or the failure to sustain the services needed to support the practice. Having emergency reserves for unexpected expenses or reduced revenue must be part of the planning conducted with financial consultants. Recognizing the pattern of reimbursement income (how often payments are received for claims submitted) is an important consideration. Submitting claims with no errors and no omissions that are supported by detailed documentation helps avoid delays in payment because of denials of third-party payers and the time required to appeal those decisions.

In addition to reimbursement and other payments for services performed, some larger practices also may receive financial support through local government taxes or bonds. These public revenues may be specifically dedicated to large healthcare organizations with missions directed at the public service rather than those that share their profits with stockholders. Endowments, gifts, and fundraising activities, such as annual balls and art shows, may support organizations' special projects. Even private practices may have the opportunity to seek funding through grants for special projects or ongoing programs to meet the needs of particular populations. The preparation of grant applications is similar to that for feasibility studies. The bigger challenge is identifying potential public and private funding sources. See Activity 10.8.

Budgets

A budget is a tool for projecting and monitoring revenues and expenses (costs) so that managers stay on course financially to meet an organization's goals. Mid-level managers in large organizations may present a departmental budget for approval, receive one for implementation, or use some combination of both approaches. Once established, a common management rule is that a 10% positive or negative change in budget lines requires investigation and

ACTIVITY 10.8
FINDING GRANT OPPORTUNITIES

As a starting point, explore potential grant funding at http://www.grants.gov/applicants/find_grant _opportunities.jsp and at http://www.scangrants .com/.

TIME-OUT FOR WRITING: Include any potential grant funding in the budget for your program proposal, feasibility study, or business plan.

perhaps managerial decisions for either immediate correction or further monitoring to determine whether a trend is developing. For example, a 10% increase in revenue may reflect a need for additional staff, and a 10% decrease in revenue may mean that a manager needs to monitor the professional development of staff members by controlling continuing education expenses.

The budget itself is an itemized listing of the approved anticipated revenue and projected expenses for an organization. Typically prepared annually, the budget serves as the outline for a profit/loss statement that is commonly updated monthly to track financial data for comparison to budget projections as shown in Figure 10.1. Most organizations rely on the more complex zero budgeting strategy. This means there is no automatic carryover of profit and loss numbers from one year's budget into the next. Instead, a strategic planning process drives a new budget each year in which both revenue and expenses are set at zero. The alternative approach to budgeting is to inflate the numbers from year to year using the prior year's budget to reflect a blanket increase in revenue and expenses. Although simpler, this inflation approach to budgeting may not lead to improvements in the organization that are more likely to occur with the planned strategy and careful decision-making about each specific component of an organization that occur with zero budgeting models.

In any organization with a budgeting strategy, budget numbers need to be consistently and frequently monitored, at least monthly. Many financial software systems linked to billing and coding systems may lead managers to a daily review of revenue data. Mid-level managers and executives discuss the numbers for short-term and long-term planning. Private practice physical therapists may consult with business managers and accountants to monitor the practice's revenue, expenses, profits, and losses. See Activity 10.9.

Other Financial Tools

Break-Even Point

Breakeven is the point at which revenues equal expenses. It is the projected point (date) at which there is no profit and there is no loss. It is the estimated point after which a practice or program becomes profitable. Breakeven may not be important for managers in organizations whose financial decisions are based on multiple factors and that probably reached their break-even point long ago. Entrepreneurs starting from scratch will find this tool important and expected in feasibility studies and business plans.

Break-even analysis is based on estimates that need to be as accurate as possible, although the figures may change over time. The break-even point before the practice opens may not be the same break-even point after the business has been running for a few months. It is hoped that the practice has reached the break-even point before expected, but more typically, breakeven is pushed back because the best-laid plans are still unpredictable.

To conduct a break-even analysis, developers need to use a treatment session as the unit of service. Managers then ask, How much does it cost to treat

ACTIVITY 10.9
THE PROFIT AND LOSS STATEMENT

Analyze Figure 10.1. Identify any additional revenue and additional expenses that might be included for a typical physical therapy practice. Remember to include loan payments as expenses.

TIME-OUT FOR WRITING: Based on decisions in Activities 10.1 through 10.9, prepare a projected budget for your program proposal, feasibility study, or business plan. Using Figure 10.1 as a guide, prepare a profit and loss statement (pro forma–calculating figures for current or future profits) for monitoring of the budget plan for at least 6 months. Prepare other financial statements as requested.

| ROSEMONT PHYSICAL THERAPY | | | | |
| From_____ To_____ 20_____ | | | | |
	Month_____	Month_____	Month_____	Month_____
INCOME				
Services Provided				
Less Deductions				
Other Income				
TOTAL INCOME				
EXPENSES				
Bonuses				
Business Licenses, Accreditation				
Clinical Supplies				
Education				
Employee Benefits				
Equipment				
Dues				
Insurance				
Office Supplies				
Other Loans				
Other Perks				
Outbound Marketing				
Payroll Deductions				
Professional Services				
Purchased Services				
Recruitment				
Rent or Mortgage				
Salaries and Wages				
Travel				
Utilities				
TOTAL EXPENSES				
NET PROFIT(LOSS)				
TAXES				
NET PROFIT(LOSS) AFTER TAXES				

Notes: Dues (professional and community organizations)
Education (in-house, subsidizing graduate work, continuing education)
Equipment (clinical and office leases, loan payments, new purchases)
Insurance (general and professional liability)
Professional Services (attorneys, financial consultants, human resource experts, etc.)
Purchased Services (billing, registry staff, laundry, janitorial, lawn and landscape)
Travel (for education, marketing, etc.)
Other perks (coffee, monthly lunches, parking fees)

FIGURE 10.1 A sample profit and loss statement outline.

the average patient in an average treatment session? This number may not stabilize for a few months—the fewer the number of patient treatment sessions per month, the greater the cost per treatment session because of fixed costs. Taking the total costs per month and dividing by the number of expected treatment sessions per month provides the average cost per treatment session per month. For break-even analysis, the next question is, What is the number of treatment sessions per month at an average revenue of $100 per session (for example) that will pay for the total combined variable and fixed costs per month? A simple example for a hypothetical new practice follows in which the fixed monthly cost is $4,500, the variable cost per treatment session is $5, and the average revenue per treatment session is $100:

Total costs per month = Fixed costs per month + (variable costs per treatment session × no. of treatment sessions per month)

Revenue per month = Average revenue per treatment session × total number of sessions per month

Profit per month = Revenue per month − total costs per month

Profit margin = Revenue − expenses ÷ total revenue (expressed as a percentage)

Formulas:

	IF 10 TREATMENT SESSIONS/MONTH	IF 100 TREATMENT SESSIONS/MONTH
Total Cost (fixed + variable)	$4,500 + $5(100) = $5,000	$4,500 + $5(10) = $4,550
Gross Revenue	$100 per treatment × 100 = $10,000	$100 per treatment × 10 = $1,000
Profit	$10,000 × $5,000 = $5,000	$1,000 × $4,550 = ($3,550)
Profit Margin	$5,000 ÷ $10,000 = 50%	None: Loss of $3,550

Breakeven is typically represented in a line chart as shown in Figure 10.2 in which revenue is $50 × number of visits. For this example, the break-even number of visits is the point at which the total revenue is about $4,000 or 80 visits per month, which is expected to happen in June if projected referrals, contracts with insurance companies, and other factors occur as expected. The major rule of business becomes obvious. Keep costs per treatment session low and the number of treatment sessions high. Profit is the business goal. See Activity 10.10.

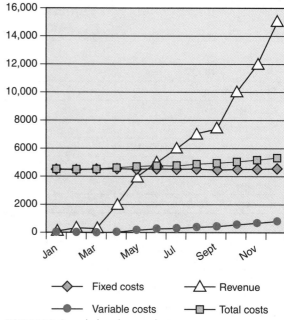

FIGURE 10.2 Sample break-even chart.

Determining Total Start-Up and Initial Operational Costs

When the financial analysis is completed, the important questions become, How much money is required to open the practice on the first day? How much more will be needed to keep the practice open until it becomes profitable (crosses the break-even point)? Good "guesstimates" are acceptable but omissions of costs are not. Failure to recognize and consider costs may be the source of more early business failures than any other factor. These start-up and initial operational costs constitute the amount of money on hand, or that needs to be borrowed, to open the doors and keep them open for perhaps several months or years. It is money needed to pay all expenses before receiving enough revenue to cover expenses. If the money is borrowed, the interest payments must be included as an expense item. The money borrowed is not shown as revenue in the budget or profit and loss statement.

In healthcare, the first reimbursement checks from third-party payers may take time as contracts are negotiated, reimbursement systems are created, and claims are submitted. Although treatment sessions are provided, payments may be delayed, especially for new providers. Without proper planning, these can seem like scary times. This is a period in which entrepreneurs are essentially paying to go to work, so they must be comfortable with this concept. For managers developing new programs, costs may be low if existing facilities and equipment are to be used and revenue has been clearly defined.

Cash Flow

Understanding cash flow is a related management tool. Although it is exciting to focus on revenue, its relationship to expenses is critical. Although a practice may be making money, whether it has enough cash to pay all of its expenses and loan payments is the more important question. Cash flow is analogous to a checking account. Determining whether there are deposits to cover the checks written is a type of cash-flow analysis. For managers in healthcare who are dependent on third-party payers, cash flow is critical because the check to pay for services provided may arrive weeks after the services have been delivered. Depending on the reimbursement model, some claims may not be submitted until the patient's entire plan of care is complete. The actual time that income from reimbursement remains an account receivable (defined as the money owed the practice from insurers or patients for services rendered that has not yet been received) becomes a major factor in operations management.

Cash flow is typically checked on a monthly basis by simply comparing the money received with the money spent. Including a simple month-by-month projected cash-flow chart like the example in Figure 10.3 in a feasibility study or business plan may be useful but not required. The two major columns in the chart are revenue and expenses. The third column is the bottom line or balance—the net increase (decrease) in cash each month. Each row of the chart represents a month or some other time period.

Expected Balance Sheet When in Full Operation

A balance sheet is another valuable financial tool. It is a documented report of a company's assets, obligations, and claims against equity at any given point in time. A balance sheet is a cumulative record of business to date. Balance sheets are used for comparisons to determine the changes in the value of the organization and whether debts and capital are increasing or decreasing. Remember that a balance sheet should balance. Assets − Liabilities = 0. Developers may wish to seek consultation or software to complete a balance sheet.

A Manager's Responsibility

Managers must carefully predict their costs and projected revenues to manage any organization. Profitability is a necessary condition for the existence of an organization, which must be accomplished in the context of legal requirements and ethical expectations for healthcare organizations. Managers who focus on controlling costs rather than generating more revenue as the means for increasing profits may be more successful in achieving their goals. Although some level of profit is an organizational goal, profits are the means to more important ends based on the vision and mission of the organization. See Activity 10.11.

DATE	INCOME	AMOUNT	EXPENSE	AMOUNT	BALANCE
					8,000
JAN 1			Rent	4,000	4,000
			Wages	3,000	1,000
JAN 10	Medicare check	5,000			6,000
JAN 15			Wages	3,000	3,000
JAN 30	United Health check	1,500	Utility and other bills	2,300	2,200
JAN 31					2,200 (to carry over)
TOTAL		6,500		12,300	

Sample Cash Flow Projection

	Cash Flow Projection				
Date	Sale	Amount	Expense	Amount	Balance
					2,000
1-Jan		3,000	RENT	1,200	3,800
5-Jan			WAGES		3,800
10-Jan					3,800
14-Jan		7,000	TAXES	3,500	7,300
25-Jan			BILLS	2,300	5,000
31-Jan					$5,000.00
TOTAL		10,000		7,000	

FIGURE 10.3 Actual and sample cash flow chart for 1 month.

ACTIVITY 10.11
TIME-OUT FOR REVIEW

The time-outs in the activities in this chapter should result in a first draft of the material needed to complete the financial section of a program proposal, feasibility study, or business plan. The final paragraph of the financial section should summarize the assumptions that underlie the information presented. It is a place to bring all of this financial information together in a clear, concise statement.

A review of vision, mission, goals, staffing, and marketing is important at this point to align all components of a proposal with financial analysis.

REFERENCE

1. Ross A, Wenzel FJ, Mitlyng JW. *Leadership for the Future: Core Competencies in Healthcare.* Chicago, IL: Health Administration Press; 2002.

WEB RESOURCES

American Physical Therapy Association. Alternative payment system information. http://www.apta.org/APS/. Accessed November 29, 2013.

American Physical Therapy Association. Coding and billing information. http://www.apta.org/Payment/CodingBilling/. Accessed November 29, 2013.

American Physical Therapy Association. Payment information and calculation. http://www.apta.org/Payment/. Accessed November 29, 2013.

CHAPTER 11

Risk Management, Legal, and Ethical Responsibilities

LEARNING OBJECTIVES

- Discuss insurance as a risk management tool.
- Compare the categories of potential risks and strategies for reducing them.
- Discuss Occupational Safety and Health Administration (OSHA) requirements.
- Discuss security of documentation, environment, and stakeholders.
- Develop a strategy to improve a practice's bad reputation.
- Determine the role of job descriptions in reducing personnel-related risks.
- Discuss the risks associated with the direction of supportive personnel.
- Determine the role of establishing patient rapport in reducing risks.
- Analyze an incident report.
- Apply root cause analysis to given scenarios.
- Identify the basic structure of the U.S. legal system.
- Discuss legal rights, duties, and remedies.
- Discuss a manager's role in contracts and professional malpractice.
- Discuss the role of managers in addressing the legal duties of organizations.

The intent of this chapter is to alert current and future managers to possible risks, related legal duties, and ethical concerns. Jurisdictions and circumstances differ. CONTENT SHOULD **NOT** BE TAKEN AS LEGAL ADVICE.

Overview

Risk management is the process of identifying potential threats that could severely damage or completely ruin an organization and taking action to reduce those risks. The increased complexity of healthcare organizations has broadened the scope and importance of risk management as a tool in achieving patient outcomes and financial goals. This specialized demand has led to the creation of risk management professionals for healthcare organizations who often report directly to the chief executive officer.[1]

Using a range of measures and data collection, often supported by computer software, risk managers are central to controlling risks so that losses are minimized. Risk management is about processes to avoid accidents, to decrease liability when incidents occur, and to improve the quality of care. Failure of risk management has serious financial implications for healthcare organizations. Risk management requires a broad scope of effort that depends on the attentiveness and carefulness of all employees at all times.

Mid-level managers provide data and implement risk management plans within their units of responsibility as part of the larger organization's plans. In other types of health organizations, risk management may not be as clearly centralized, or it may be among the responsibilities of the upper management team as a whole. Private practitioners in physical therapy also must consider the importance of risk management to the financial success of their businesses because they typically assume responsibilities for these duties themselves.

Managers, particularly in developing program proposals, feasibility studies, or business plans, may use risk management as a "big picture" opportunity to address all components of the business from the somewhat negative perspective of potential losses as shown in Activity 11.1. This process may identify insurmountable barriers or risks that could destroy an exciting or promising business venture. More likely, it may result in a more impressive, well-thought-out plan.

Managers in healthcare also face a variety of legal and ethical responsibilities. A brief overview of the U.S. legal system is presented in Figure 11.1. The relationship of the four sources of law of the U.S. legal system to healthcare shows the complexity of these issues. Managers must focus on the legal duties of their organizations and employees as well as on the rights of employees and patients. Laws, contracts, and the ethical duties of professionals to behave reasonably and responsibly in meeting the needs of society all impose on the responsibilities of healthcare managers.

This chapter introduces a few selected risk management, legal, and ethical issues to raise awareness of their complexity. Because the failure to manage risks may result in legal or ethical consequences, the categories of potential risks are presented first:[2]

- Hazard
- Market
- Reputation
- Operations
- Human capital

Hazard Risks

Because they are beyond the control of managers, the risks of natural disasters demand property damage insurance coverage. Depending on location, managers may identify the need for extra protection against hurricanes, fires, or floods, for example. In areas where hazard risks are particularly high, business interruption insurance that will cover the losses that occur while the business is temporarily unable to operate also reduces the risk of lack of revenue should the business be forced to close.

Managers in smaller organizations may rely on the skills of insurance agents for these policies and other policies such as professional insurance and general liability insurance, which are discussed in other sections of this chapter. Managers who are part of the upper management team in large healthcare systems may negotiate all categories of insurance policies for their organizations in consultation with professional risk managers. Both types of organizations need to establish ongoing review of their insurance policies to ensure compliance as new governmental regulations are imposed.

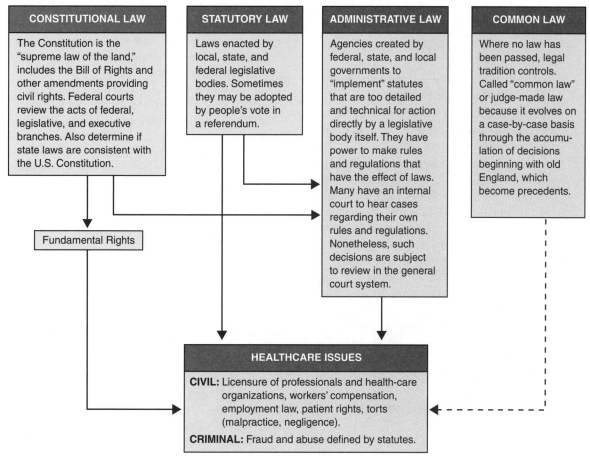

FIGURE 11.1 Overview of the U.S. legal system and its effect on healthcare.

Hazardous Materials

Another risk in this category is hazardous materials. Although not as critical in outpatient physical therapy practices as in other practice settings, the identification of risks related to infections, bloodborne pathogens, the disposal of sharps and other waste, and the provision of protective devices assures the safety of employees and patients.

Hand washing between patients, disinfecting surfaces and equipment, and supplying fresh or disposable paper linens contribute to a safe and healthy environment. Policies and procedures in compliance with universal precautions and required absences for staff who are infectious are equally important for reducing contamination. Patients who are infectious should be rescheduled for outpatient therapy or isolated during treatment to lower the risk of disease transmission.

Failure to identify and reduce hazards in the broad categories such as environmental safety, patient handling safety, and chemicals and radiation exposure may result in serious violations of federal mandates under the Occupational Safety and Health Administration (OSHA). See Web Resources for more detailed OSHA information on requirements and recommendations.

Market Risks

Changes in the target markets served by an organization may seem to be the biggest financial risk, particularly for independent practitioners in healthcare. Defining a market as a specified category of potential buyers, managers of private (independent) physical therapy practices face the possibility of revenue losses if:

● Employers in the community change healthcare policies for their employees so that coverage for rehabilitation services is more limited or eliminated.

- Insurers reduce the reimbursement for services that are covered.
- Physicians who refer to the practice relocate, retire, or choose other providers.
- Insurers reduce the number of contracts offered to independent practitioners to control their administrative costs.
- Populations shift so the percentage of people who seek rehabilitation services changes. (For example: a factory closes so that patients treated who receive Medicare become a much larger percentage of the total number of patients. Conversely, many older Medicare patients may give up their second homes in retirement areas and no longer make up a large percentage of the patients at certain times of the year.)
- Technological advances in medicine reduce the number of people with disabling conditions and diseases who would otherwise require intensive rehabilitation, or the amount of rehabilitation services required is decreased as surgical procedures become less invasive and disease processes are better controlled.
- Healthcare policy changes such as accountable care organizations (ACOs) and reimbursement bundling models reduce patient referrals if a practice is not included in these business arrangements.

Avoiding most of these risks is beyond the control of managers, and there is no insurance protection for market changes. The ability of managers to develop contingency plans for market changes may be critical to the survival of their businesses. Diversification of services, new collaborations and partnerships with other healthcare providers, and alternative sources of revenue are some possibilities that may be considered. Seeking legal counsel may reduce the potential risks associated with the contract negotiations necessary in entering into new types of relationships with other organizations.

Cash Flow

Another risk related to the market is one that is under the control of a manager—the stability of the organization's assets, resources, and expenses. Managers soon discover that hands-on, ongoing, diligent attention to the flow of money in the organization is essential to reduce the risks of spending too much, or not collecting enough, money. These efforts require coordination with an organization's accounting office or reliance on the services of a certified public accounting firm.

Managers often set "payment due when service is rendered" procedures to reduce the risk of patients who fail to make co-payments or fail to pay their bills on time. Because most patients have to make co-payments, failure of a large number to pay may be ruinous, particularly to a small practice. Establishing accounting practices and preparing staff to follow clear policies and procedures related to the collection of fees and the payment of bills reduces uncertainty, confusion, and financial risk.

Reputation Risks

A bad reputation has the potential to severely damage or shut down an organization. It is extremely difficult to earn a good reputation, and even harder to restore one that has been compromised—regardless of the reason. Managers in large organizations may not even know until it is too late that the organization's reputation or the reputation of someone in the organization is tarnished because of poor patient outcomes, suspicious accounting, fraud, false advertising, or unprofessional behavior. Some reasons for a tarnished reputation may be beyond the control of a manager whereas others are avoidable. At least the potential impact of negative actions should be identified to reduce risks.

In any case, managers may discover that restoring a reputation requires starting all over—essentially wiping the slate clean. Strategic planning may be vital to tackling this restoration, one of the most difficult managerial challenges. A bad reputation affects interactions with all stakeholders and can be financially devastating. Transforming a "good reputation" into measurable, objective terms takes work. Managers must resist tackling a bruised reputation with quick fixes or jumping to conclusions without a thorough analysis of the current situation and a clear definition of where it wants to be.

Operations Risks

Operations is the way work is conducted. The risks of operations are most likely to be related to the safety and security of workers and patients.

Clinical Equipment and Other Furnishings

Regular maintenance of all equipment used in patient care reduces the risk of adverse effects that are possible, particularly if electrical equipment requires calibration. Managers are responsible for establishing maintenance schedules and service agreements to ensure necessary repairs are completed and documented in a timely manner by qualified people. Operations manuals must be conveniently available for reference by everyone using the equipment, and managers are expected to answer or find the answers to questions that arise about effective use of equipment and warranty agreements.

Using Equipment

In addition to routine maintenance, managers must *demonstrate* the importance of inspecting equipment before *each* use and proper usage of equipment. Should harm come to a patient because of failure to do so, there is little defense in a potential legal action. It is dangerous to modify exercise equipment or use it in ways other than that for which it is intended. Wheelchairs, treatment tables, office furniture, and even chairs in the waiting room require ongoing inspection for signs of instability or wear to prevent breakage. Broken or damaged equipment is better removed than repaired, especially if amateurs are making the repairs. Temporary fixes may lead to permanent losses to the organization.

Not only are frayed electrical cords, loosened connectors, parts held together with tape, and missing parts potentially dangerous, but they also project a negative impression that may undermine confidence in the services delivered and the practice's reputation. For example, using extension cords is electrically dangerous, and extending electrical cords across large spaces presents a hazard for tripping and falls.

Ergonomics

Ergonomic analysis of office staff and their workspace is another important consideration for reducing the risk of workers' compensation claims or simply loss of work time and pain of injured parties. Depending on the size of the organization, managers may have workers' compensation insurance

that defers related costs. With or without workers' comp, managers must be concerned about ongoing repetitive injuries and sudden accidents that may profoundly affect a person's life. Placement of heavy boxes to decrease frequent bending and lifting is one example of factors to consider. Managers must also consider implementing safe patient-handling guidelines to address the challenges of lifting and moving patients who are dependent or obese. To avoid both mental and physical fatigue, employees should be encouraged to change positions and to take short walks during the day.

Environmental Safety

Managers are not only responsible for complying with the requirements of the Americans With Disabilities Act for accessibility to services, but they are also responsible for external and internal environment safety. Managers obtain general liability insurance policies to defer the risk of injuries that may occur on their property, and they reduce risks in an environment by making sure of the following:

- Entryways, streets, and parking lots are free of debris, obstacles, ice, and snow.
- Commonly used traffic paths within a practice are clear of obstacles.
- Floor coverings are tightly adhered to prevent tripping or falling.
- Spills are cleaned up immediately.
- Adequate space is available for patients and staff to move about easily without bumping into walls or equipment.
- Stairways and steps used for gait training are well lit, are free of obstacles, and have nonslip surfaces.
- Storage areas include sturdy shelving and other receptacles to clear floor space and prevent falling objects.
- Fire alarms and extinguishers are conveniently placed and functional.

Security and Personal Safety

Building security not only reduces the risk to personal safety and belongings, but also reduces loss of inventory and property damage. Electronic passes and identification badges are commonly required for access to buildings and units. Although property insurance shifts the risk, the potential danger compels people to follow procedures for locking doors and reporting suspicious behavior.

To reduce risks to both employees and patients, managers need to consider assignments that do not result in people working alone in a building or office. Paths and parking lots must be well lit. All staff must be alert to patients and coworkers who present a danger to themselves or others. OSHA includes workplace violence as a work hazard that managers are required to address. Increased visibility of security staff in healthcare organizations is a reflection of these safety concerns. Having a plan to call for assistance is as important for the receptionist as it is for the therapist. Emergency numbers should be clearly posted by phones and in other conspicuous places.

Patient Care Safety

Foremost, managers are responsible for the safety of patients during their care in any organization. Managers who establish procedures to be performed without fail may help reduce the risk. For instance, consistently monitoring vital signs to determine physiological responses to exercise may also lead to the identification of previously undetected cardiopulmonary problems. All staff should be certified in basic life support and in the use of automated external defibrillators that are made available in convenient locations. First aid kits should be readily available.

Generally, as the number of patients with complex conditions continues to increase, staff in all practice settings must be increasingly vigilant and knowledgeable to reduce risks related to as the following:

- The effects and adverse side effects of medications
- Proper identification of each patient
- Balancing the use of restraints against the rights and dignity of patients

Managers rely on the skills and decisions of physical therapists and physical therapist assistants involved in patient care to do no harm, or at the least do what any other physical therapist (or physical therapist assistant) would do in similar situations. Patients expect that their caregivers are competent and caring in providing care that is safe and results in a positive outcome.

Documentation

Documentation of care provided consumes a great deal of time in the operations of clinical practices. The medical record assists in protecting the patient, practitioners, and healthcare organization when questions about a patient's care arise. *It is a legal document* that demands managers attend to the production and maintenance of clear, complete records that can meet legal challenges if harm should come to a patient.

The medical record serves as the basis for planning patient care and reflects the continuity of decisions and the implementation of those plans. It is the evidence of the course of a patient's care, including communication among all caregivers. No one wants to be summoned to give a deposition to explain what happened with a particular patient only to be placed in the embarrassing position of having incomplete or inaccurate documentation. No one wants to be denied reimbursement because documentation reflecting the medical necessity and goals achieved by patients is missing in the medical record. Documentation is a powerful risk management tool.

Regardless of whether or not the medical record is a hard copy or electronically generated, if some basic principles of documentation are followed, the risk of lawsuits (for any reason) may lessen. These principles* include the following:

1. The patient record is presumed to be true. Licensed health professionals are trusted to be honest in their documentation unless proved otherwise.
2. Documentation of a physical therapist is the single most important evidence of the physical therapist's judgment, actions, skills, and decision-making.
3. Only the person who delivers care can, and must, document that care. One person cannot write notes for another or sign (verify electronically) notes written by another person.
4. The record must be detailed enough so that another practitioner can assume the care of the patient with no questions to be asked.

*Based on the booklet *The Practical Approach to Documentation* developed by Catherine G. Page and Debra F. Stern, 1994.

5. Information included should clearly identify important characteristics of the patient, support the diagnosis, justify treatment, and establish outcomes reached.

6. All significant information about the patient should be included in the medical record. A parallel set of informal notes is not considered part of this legal document.

7. Entries need to be timely. Writing the notes as part of the session can be important. Other members of the team may need to refer to the notes written earlier in the day before taking action with a patient.

8. Waiting until later in the day to complete documentation increases the risk that the notes may not be accurate because memory fails, particularly after a busy day when the therapist may be fatigued. Also, it is inefficient. Time spent trying to recall what happened earlier in the day lengthens the time needed to complete documentation.

9. Although the use of electronic documentation is increasing, written documentation must be legible to be of value to others as well as to the writer. It may be hard to convince others of one's credibility if a person cannot read his or her own writing.

10. All spaces on a standardized form must be completed even if the only item to enter is N/A or a line through the space. Readers need to know that the person documenting attended to all of the details without having to wonder whether the item was addressed and simply not documented. Blanks also provide the opportunity for others to modify documentation in ways that the person who made an entry may not intend.

11. Each entry in the medical record must be signed (legible, legal signature) or verified electronically, and dated. Managers need to clarify if the time of day entered is the time of the treatment session or the time the note is written. Documentation must be completed by the end of the day, or staff needs to stay until all documentation is completed. Hard-copy records should never leave the facility because the risk of loss and the potential breach of confidentiality and privacy are too high.

12. All sources of documentation must withstand audit. Treatment notes, attendance grids, appointment books, billing, and the like must all match. Inaccuracies reduce credibility, and they increase the likelihood of denial of payment.

13. The need for good spelling and grammar may be obvious, but the need for consistent use of abbreviations is often less so. Managers need to adopt a list of acceptable abbreviations for use by all, and a list of professional jargon that everyone should avoid. The fewer the number of abbreviations used, the better the communication. Some electronic systems automatically correct or select appropriate terminology.

14. Corrections must be clearly identified with a line through or an addendum to explain the error. Patient records cannot be deleted, erased, or obliterated with whiteout.

15. Keep the content of entries pertinent. Do not include information that is not of value in clinical decision-making. Do include *all* information that supports a patient's need for services. Do have space for additional comments on electronic forms so that information is thorough enough to present a complete picture of a patient's care.

16. Do not complain, criticize, or argue about the patient or other members of the team in the patient record. These entries raise concern about the quality of care provided if members of the team are in disagreement.

17. The patient record also serves as a record of all communication among caregivers including phone calls, faxes, and verbal orders. Missed appointments and the reasons for them need to be noted so that huge gaps in care do not place reimbursement at risk. Many systems electronically link documentation, scheduling, and payment to reduce the possibility of omissions and other errors.

18. Documentation must reflect reasonable and necessary care to accomplish patient goals.

19. Treatment notes reflect what care the patient received and the patient's response

to it. Progress notes refer back to the initial examination and goals set to demonstrate that the patient is moving toward their accomplishment.

Other Important Documents

Patient records are not the only the sensitive material that managers must secure. Patient record storage must comply with state and federal regulations related to access and to the length of time they must be kept available after patients are discharged. If staff takes informal notes to assist their memories of facts gathered during patient care for documentation in the medical record at a later time, these notes also must be secured or destroyed when they are no longer needed. Active records should be accessible only to those personnel who are involved in the patient's care and comply with all legal requirements.

Personnel records, contracts, leases, meeting minutes, and incorporation documents should be stored in a locked, fireproof box or safe. Passwords for access to computer-based documents need to be protected. Managers need to implement some system to keep both computer and hard-copy files organized so that authorized personnel may easily retrieve them.

Human Capital Risks

Organizations begin the management of human capital risks with current job descriptions that include qualifications, duties, reporting relationships, and key indicators of quality performance. Objective performance appraisals that align with job descriptions are the other key documents related to personnel management.

Should a person for some reason be unable to perform his or her duties, another person or persons must be ready to continue the critical functions so that the integrity of the organization is not compromised. To be taken seriously, these backup duties should be formally included in a job description rather than left to the nebulous "other duties as assigned" section. For example, a physical therapist assistant may be the backup for a business manager who obtains prior authorizations required for patient care. The business office manager may be the backup for scheduling patient appointments.

The manager of laboratory services may be the backup for the payroll responsibilities of the rehabilitation manager in a large organization.

Identifying the key responsibilities that must be sustained is a first, important step. Status reports also serve as a formal check that additional duties and responsibilities are not deliberately or unintentionally built on until job expectations become unrealistic and performance goals are impossible to meet. Finally, the risks presented by ineffective or suddenly dangerous employees and their effect on an organization must be controlled and eliminated.

Workforce Shortages

Not having enough people to do the work often leads to unhappy, stressed employees and dissatisfied patients. Patients on waiting lists for appointments or those who are simply not scheduled because of lack of personnel result in lost revenues. More important, the risk of worsening patient conditions owing to lack of, or delay in, treatments is a serious concern. Managers may need to identify other actions to take to improve efficiency and effectiveness in lieu of additional help. For example, they may decide to limit the growth of the practice by rejecting new referrals.

Contracting with outside agencies to fill positions temporarily is also risky. Temporary workers or "temps" do not often receive the same orientation, and they may not have the same commitment to the vision and mission of the organization as full-time employees do. They may bring ways of doing things from other experiences that are not consistent with the culture or goals of an organization. Should harm come to a patient at the hands of the temp, the legal responsibility may fall on the supervisor. The bigger risk is inconsistent care as temps come and go every few weeks. Managers have to weigh the risks of this constant turnover against the risks of a personnel shortage.

Recruitment

The risk of loss in the recruitment process is the investment in the costs of employment recruiters, want ads (newspapers, direct mail, online), or bonuses to current employees that may not lead to a new hire. The risks of workforce shortages are compounded by these additional losses. When the number of additional employees required has been determined, the next step may be to shift the analysis to identification of the factors that make the organization the employer of choice. If the supply of employees is small, then encouraging people who are employed in other organizations to change employers may be the only strategy that reduces the risk of loss. Potential employees need to be wary of offers too good to be true, and managers need to be concerned about risks to their reputations that may result from aggressively recruiting employees from competitors.

Hiring

Managers must determine the accuracy of credentials submitted at the time of hire. One of the greatest risks is a staff member who falsely represents his or her license to practice or other credentials. Conducting background checks of all healthcare employees has become another requirement to determine whether any criminal offenses had been committed or whether any disciplinary actions against a licensee were made in other jurisdictions. Because of this requirement, job applicants are more likely to divulge potential areas of concern than they have been in the past. The risks involved are that billing charges submitted by someone who is not licensed to practice may be retroactively denied or, more important, the knowledge and skill required to perform the job may be lacking. The result may be harm to patients and the organization's reputation.

Particularly when there is a shortage of workers, managers cannot risk being hasty to hire any available person. Scrutiny of credentials may, in fact, become even more important. Checking references and work history to verify information is as important for solo practitioners as it is for human resource professionals in large organizations.

Employment

Once workers have been employed, risks may be associated with personnel who fail to perform their professional duties. Although not intentional, injuries to patients in physical therapy may include burns, fractures, or the deterioration rather than improvement of their conditions. Typically, injuries result when staff fail to identify complicating factors, precautions, and contraindications. The failure of staff to closely monitor patients' ongoing responses

to treatment is another cause of unfortunate incidents. Failure to modify or correct interventions to assure patient safety during treatment sessions may also lead to injuries.

Costs of potential malpractice are typically deferred through professional liability insurance policies. Physical therapists who are employees need to determine whether they should obtain individual liability insurance policies, although the organization's insurance includes their work. Employers are responsible for the actions of their employees—vicarious liability. This does not mean that the employer will be sued and the employee will not. Attorneys will bring action against both parties on behalf of patients. If an employer believes an employee failed to perform his duties in a manner expected of professionals, the healthcare organization may decide not to support the conduct of the employee and assume no liability, or it may decide to take legal action against an employee as compensation for damages the organization was liable to pay.

Volunteers, independent contractors, even students in healthcare organizations are potentially liable for their actions that result in injury to others. They therefore need to decide the value and need for their own liability insurance. The perceived disadvantage to holding individual liability insurance is that professionals with individual insurance are more likely to be named in a suit along with the employer because the insurance provides more opportunity for a plaintiff to collect damages. The advantage to holding an individual policy is that an employee who is sued with or by an employer has some protection against the loss of personal assets. A rise in complaints, regardless how frivolous, may result in a rise in insurance premiums as well. Because insurers seek to control their costs, they may decide to reach a financial settlement rather than face the legal expenses of a trial. Professionals may be disappointed that the opportunity to clear their good names is not as important to insurers as actions that reduce the costs of claims. Physical therapists must consider the details of their liability insurance policies to understand their role in settlement decisions made by the insurer, and the potential risks to their reputation that the policies present.

Direction and Supervision

The inappropriate direction and supervision of physical therapist assistants or other supportive personnel are other key factors in professional liability. Managers must promote an organizational culture through policies and procedures that support the independent decision-making of physical therapists in directing and supervising others. Physical therapists need to decide for each patient in each treatment session when and what components of care may be transferred to the care of a physical therapist assistant. Because the patient's condition and the skills and expertise of physical therapist assistants vary, blanket policies about the work assignments of physical therapist assistants should be discouraged.

Managers must scrutinize the duties of non-licensed personnel as well. The type of direction and training they receive must be formalized to reduce the risks of illegal activity or the potential of harm to the patient. Because levels of delegation and supervision are included in many state statutes governing the practice of physical therapy, any harm to a patient because of failure to direct or supervise appropriately may not only lead to a lawsuit for damages, but may also place physical therapists at risk of disciplinary action against their licenses to practice. Harm that occurs during care that was delegated to others remains the responsibility of the physical therapists, and managers must make sure that all staff thoroughly understand this. Because the standards of practice vary from state to state, managers must also be certain that policies and procedures for staff mix, and the direction and supervision of supportive personnel promote compliance with the professional regulations specific to their state laws.

Patient Rapport

The most powerful risk management tool is establishing a professional rapport with patients. People may not take legal action when unintentional or unavoidable harm occurs if they feel they have been treated with respect and dignity in a caring manner. Patients may even decide *not* to take legal action when they feel the organization has made appropriate amends although the physical therapist or physical therapist assistant was obviously not careful enough. The truth is that mistakes happen. Unavoidable adverse incidents occur with the best intentions and skills. Taking immediate action when an injury occurs may deflect legal action. Patients expect the truth and resent actions taken to cover up mistakes. Being honest and calm in

developing a plan to manage the recovery from an injury that is the result of treatment is an important first step. Focusing on the patient's best interest often leads to more positive outcomes than efforts to minimize a problem or attempts to protect reputations.

Making follow-up calls and assuring patients that the physical therapist is available at any time should problems arise are other helpful risk management tools. Many patients have increased pain or new symptoms as a normal response to therapy interventions, so encouraging patients to call if they have any questions or problems after they leave a treatment session is good risk management. Reassuring patients that what they are feeling is expected and normal is often all that is needed to reduce many concerns about potential harm as a result of treatment. Staff must identify adverse reactions as such and address them immediately and appropriately.

Managers need to be sure that staff is prepared for patients with whom it is difficult to establish a rapport. Conflicts arise despite the best efforts of therapists to establish a professional relationship. Documentation of issues that arise and action taken is important. If conflicts cannot be resolved, transferring patients to another therapist or termination of care may be the only alternative. These situations must be handled carefully to avoid abandonment—unilateral severance of a professional relationship. Should harm come to the patient because of lack of care, there is also a risk of a lawsuit. Transfer of care or discharge plans must be acceptable to a patient, and therapists need to follow through on these actions to completion.

Another critical aspect of patient care for physical therapists arises because of their intimate contact with patients. Many physical therapy interventions involve a great deal of physical touching. If not clearly explained, and if permission to touch is not obtained, patients may misinterpret touching as sexual advances. **Inform before you perform** is a particularly important mantra in physical therapy practice. Patients need to be told where and why they need to be touched, and their permission obtained. Because sexual offenses are taken very seriously, any suggestion of impropriety by the therapist or patient must be thwarted. Discouraging sexual innuendos from patients without destroying rapport must be handled carefully. Transfer of care to another therapist or the presence of others during treatment sessions may be necessary.

Although managers cannot control affairs of the heart, avoiding personal relationships with patients is vital. Such associations suggest impropriety because of the power role of the caregiver, and they give other patients the impression of special or preferred treatment. Managers may need to be alert to these situations and take action to separate personal relationships from professional relationships by transferring the care of the patient to others. Similar relationships among staff may be equally difficult. There is a risk that other staff members may perceive these relationships as favoritism or leading to unfair decisions about assignments and performance evaluation. Their concerns may affect patient outcomes and job satisfaction.

Many patients are already involved in litigation because their need for rehabilitation results from work-related injuries, car accidents, or falls in public places. Managers need to pay particular attention to review their medical records for accuracy and completeness because the records will surely be presented as evidence for recovery of damages in court.

Professional Development

Professional development plans that address specific goals of each employee reduce risks because addressing the specific needs of individuals to improve knowledge and skills is more effective in reducing errors and harm than providing blanket courses directed to all. Employees need to justify their requests for approval of continuing education courses in terms of their professional development and the goals of the organization. This strategy helps to establish the costs for classes as an investment in the organization through its personnel. Managers need to direct attention to courses related to sociocultural issues, reimbursement, and other nonclinical topics. Without this need analysis, the investment in the development of continuing clinical competence may have no impact on the quality of care and patient outcomes.

Termination of Employment

Disagreements about promotions, salary increases, harassment, and discrimination may surround the termination of employment. Related lawsuits may be costly and disruptive, as are wrongful termination suits. Most states recognize that employment may be terminated at the will of the employer. Personnel policies must be clear and reviewed for compliance at least annually because of these complex legal relationships. Fairness, good faith, and communicating the rights and responsibilities of employees upon hire may avoid disagreeable terminations of employment. See Activity 11.1 for the opportunity to address all categories of risk.

Identifying Risks

Like the care given to keep policies and procedures current and relevant, *all* organizations need to formally review the effectiveness of efforts in preventing and controlling risks in detail, at least every 6 months. This review should be documented and

---

ACTIVITY 11.1
TIME-OUT FOR WRITING

Consider each category of risk as you review your program proposals, feasibility studies, or business plans. Some general questions are posed to begin the review process. Are budget modifications necessary because of identified risks? Are there changes in other components of the proposed document?

Hazard Risks	General liability and hazard insurance?
	Location and environment safe and secure?
	Costs?
Market Risks	Target market?
	Inbound marketing?
	Outbound marketing?
	Revenue? Costs?
	Backup plans?
Reputation Risks	Vision, mission, values, goals?
	Patient outcomes?
	Revenue?
Operations Risks	Safety?
	Documentation systems?
	Security of records?
	Revenue?
	Costs?
Human Capital Risks	Staffing mix?
	Credentials?
	Scheduling staff and patients?
	Professional development?
	Professional liability insurance?
	Contracts?
	Revenue?
	Costs?

the actions recommended should be implemented. This process may include a retrospective review of documents, such as committee minutes, quality assurance and safety reports, performance measures, peer reviews, benchmarks, qualitative data, process reviews, and submitted incident reports. The following questions raise the awareness of managers about potential professional liability risk factors. They may be used to identify areas that require risk management interventions as staff plan their professional development.

- Do therapists limit treatments of patients to those they are qualified to handle?
- Do therapists know their legal duties to their patients?
- Are therapists careful of being overly optimistic when discussing goals or prognosis with patients?
- Do all patients participate in rehabilitation with informed consent?
- Would the organization be embarrassed or prejudicially affected by its patients' records?
- Would the medical records give the organization and the individual maximum protection in a lawsuit?
- Do therapists take special action if a patient does not follow directions or discontinues treatment?
- Are therapists tactful with patients and families?
- Do therapists consult with each other and other health professionals to protect the patient?
- Are instructions to patients and families complete and understandable?
- Are patients notified when therapists will be away and that other arrangements have been made for their care?
- Is expert legal advice sought whenever the possibility of negligence is suggested?
- Do therapists refrain from making any statements about a case unless they have legal advice?
- Are all equipment and the environment in the safest condition possible?
- Are all therapists technically prepared to use all equipment?
- Are all employees qualified? Capable? Courteous?

- Do therapists keep current with courses and publications?
- Do therapists refrain from adverse criticism of other healthcare workers?
- Are disagreeable misunderstandings about fees avoided?
- Is special care taken in documentation on patients with work-related injuries, who are indigent, and all others who may be involved in litigation?
- How do the professional skills and experience of therapists compare with others in the profession?
- Are patients advised if treatments may be of doubtful efficacy?
- Are therapists always attentive and thoughtful so that patients feel confident and secure?
- Is consideration given to social, religious, and economic factors affecting patients?

Incidents, Occurrences, and Sentinel Events

Although these terms may be used interchangeably, an *incident* is anything that is not consistent with routine care or normal operations.[2] The word *occurrence* may be used for clinically related incidents. In healthcare, *sentinel events* is another term for incidents or occurrences that signal that a death or serious physical or psychological injury or risk thereof has occurred. Any poor outcome may be labeled as a sentinel event to emphasize that healthcare organizations are to be held accountable for them.

The problem is that the identification of these threats is dependent on reporting events. People may be reluctant to report because of perceived negative personal consequences or because they do not want to be known as whistle-blowers or troublemakers. Perhaps they simply do not realize that what happened is an actual incident to be reported. Often significant issues that are nonclinical are simply overlooked.[2] To make reporting easier, organizations typically have a standardized reporting form. The basic content of an incident report consists of the following:

1. Date and time of incident
2. Names of persons involved
3. Age, sex, diagnosis, and physician (if patient involved)

4. Description of the event
5. Name and contact information of witnesses
6. Witness's description of the event
7. Treatment offered or rendered
8. Name, title, position of person completing the report
9. Signature and date of person preparing the report

Incidents should include only the facts, very detailed facts, while avoiding personal opinions or judgments. Whenever possible, the person involved in the incident should complete the report rather than having it completed by someone using secondary information. The typical procedure is that the report is submitted to the immediate manager first. Managers may find that they must suggest revisions and closely monitor the completion of all components of incident reports so that information is accurate. Immediate action may be necessary, but it should not mean that managers forgo more analysis of the incident. Managers are responsible for frequently reminding the reporter that the incident should not be discussed with anyone else, whether other people were involved or not, to preserve accurate presentation of facts without bias.

Because incident reports are treated as confidential information to be used internally for quality assurance and other administrative action, they should never be referred to in the medical record. A reference to an incident report may result in an inadvertent disclosure of the incident report during legal proceedings. Confidentiality of reports is critical to protecting the parties involved and the organization itself. Most states protect this information as part of an organization's quality assurance process so that people and organizations use the process without fear of repercussions. See Activity 11.2.

Analyzing Risks

Risk managers are challenged to analyze the data about potential risks and incident reports to arrive at a root cause. The root cause is the factor that, if eliminated, the incident or potential risk will not recur. Root cause analysis focuses on systems and processes to determine the what, how, why, when, and where of an unwanted event.

Healthcare organizations require a more complex approach to risk analysis that focuses on the

---

ACTIVITY 11.2
AN INCIDENT REPORT

Critique this completed incident report.

INCIDENT REPORT
GREENDALE HEALTH CARE

WARNING: The information in this quality assurance report is confidential and subject to privilege as defined by state and federal statutes. Penalties may apply for unauthorized release of this information. Do not file or refer to this report in the medical record.

Date and time of incident: *October 1, 2007   3:15 P.M.*

Names of persons involved: *Brenda Jones, PT, and Ethel Walker, patient*

Age, sex, diagnosis, and physician (if patient involved): *88-year-old female patient of Dr. Creighton*

Description of the event: *Patient fell in hallway when walking with the PT*

Name and contact information of witnesses: *none*

Witness's description of the event: *none*

Treatment offered or rendered: *X-ray of right hip*

Name, title, position of person completing report: *Richard Ricardo, OTR, Rehab Manager*

---

many interacting system processes rather than people as the major source of most patient care risks or incidents. Although the format may vary, an expanded root cause analysis is commonly used for more formal, detailed analysis in healthcare. Figure 11.2 provides one example of the steps involved in risk analysis.

Not all of the components of the organization may need to be addressed in the analysis of any incident. More likely, some combination of factors, or other factors not included in Figure 11.2, may be identified in the process. This multifactor model is more conducive to examining possible alternative root causes. In healthcare, the added dimension, particularly for sentinel events, is often to demand evidence to support the identification of the root cause, alternatives, and actions selected. Rather than relying on what may be personal biases in the process, a focus on reliable sources of information that support the cause and effect relationships identified

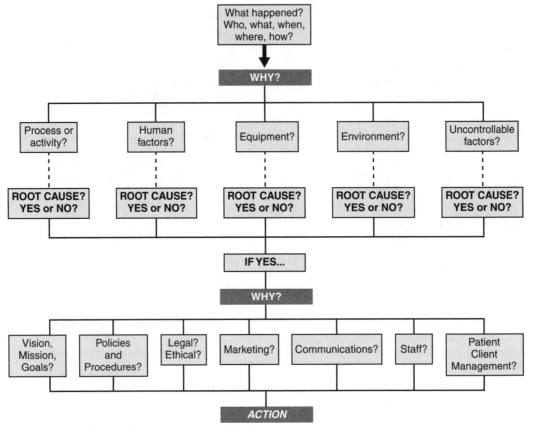

FIGURE 11.2 Root cause analysis.

increases the power and acceptance of action to be taken.

Legal Responsibilities of Managers*

The Legal Responsibilities of Managers section was prepared in consultation with John P. Page, Esq.

Managers must understand that every legal right includes a duty for themselves and others. The classic example is that the right of free expression does not include the right to scream "Fire!" in a crowded theater when there is no fire. As another example, a person's right to swing her arms ends when one of them touches another person. The person swinging has a duty to take reasonable care to avoid the danger of hitting someone else. As a healthcare example, managers may have the legal right to hire and fire employees at will, but they also have the duty to take such actions seriously by following guidelines promulgated to enforce employment laws.

Another basic legal principle is that "every wrong has a remedy." Managers may become involved with criminal, civil, and administrative actions. Courts enforce violations of criminal laws by closely following legal remedies such as fines and/or imprisonment by enforcing a right, imposing a penalty, or making a new court order. Civil law violations may involve both legal and equitable remedies. When there is no adequate legal remedy, the court creates equitable remedies (often monetary) that are at the discretion of the judge. *Equity* is broadly defined as fundamental fairness. Violations of statutory laws such as practice acts governing healthcare professionals in each state are "remedied" through penalties and fines established by these statutes. They are heard by internal courts within state administrative agencies.

Managers require expert legal advice for many of the complex decisions they face. In many healthcare organizations, in-house legal counsel and risk managers provide advice to managers as issues arise. Independent practitioners also need access to legal counsel for many decisions. This section serves only to highlight two legal concerns that most often impact mid-level managers—contracts and malpractice. These general discussions should be used as the basis for consideration of any specific experiences, which should be left to consultation with legal counsel.

Contracts

Contracts that are of most interest to healthcare managers include:

- Service and equipment maintenance contracts
- Contracts for employee benefits
- Contracts with third-party payers
- Contracts with registries, placement agencies, or independent contractors
- Employment contracts
- Implied contracts with patients
- Clinical education agreements

Contracts are legally enforceable agreements created when an offer by one party is accepted by another. They may be oral or written and they must include some benefit or consideration for each party. Some provisions of all contracts are implicit (e.g., each party must act in good faith and deal fairly). Each party in a contract is entitled to the benefit of its bargain under the contract; therefore, managers have a duty to perform exactly as a contract provides. Although a party may be excused from a duty if it becomes impossible (frustration of performance), a court may compel a party to keep an exact promise to a specific performance or to pay money damages. Only the court can decide that the substitution of damages is fair.

Both oral and written contracts are a legally binding exchange of promises or agreements between parties, enforceable as law. Managers should rely on attorneys to negotiate contracts to assure that their legal interests are protected. For example, restrictive covenants in employment contracts prevent an employee from doing certain things after employment ends. Can the employee work for a competitor? How soon? How nearby? Are any business secrets at risk? Attorneys ensure such contracts conform with state law, or in some cases select which state's laws will be used in contract negotiations. Attorneys are also consulted when there is a breach of contract and identify the remedies available to employers.

Managers need to be cautious about promises they make to employees that may be interpreted as contracts. They also need to remind staff about inadvertently making promises about outcomes to patients that may be taken as verbal contracts. For example, physical therapists working with professional athletes may need to be careful in their discussions with these patients because conversations meant to be casual could be heard as contracts. In this example, a physical therapist should think twice before responding with, "No problem, you will be as good as new by Saturday."

Torts

A tort is an injury or wrong—other than breach of contract—committed on another person, his or her property, or reputation for which the injured party is entitled to seek compensation. For example, damages sustained in an automobile accident may be a tort of negligence because there is a duty to avoid hitting another car. In healthcare, the duty to respect and protect patients and their privacy is probably the most important duty. Failure to do so is taken very seriously by the law. If reasonable care is not exercised, that failure in duty constitutes the tort of negligence and creates liability for any resulting injury.

Negligence is the failure to exercise that degree of care that a reasonable person would exercise under the same circumstances. Other torts may be based on intentional injuries or wrongs, which also may be criminal acts. Distinguishing whether an action was negligent or intentional is important in the law because of the difference in damages that might be awarded. Intentional torts may include additional punitive damages beyond the actual losses that are the direct result of negligence. Intent is sometimes implied from the acts of the parties.

Professional Malpractice

Malpractice is a particular tort based on negligence and of special interest to healthcare managers. The tort of professional malpractice consists of the following elements:

- The duty to conform to a certain *standard of care*.
- A failure to conform to the required *standard of care*.

- Actual injury or damage.
- A legally sufficient causal connection between the conduct and the injury.

Standard of care is a legal term with a precise meaning. Practice acts that govern professional practices usually include a statement similar to the one below that is the accepted legal definition of standard of care:

> *A given healthcare provider must provide the level of care, skill, and treatment that, in light of all relevant surrounding circumstances, is recognized as acceptable and appropriate by reasonably prudent similar healthcare providers.*

Although definitions may vary in detail, confusion will result from attempts to paraphrase the term or apply it for purposes other than legal analysis. For instance, most important, the legal standard of care does not necessarily equate with professional practices, guidelines, or other clinical "standards."

Because of the variables involved, the standard of care, and whether a physical therapist negligently failed to comply with that standard must be determined case by case. It is *not* malpractice if the patient received appropriate care, but the outcome was not as expected because of other factors. These determinations can be established only by competent expert testimony at trial. Because expert opinions may vary, the result is often a "battle of the experts." Consider the following scenario:

> *A physical therapist might follow and then modify a postoperative plan of care for a patient with a total hip replacement as necessary to accommodate an individual's current status. That patient may remain unable to walk independently as expected because of circulatory deficits or the patient's fear of falling. In this case, the therapist performed as another therapist would with the same patient and performed carefully so that harm or injury to the patient was avoided during that plan of care. The failure to achieve the patient's goal of independent ambulation is, most likely, not professional negligence.*
>
> *Conversely, using the same scenario, if the therapist failed to address the patient's circulatory problems and fears, resulting in the patient's inability to walk, that may be considered malpractice because a prudent therapist in similar circumstances would have taken all of these important factors impacting performance into consideration.*

Managers and Harm to Patients

Unfortunately, managers may face incidents that result in harm to patients. When an incident occurs, managers must ensure that employees avoid discussions of the incident. The incident is reported first within the organization according to its procedures. In the absence of a risk manager, the organization may report directly to the insurance company that is providing professional or general malpractice insurance or to an attorney. In many states, organizations must report any harm to a patient to the appropriate practice board(s) for investigation of potential violation of a practice act(s). Managers must be certain that documentation is thorough, is accurate, and held as confidential during these investigative and legal processes. Managers must insist that employees involved in incidents seek assistance from and follow the instructions of risk managers and attorneys during these difficult times.

Receiving subpoenas to provide legal testimony and records can be disruptive to an organization's operations and can cause personal distress to employees. When an employee with a good performance history is involved in a negative incident, managers may need to be supportive to avoid the devastating effect on the employee. Conversely, managers have other challenges if there is a history of questionable performance that has now resulted in harm to a patient. Documentation of employee performance becomes critical, and documentation of patient care is equally essential to provide accurate information during malpractice suits.

Lawsuits are expensive and disruptive processes for the people directly involved and the organization as a whole. Managers must attend to the seriousness of these lawsuits while maintaining the smooth operations of the organization. These situations may evolve into adversarial situations as employers and employees each retain their own attorneys to represent them in lawsuits. Managers must continue to uphold their duties to employees and patients in these difficult situations with consideration for reputation risks.

Duties of Organizations*

*The Duties of Organizations section was prepared in consultation with John P. Page, Esq.

Managers also must attend to laws that apply to the organization as well as persons. Healthcare organizations must comply with many federal, state, and county laws that affect a wide range of their responsibilities for safety, payments of taxes, and the like. Wrongful actions by healthcare organizations may be prosecuted under any or all jurisdictions just like the actions of individuals. Some examples are:[3]

- False Claims Act of 1986: prohibits knowingly submitting false claim for reimbursement to the government, getting paid for a false claim, or falsifying a record to get paid.
- Medicare and Medicaid Patient Protection Act of 1987: prohibits solicitations or receipt of remuneration for anything of value in return for referring a person or furnishing products to a healthcare organization (anti-kickback legislation).
- Health Insurance Portability and Accountability Act of 1996 (HIPAA): reduces fraud through a coordinated national program of federal, state, and local law enforcement. Examples of healthcare fraud include billing for services not rendered, falsifying a diagnosis to justify tests and treatment, misrepresenting procedures (cosmetic surgery), upcoding services and supplies, unbundling a procedure so that each stage is a separate procedure, billing for medically unnecessary services, waiving co-payments or deductible payments, overbilling an insurer.
- HIPAA Title II: provides national standards for electronic healthcare transactions; national identifiers for providers, health insurance plans, and employers; standards for security and privacy of health information.

Organizations are responsible for implementing policies and procedures systems to assure compliance with these and many other laws. Failure to do so compromises professionals who are required to meet these legal obligations as part of their professional duties.

Respondeat Superior

Under the legal theory of *respondeat superior* ("let the master answer"), employers are held legally responsible for the actions of employees during the course of their employment. Patients may take legal action directly against the health professionals who harmed them and against the healthcare organizations that employ the health professionals. This concept reflects vicarious liability in which one party can be liable for the actions of another. This liability becomes more complicated when contingent employees are involved in an adverse incident.

The actions of the employer, conversely, may negatively impact the duties and professional responsibilities of employees. From the failure to provide a safe and secure environment to lack of accountability for coding and billing, executive actions may lead to adverse effects on employees and patients. Failure to meet an organization's licensing requirements also may negatively affect the safety and health of employees.

Ethical Responsibilities of Managers

Some healthcare managers may be former clinical healthcare professionals. Their understanding of ethical responsibilities may easily transfer to their new managerial roles. Other managers may adopt codes of ethics developed through professional associations for healthcare managers. An example may be found at the webpages of the American College of Healthcare Executives. See Web Resources. In either case, the expectations of employees are that managers meet their obligations to patients and other stakeholders as moral advocates and role models for the values necessary for the delivery of quality healthcare.

Healthcare ethics span professional ethics that guide what is right or wrong in patient care, managerial ethics that guides what is right and wrong for the organization, and social responsibility that guides what is right and wrong for the good of society. Examples of healthcare issues that require ethical consideration are patients who cannot afford expensive medication or treatments to control their conditions, marketers that exaggerate benefits of new programs, a human resource director who thinks a supervisor is discriminating against older workers, an employer who fails to keep promises made to a new employee during a job interview, a maintenance director who is taking kickbacks from suppliers, managers who decide which employees will be laid off, and those who provide needed community services that are not profitable.[4]

Healthcare ethical decisions have more far-reaching implications than individual, professional clinical decisions. For instance, managers have broader responsibilities for enhancing the overall quality of life in a community and the dignity and well-being of patients, and for creating an equitable, accessible, effective, and efficient healthcare system. A careful, ethical assessment of the impact of their decisions is important to safeguard the rights of patients and employees and the interests of the organization as a whole. Healthcare organizations must consistently make efforts to demonstrate their willingness to be held accountable for their important role in society. These efforts include:[5]

1. Enforcing standards that are followed every day while remembering that a standard is the floor and not the ceiling of performance that may be required for excellent quality care
2. Positive responses to errors and problems rather than finger-pointing and blame-fixing
3. Celebrating rather than punishing the reporting of errors and problems
4. Eliminating immunity for wrongdoing or misbehavior (including actions of trustees and executives)
5. Transparent public sharing of information about the organization, including mistakes
6. Honesty and trustworthiness that cannot be broken

Conflicts of Interest

Managers may need to be particularly sensitive to potential conflicts of interest. Conflict of interest is a matter of degree and often difficult to identify. Because there may be legal implications, managers must be careful to avoid the benefits that result from using their positions of authority to gather information, to use information to adversely affect an organization, or to accept gifts in exchange for influence. Failure to inform their organizations of involvement in or affiliations with other organizations that may impact their decisions may raise legal and ethical issues.

A Manager's Responsibility

Risk management, legal, and ethical responsibilities underlie all other managerial responsibilities. Managers who view these foundations as consultative rather than punitive are more likely to have others assume these responsibilities as part of their own work. Preventing, reducing, and eliminating risks requires managers to be alert to a wide range of possible occurrences and decisions. They must also be alert to the potential legal implications of their actions, the actions of employees, and the actions of their organizations to protect patients in the context of ethical duties of healthcare providers. They need to seek legal advice rather than make assumptions that may result in more complex situations than necessary. Although it may be tiresome and unwise to be on the defensive, it is also important to seek risk management advice to identify red-flag situations that may arise with employees, patients, or even executives. Managers may need to remind staff of the following catchphrases that may help reduce risks and legal action:

- Clean Up, Don't Cover Up
- Defect Prevention, Rather Than Defect Detection
- Inform Before You Perform
- Listen, Listen, Listen
- No Second Chances
- Actions Speak Louder Than Words
- Treat Others As You Expect to Be Treated
- Under Promise and Over Deliver
- Follow Up and Follow Through

Activity 11.3 provides the opportunity to engage in decision-making to reduce hazard, market, reputation, operations, and/or human capital risks. Each scenario marked with an asterisk is a synopsis of an *actual* complaint presented to a physical therapy board as required in some jurisdictions (states) when legal action involving a licensed physical therapist or physical therapist assistant and harm to a patient occurred.

ACTIVITY 11.3
ANALYZING THE RISK

For each of the scenarios, identify the risks, legal concerns, and ethical issues. Did a violation of the practice act or rules of practice in a given state occur? If you were on the board of physical therapy practice, what action might you recommend to the other board members? Were the professionals involved negligent? What ethical concerns should be addressed? Refer to the root cause analysis chart in Figure 11.2 and consider strategic planning to explore the important issues in each scenario from a managerial perspective: (1) What is the current situation? *Adverse event or problem,* (2) Where do we want to be? *No recurrence nor specific improvement,* (3) What do we have to work with? (4) How will we get there?

SCENARIO 1*

A patient's ambulatory ability at 3 weeks post–total hip arthroplasty had improved enough that the physical therapist coordinated with nursing staff to have the patient use a walker with standby supervision anywhere within the nursing home. While walking to the dining room the next day, the patient reported sharp hip pain and began to collapse. The nursing assistant walking with him was able to break his fall and he was seated in a chair. He reported that he was fine.

The next day, his hip pain limited his ability to walk at all. The nursing supervisor ordered an x-ray that revealed dislocation of the hip prosthesis. His recovery period was significantly lengthened because of the physical stress of a second surgery and the development of pneumonia during his second hospital stay.

The patient sued the rehabilitation center and the physical therapist for failing to properly instruct and supervise the nursing assistant about the correct gait instructions.

SCENARIO 2*

A woman with a history of osteoporosis was receiving physical therapy for a fracture of the right wrist. Because her function was also limited by back pain, the physical therapist added hot pack and massage to the spine to her treatment plan. The patient reported temporary relief from the back treatments.

The patient called to cancel her 12th appointment and told the receptionist that she had a fracture of one of her vertebra from the massage and would be unable to continue treatments. The receptionist documented the phone call as "cancellation."

The patient sued the physical therapist because of the new injury, which also led to her inability to continue therapy for her wrist. She developed contractures of the wrist that severely limited her ability to use her hand. She also claimed that the physical therapist violated the practice act because he did not have doctor's orders to treat her back in the first place.

SCENARIO 3*

A patient who has a reputation for making constant demands during her treatment sessions is treated with hot packs to her right shoulder for pain related to her right hemiplegia. She was given a bell to signal if she needed anything. She was left unattended throughout the treatment session, although several people in the department heard her yelling that the hot pack was too hot and she could not move it. She rang the bell many times. The physical therapist assistant, from across the room, asked her to please be quiet, and reminded the patient that she complained at the last treatment session of not enough heat.

When the physical therapist assistant removed the hot pack at the end of the 20-minute treatment, the patient insisted that she look at her skin because the hot pack was placed over her clothing. The physical therapist assistant discovered a burn that had already begun to blister and applied ice. The patient required a skin graft and sued the physical therapy organization, the physical therapist, and the physical therapist assistant.

SCENARIO 4*

A physical therapist asked a new coworker who had just completed a certification in mobilization to consult with him on a patient who continued to have severe pain and limited spinal range of motion after 2 weeks of daily physical therapy sessions. The patient agreed to be seen by the coworker at the next treatment session. At the beginning of that session, the physical therapist was called away to care for another patient after giving brief

continued

ACTIVITY 11.3
ANALYZING THE RISK—cont'd

introductions and providing the new therapist with a brief summary of the patient's problem. The coworker proceeded with his intervention.

The patient experienced a severe increase in pain during the mobilization procedure. The patient asked that the treatment stop immediately and she left the clinic.

She sued both physical therapists and the physical therapy corporation because she claimed the treatment caused an exacerbation of her problem that required several unsuccessful surgeries. The primary therapist admitted that he did not discuss the patient's history with his coworker. The coworker admitted that he did not review the medical record or conduct his own history and examination before initiating treatment.

SCENARIO 5*
A patient with severe knee pain for an extended period reluctantly agreed to an arthroscopic procedure and he was referred to a physical therapy center for a standardized postsurgical regimen. Because of a waiting list, there was a 2-week delay in initiating physical therapy. The patient did the best he could at home with the exercises the surgeon's nurse gave him to follow.

The physical therapist conducted the initial examination and decided to begin the regimen as though the patient had already had 2 weeks of physical therapy. She assigned the physical therapist assistant to continue the regimen and to report to her every third session.

The physical therapist assistant, new to the center and the protocol, included passive stretching of the knee and continued to stretch, although the patient complained of a great deal of pain and heard a pop in the knee.

The patient asked to see the physical therapist and reported that he had a great deal of pain and that he had never been stretched to that extreme before. Without examining the knee, the physical therapist applied a cold pack and instructed the patient to apply cold several times a day.

The patient never returned for treatment. The patient sued the physical therapist, the physical therapist

assistant, the physical therapy center, and the surgeon for making the referral. The patient required additional surgery and extensive rehabilitation to repair the reinjured knee. The documentation includes only checks on a flow sheet.

SCENARIO 6*
A child had been progressing well with his exercise program for the past several months and his parents were very pleased. As a reward for good behavior, he was allowed to jump on the small trampoline in the department for a few minutes at the end of the treatment sessions.

During one trampoline play session, although the physical therapist was guarding him, she turned her attention away for a second. The child fell, suffering a concussion and fracture of the left humerus. The immobilization of the arm resulted in an elbow contracture and prolonged physical therapy in another center. The care was complicated by the child's new fears and confusion, although the physician reported no evidence of brain damage resulting from the head injury. The family sued the physical therapist and the center.

SCENARIO 7*
A patient reported increased numbness and tingling down the right upper extremity that had been getting progressively worse during the 2 weeks she had been receiving physical therapy, although her cervical spasms and headaches were reduced. The physical therapist urged her to see a neurosurgeon as soon as possible.

The patient returned to her family physician for a referral to a neurosurgeon. Instead of a referral, the physician told her just to continue the physical therapy.

Physical therapy continued for another week until the physical therapist decided that she should discontinue therapy because the treatment was having no impact on the numbness and tingling. She discharged the patient, again advised her to see a neurosurgeon, and even suggested the name of someone to call.

Two weeks later the patient had an MRI that revealed herniation of two cervical intervertebral discs. Although surgery was successful, the patient was left with residual weakness and numbness in the right upper extremity.

She sued the physical therapist and her family physician for failing to assess her condition correctly and in a timely manner.

SCENARIO 8*

A patient signed a financial responsibility form that all patients sign in a certain outpatient center. He understood that he was agreeing to pay 20% of the total bill and the office manager assured him it would not be more than $20/visit. At the end of his course of rehabilitation, the patient had paid $1,000 for 50 visits and the insurance paid the center $5,000 ($100/visit) as their contract permitted, although the center had billed for $300/visit.

The patient's doctor ordered 16 additional physical therapy visits. The business manager/receptionist advised the patient that the insurance company might not approve the additional visits. He signed an agreement stating he would pay for the 16 visits if the insurance company denied the claim. He was assured a fair payment plan would be established to pay for these additional services as they were for his previous payments.

The insurance company offered to reimburse the physical therapy center for the 16 additional treatment sessions at $57/visit. The physical therapist rejected the offer because it was too low and advised the patient of his action.

The patient reported the physical therapist to the Board of Physical Therapy Practice in his state, charging that the physical therapist committed fraud, which is a violation of the practice act. He claimed it was dishonest to charge him the full $300 amount that was billed to the insurance company when the therapist accepted less for the same treatment previously. He felt that he should have been charged the $120 that was collected from him and the insurance company for the first 50 visits. He did not pay, and refused to pay until this matter was settled. He reported that the physical therapist's business manager was harassing him for the money.

SCENARIO 9*

A woman had been receiving the same outpatient treatment for pain relief three times a week intermittently during the past 6 months since her spinal surgery after a car accident. One day she received her usual treatment, which included interferential electrical current with the electrodes placed along the lumbar spine and at the right lateral ankle. Her usual therapist had set up the treatment and left to care for an inpatient in the hospital.

Another physical therapist removed the electrodes at the end of the treatment. He noticed more than usual redness at the ankle. He asked the patient whether she felt any discomfort and the patient said that she really did not ever feel anything because of the numbness in her leg. The therapist became very excited and said that this electrotherapy treatment should never have been administered.

The patient also reported that her therapist had shown her how to adjust the current and maybe she (the patient) had turned it up too high this time.

A burn was noted at the right ankle during the next treatment session, and the patient was referred to the emergency room. The patient eventually required surgical débridement and a skin graft to repair the wound. She sued the physical therapy center and the physical therapists.

SCENARIO 10*

A patient had a left total knee replacement, which became infected and was rejected. The prosthesis was replaced and he began a usual regimen of physical therapy. About 8 weeks later, he was discharged from physical therapy because he had reached his goals. The office manager told him he would have to pay for further treatment himself because reimbursement for more than 8 weeks of therapy would be denied.

He returned to his physician, who was persuaded by the patient that he could make more gains with additional therapy, which the doctor then ordered. The patient went to a different center to continue treatment.

continued

His new physical therapist noted at transfer of care that the patient continued to have edema, decreased strength and range of motion of the left knee, and an antalgic gait.

The plan of care in the new center included isokinetic exercises, which he had not had before, followed by passive static hamstring stretch and ice application. All interventions in the first two treatment sessions were completed without complaint. Three days after the second session, the patient went to the doctor because of increased pain that he attributed to the new exercises. An x-ray revealed no problems, but pain was elicited at the lower pole of the patella. The doctor noted how well the patient was walking. The doctor discontinued physical therapy and the patient was advised to swim for exercise.

Two weeks later, the patient returned to his doctor because the pain had worsened and he was unable to walk. There was no loosening of the prosthesis and the doctor told him to come back in a month. Three weeks later, his condition was unchanged and exploratory surgery was scheduled. It was discovered that the patellar tendon was ruptured at the tibial tubercle. The revision and repair of the tendon that were done at that point were unsuccessful because the patient could not tolerate any knee flexion. An arthrodesis was performed 3 months later.

The patient sued the second physical therapy practice, claiming that his knee was hyperflexed on the isokinetic machine, resulting in the tendon tear.

SCENARIO 11*

The patient was an 88-year-old resident in a skilled nursing rehabilitation center at the time of the incident. His poor medical condition (general debilitation secondary to pneumonia) was complicated by dementia for which he was receiving medication. The rehabilitation team reports on the medical record reflect the decision that the patient required restraints except under limited, supervised conditions because of his high risk for falling.

The patient was transported to the therapy room in a wheelchair with a restraint properly applied. The occupational therapist assistant removed the restraint, draping it around the handgrip of the wheelchair, and attempted to work with the patient, who was too lethargic to participate.

The patient's occupational therapy was to be followed directly by a physical therapy session. The physical therapist assistant who had been assigned to work with the patient for his session was working with another patient in the same room. The occupational therapist presented the patient to the physical therapist without reapplying the restraint belt and reported that the patient could not be awakened. The occupational therapist then returned to the staff office, and the occupational therapist assistant left the room to escort a patient to her room.

The physical therapist immediately tried to awaken the patient, without success, and left the room to report her findings to the nurse. The physical therapist assistant left the treatment area to transport another patient to his room.

Shortly thereafter, the occupational therapist and occupational therapist assistant in the adjoining staff office heard a loud bang. The patient had stood up and fallen to the floor. While in other areas of the nursing home, the physical therapist and physical therapist assistant heard the coded announcement on the loudspeaker indicating a patient had been injured in rehabilitation. They hurried back to the therapy room. The physical therapist's initial examination of the patient suggested that he had broken his hip.

The patient was transported to an emergency room where it was confirmed that the fall had resulted in a fracture of the left hip. Surgery to repair the hip was performed. The patient died a few weeks later. The family sued the nursing home, the physical therapist, physical therapist assistant, occupational therapist, and occupational therapist assistant.

SCENARIO 12*

Eric Walters feels fortunate that he was finally able to hire Candace Dumar, a physical therapist assistant with almost 20 years of experience in acute care and nursing homes, although he was hoping to hire another physical therapist in his outpatient practice. After a few weeks, Julie Spencer, one of the physical therapists on staff,

ACTIVITY 11.3
ANALYZING THE RISK—cont'd

approaches Eric to discuss her concerns. She feels that Candace is not transitioning to the outpatient setting very well. Candace has been modifying plans of care routinely without consulting with Julie, and she had heard Candace giving patients inaccurate information about their conditions and goals. When Julie discussed her concerns with Candace, she told her she has 20 years of experience and knows what she is doing. Her last employer had insisted that she take on more responsibility for patients that she was assigned and she does not want those duties curtailed.

SCENARIO 13
Unfortunately, one of the physical therapists on staff, George Prego, at one of the St. Barnabas Hospital outpatient centers had received a second verbal warning about his unprofessional behavior including rudeness, tardiness, and disregard for patients' concerns and well-being. Before the manager, Sam Zacharias, fired him a week later, George's reputation had already had a negative effect—loss of referrals from several physicians, patient cancellations—and it provoked anger among the staff who felt that Sam should have acted sooner.

SCENARIO 14
Determine the legal requirements for documentation in the model practice act found at the webpages of the Federation of State Boards of Physical Therapy (https://www.fsbpt.org/RegulatoryTools/ModelPracticeAct/index.asp). Compare with the actual licensure statutes in selected states. What are the potential risks addressed by the statutes?

SCENARIO 15
Vincent Valler is the manager of a large satellite outpatient clinic within a multicenter regional healthcare system. The patient waiting list is out of control, with the average wait time to begin therapy at 15 calendar days and between 12 and 18 patients on the list at any time.

SCENARIO 16
Erma Nguyen has heard the rumbling of discontentment among her staff. They are trying to understand how profits of their healthcare system have increased 23% in the past year (as reported in the local newspaper) but their salaries have remained frozen for the past 2 years.

SCENARIO 17
Carla Morsetti, the manager at Snow Valley Nursing and Rehabilitation Center, is so saddened that she has difficulty performing her job. Several weeks ago, a patient was injured while in the physical therapy department. Although she, her staff, and the administration took all appropriate action, the patient died and the family is suing for damages. They contend that the accident in therapy contributed to her death. The staff involved in the incident is not handling the patient's death well, and Carla is becoming increasingly concerned as the person in the middle of this situation.

It seems that the patient's death is the principal topic discussed in the nursing home and she cannot seem to get anything else done. The staff is divided between those who are defending the actions of the therapists and assistant involved in the incident and those who are demanding that Carla fire all staff involved. The attorney for the nursing home has advised her to avoid talking about the situation, and she has been advised that subpoenas from attorneys for the therapists to appear at deposition hearings have been received by the nursing home administrator. Sorting out the facts of the incident at the time from all of the conversations and rumors circulating since then has distressed Carla.

SCENARIO 18
Stephanie Morgan is concerned that her therapists do not wash their hands consistently as they move from patient to patient. There is a sink in one corner of the exercise room, in each public restroom, and in the staff bathroom. Staff has reported the locations are inconvenient as the major reason for failing to wash their hands.

REFERENCES

1. American Society for Healthcare Risk Management (ASHRM). http://www.ashrm.org/ashrm/about/index.shtml?page=index. Accessed July 28, 2013.
2. Carroll R. *Risk Management Handbook for Health Care Organizations.* San Francisco, CA: Jossey-Bass; 2001.
3. Pozgar GD. *Legal Aspects of Health Care Administration.* 11th ed. Sudbury, MA: Jones & Bartlett; 2012.
4. Olden P. *Management of Healthcare Organizations: An Introduction.* Chicago, IL: Health Administration Press; 2011.
5. Friedman, E. A question of accountability. In: Hofmann PB, Perry F, eds. *Management Mistakes in Healthcare.* New York, NY: Cambridge University Press; 2010.

WEB RESOURCES

American College of Healthcare Executives (ACHE). Code of ethics. http://www.ache.org/abt_ache/code.cfm. Accessed November 22, 2013.

American Physical Therapy Association (APTA). Legal topics of interest to physical therapists and physical therapist assistants. http://www.apta.org/Legal/Topics/. Accessed November 22, 2013.

American Physical Therapy Association (APTA): Risk management. http://www.apta.org/RiskManagement/. Accessed November 22, 2013.

Cornell University. Constitutions, statutes and codes. http://www.law.cornell.edu/statutes.html (Note: Links to individual U.S. States.) Accessed November 22, 2013.

The Joint Commission. Facts about the Sentinel event policy. http://www.jointcommission.org/assets/1/18/Sentinel%20Event%20Policy.pdf. Accessed November 22, 2013.

Library of Congress. Administrative law guide. http://www.loc.gov/law/help/administrative.php. Accessed November 22, 2013.

Bureau of International Information Programs. Clack, G., Executive Editor. About America: How the U.S. is governed. http://photos.state.gov/libraries/korea/49271/dwoa_122709/Outline-of-the-U_S_-Legal-System.pdf. Accessed November 22, 2013.

U.S. Department of Health and Human Resources. Inspector General. Hospital incident reporting. http://oig.hhs.gov/oei/reports/oei-06-09-00091.asp. Accessed November 22, 2013.

U.S. Department of Health and Human Services. Patient safety primers; root cause analysis. Available at http://psnet.ahrq.gov/primer.aspx?primerID=10. Accessed November 22, 2013.

U.S. Department of Labor. Occupational Safety and Health Administration (OSHA). http://www.osha.gov/SLTC/healthcarefacilities/index.html. Accessed November 22, 2013.

U.S. Small Business Administration. Contract law. http://www.sba.gov/community/blogs/contract-law-%E2%80%93-how-create-legally-binding-contract. Accessed November 22, 2013.

CHAPTER 12

Communication Responsibilities

LEARNING OBJECTIVES

- Determine oral and written communications commonly used by managers.
- Apply strategies for formal and informal meetings.
- Discuss telephone communication.
- Prepare for a business meeting.
- Prepare for a presentation to a group.
- Prepare selected written communication.
- Distinguish general literacy from health literacy.
- Address common communication hurdles in healthcare organizations.

Overview

The importance of communication in meeting managerial responsibilities has been addressed throughout Section 2—sharing an organization's vision and mission, outbound marketing, interviewing potential employees, and incident reports. Communication is a broad and complex topic that is viewed from a wide range of perspectives. Scholars in fields from sociology and psychology to digital technology, art, media, and literature use different lenses to study the transfer of information from a sender to a receiver. This chapter focuses on a small component of this broad topic by addressing selected oral and written communication skills important to managers.

Effective, understandable communication, formal and informal, is crucial to the life of an organization and dependent on mid-level managers who act as the intermediaries of organizational communications. Because communication even at its best is imperfect, managers, at the least, need to minimize misunderstandings. It is not desirable or possible to analyze every communication, but managers need to identify communication methods that are most effective for reaching an organization's goals through the work of its employees. Managers balance limiting information so they do not overwhelm their employees with unnecessary messages while encouraging an open, trusting environment for sharing information.

Effective communication depends on several factors. Senders and receivers of information compete for attention and time to communicate in busy organizations. Oral and written communications are often blocked, dropped, rearranged, and inappropriately filtered as they travel through organizations in all directions through many levels. The use of professional jargon and the shorthand speech of in-groups complicate communications within and among interdisciplinary team members as well. A commitment to open sharing of accurate information depends on managers willing to spend the time to correct distorted communication and reduce barriers. These barriers include the use of formal communication channels only, making themselves physically unavailable, withholding or limiting time for communications, disregarding messages that require action, or promoting a culture of anger and fear of reprisals so that people are uncomfortable disagreeing with managers.

Managers must also be sensitive to individual factors that influence communication. For instance, when interpersonal relationships are strained or one party provokes negative emotions in the other, it may be difficult to communicate. If messages are filtered because of whom the sender is, it may never be received. Ignoring an important message from a particular sender may result in disastrous consequences for others and the organization.

Individuals base their communications on prior experiences that may cover a wide range of socioeconomic circumstances and interactions that make people more likely to be angry, fearful, gullible, shy, jealous, or self-aggrandizing. Managers need to recognize that these behaviors raise barriers to communication.

Other people may simply not understand the message or its frame of reference because they have had no prior experience with the issue at hand. People also bring, intentionally or not, values and prejudices that can negatively influence messages. Even if all of these factors were equal among communicators, managers must be sensitive to selective listening—hearing what we want to hear rather than the actual message—which seems to be human nature. People tend to filter out the negative and amplify the positive in messages affecting them.

Oral Communications

Individual Meetings

For managers, formal oral communication most often takes the form of scheduled one-on-one meetings with an employee. All of these meetings are documented in the person's employment record. They are fairly standardized in format to reduce the risk of legal consequences should employees and managers disagree about the message sent or received. These formal meetings may be called when:

- Regularly scheduled, formal performance reviews must be conducted.

- Opportunities arise to reinforce and reward employees who are on track with their professional and personal goals that are aligned with the organization's goals.
- Work performance demands immediate attention because the goals of the organization are not being met.
- Work performance demands immediate attention because it places the worker or others at risk for injury or other negative consequences.

Meetings to discuss jobs well done when performance expectations are met or exceeded may be one of the highlights of a manager's responsibilities. Managers take pride in commending good employees, and should take care to document these achievements. These meetings may occur only annually because they involve employees with no performance issues. However, employees may find time with a manager for more frequent one-on-one meetings to praise performance to be a powerful reward.

Meetings held because of performance concerns may demand more careful planning of the message and its delivery. Managers must prepare in advance for these meetings and establish a meeting environment that reflects their importance—uninterrupted and businesslike. The more that managers limit these discussions to performance behaviors related to job descriptions, the more likely the result will be an improvement in work performance and agreement on current issues. Focusing on behavioral issues rather than on characteristics or personality helps motivate an employee to perform her duties.

This type of performance review meeting needs to be separated from that in which the person does not know how to perform. Formal meetings to address clinical expertise or professional socialization issues may identify the need for counseling or teaching. In these situations, managers may decide to refer employees to other professionals who are better able to meet their needs. These difficult meetings are successful if both the manager and the employee believe that they have learned something and can move ahead without anger. See Activity 12.1.

Managers are also on the receiving end of formal performance meetings with their supervisors. In

Managers may be surprised at how often they become the informal referee in personal conflicts among employees. Disagreements may arise over anything: time-off requests, lunchroom use, parking spaces, tardiness, phone use, patient assignments, to name just a few. Managers need to decide when to intervene (when behaviors disrupt operations), when to let people resolve issues for themselves, and when to accept the fact that people just may not get along with each other but are still able to do their jobs effectively. Sometimes employees are simply not a good match with coworkers, although they are a good match with the organization. Resolving these interpersonal issues requires managers to remain neutral and stay focused on the impact of these behaviors on performance and the goals of the organization. See Activity 12.2.

Telephone Communications

It is not unusual for large organizations to monitor telephone communications because of their importance in presenting the organization in a positive way. Even the smallest organization may require that employees receive training in effective telephone communications because a phone call is often the first impression of an organization. Managers are responsible for establishing guidelines for all

advance of the meeting, it may be prudent to prepare a written report of strengths and weaknesses. Assuring that their positive efforts are recognized during the meeting and then documented may be important, particularly if formal one-on-one meetings have been infrequent. Preparing a follow-up "report of the meeting" including new performance goals and asking that it be included in a personnel file are other options.

Informal Conversations

Informal conversations provide managers with the opportunity to survey current outlooks of the organization and its employees. They are the means for becoming better acquainted with coworkers and may provide the opportunity to reward performance, meet employee needs, or resolve performance or organizational problems before these issues need to be addressed formally. These unscheduled, spontaneous interactions are not documented. They may be referred to in the documentation of more formal meetings as they possibly evolve into the need for more complex problem-solving or conflict resolution.

employees when answering the phone, responding to messages received, and documenting calls made and received. They have several important decisions to make: Should callers select from a menu of connections? Should automatic transfer to a message box replace a receptionist?

With a receptionist responsible for screening telephone calls, staff may avoid interruptions in patient care, managers may use their time more effectively, and callers may receive immediate attention. Such a point person must be trained to establish priorities to know when it is important for clinicians to come to the phone immediately, as soon as possible, or after all patient care is completed. Managers must weigh the costs of such a position against the risks of reputation and communication failures with automated systems and callbacks. Organizations are at a disadvantage when callers do not leave messages because of their frustration or when patients miss returned calls from healthcare providers. Incoming messages that are unclear or directed to the wrong person result in delays that may negatively impact patient satisfaction and referrals for new patients. See Activity 12.3.

The use of personal cellular phones or other electronic devices during patient care is disruptive and impolite, even if they are used to answer business calls. Managers may be required to establish and enforce policies and procedures limiting personal use for calls, tweets, text messages, and so on. Patients expect the undivided attention of their caregivers. Establishing professional relationships with patients may be compromised if they overhear personal phone conversations that caregivers are having with family or friends. Having phone conversations about other patients during treatment sessions places patient confidentiality at risk. Clinicians should set a good example so that patients are also discouraged from using phones during their treatment sessions.

Conducting Business Meetings

Business meetings bring people together for discussions to address resolution of problems or to work on mutual tasks and projects that require face-to-face meetings on a regular basis. Providing participants with information they need to review in advance conserves meeting time. Presentation of background information is reduced so that time is more wisely spent on discussion and decisions. A purpose supported by a clear agenda is a powerful start for any meeting. Encouraging active participation is equally important for effective, comprehensive decision-making.

Several actions of managers can limit the effectiveness of meetings. These include:

- Holding regularly scheduled meetings for the sake of meeting. This action can be a source of aggravation for staff. It may be wise to block out time on the calendar for meetings to be held so that staff do not schedule patients or other activities during those times. When the meeting time is not needed, these blocks of time can be used for completion of non-patient care assignments or for informal socializing or discussions related to clinical decision-making.
- Taking too much of the meeting time for announcements or reports that people might receive through other channels on their own time (e-mails, memos, bulletin-board posts).
- Requiring attendance of people who become observers because they are not involved in decisions to be discussed.
- Giving short notice to attend a meeting that results in a disruption or failure to complete their assigned duties.

ACTIVITY 12.3
A TELEPHONE PROBLEM

Carterville Physical Therapy receives 25% of its referrals from Dr. Costello. He has just called Barbara Benton, the owner of the practice. He says he had no choice but to call her cellular phone because he cannot get through via her office phone system to talk to her or the other staff about patients and referrals. He is very frustrated and does not even bother to leave messages. He admits referring patients to another practice just because it is easier. Her staff requested she put in this new system because they were so frequently taken away from patients to answer the phone. What should Barbara do? Consider: Where is the phone situation now? Where does it need to be? What does Carterville Physical Therapy have to work with? How will it get to where it wants to be?

Managers should provide the opportunity for participants to suggest additions or revisions to the agenda in advance of the meeting. By providing time for informal discussion and socializing before or after a meeting, managers may be more successful in calling a meeting to order to address the agenda. Follow-up reports on action items may be provided to staff through memos, e-mails, or announcements. Minutes should be distributed by the assigned recorder as soon as possible after a meeting to everyone who attended with a deadline for feedback and correction. Typically, the first item on any meeting agenda is approval of the minutes of the last meeting so that accuracy can be documented.

In summary, the chairperson of the meeting is responsible for:

- Establishing and announcing the agenda
- Following the agenda during the meeting
- Focusing discussion on the goals to be achieved
- Encouraging everyone's participation
- Summarizing decisions and actions taken
- Assuring that agreement was reached
- Assigning a recorder to record and distribute the minutes, and a timekeeper

Meeting minutes should include a list of attendees, date and the time span of the meeting, a focus on action taken and assignments made, and a list of new items for future discussion. Managers should consider the use of templates for meeting agendas that are available in word-processing programs and other sources. An agenda template can also serve as the outline for minutes of the meeting. Agendas and minutes provide a historical record of decisions and actions of an organization. See Activity 12.4.

ACTIVITY 12.4
MEETINGS

Despite his best efforts, Jim Muncie cannot control staff meetings. First, getting everyone together to start on time every week seems to be impossible. Second, the side conversations, texting, and eating during the meeting are all very disconcerting. He does not feel he can get anything done without the group's attention. What should Jim do? Consider: What is the situation now? What does it need to be? What does Jim have to work with? How will it get to where he wants it to be?

Group Presentations

Managers often are involved in formal presentations that serve to introduce a group to new information or to provide training and education. These presentations require the same attention to communication, and they are often enhanced with the use of visual materials. The basic rules of presentations are to:

- Determine the needs of the audience and the goal(s) of the presentation.
- Prepare an outline or guide for the presentation.
- Plan what you are going to say, but do not memorize it.
- Keep the meeting to 20 to 25 minutes, which is the limit for holding the audience's attention.
- Have a beginning (present what you are going to say), a middle (say what you have to say), and an end (tell the audience what you said).
- Use slides or handouts. A picture is worth 1,000 words. Visuals reinforce, but do not substitute for, the message.
- Use visual material to make a point rather than to provide as much information as possible.
- Avoid cluttering visuals with a variety of fonts, colors, or other distracters. Visuals should be simple and consistent.
- Be clear, confident, and friendly to engage the audience
- Get up, say what you have to say, sit down.

Communication technology has enabled multisite, long-distance virtual meetings and presentations. The same principles of communication apply in the virtual world with additional considerations for effective positioning and use of cameras, microphones, and recording devices.
See Activity 12.5.

Written Communication

A manager's credibility is enhanced with written communication that is clearly organized and free of spelling, grammar, and punctuation errors. Poor writing not only detracts from the message, it also raises questions about the ability of the manager to formulate ideas in a logical, reasonable way. Written communication is at least as important as

ACTIVITY 12.5
A PRESENTATION

Select any recent presentation that you attended in the classroom or elsewhere to critique. Consider the basic rules of presentations given above and present a plan for how the speaker might improve. Consider: What is the current status of the presentation? What does it need to be? What does the speaker have to work with? How would the presentation be improved?

oral communication for all managerial responsibilities on a daily basis. As legal documentation, it may be even more important to an organization's accounting of its decisions and actions.

Memoranda and Letters

Templates in word-processing and other software programs are available to format memoranda (memos) and letters for consistency in appearance. Memos are different from letters. Letters are more formal, are used for external communication, and convey more sensitive and important messages. Memos are used internally to communicate short and direct messages. Memo formats include lines for "Date," "To," "From," and "Subject," which are followed by the body of the memo. The first line should begin with the point of the memo. The rest of the memo should be clear and concise and provide a statement of the point. If there are attachments, they should be mentioned in the memo. There is usually a heading, MEMORANDUM, which includes the organization's logo or other information. Managers should use memos when they want to inform or recommend something in a concise way that is important but not critical either in hard copy or electronically.

Business letters follow formal formats with inside addresses, salutations, and closings. They suggest an important message that demands the attention of the recipient. Because they may typically become part of the organization's records, they should reflect the sophistication and writing ability of the sender. Business letters should be taken seriously and reviewed carefully because they document an important issue communicated between two parties. Templates in word-processing programs are helpful for new letter writers. Managers may generate letters for a variety of reasons to employees and other stakeholders—a follow-up to an important meeting and an offer of employment are examples. Determining the goal of the letter and rereading to be sure the goal has been met is important to this form of communication. See Activity 12.6.

E-communication

Electronic communication (e-mail, text messages, tweets, and the like) in healthcare is meaningful only if it is read. Reading often means that the message must be easily separated from the uninvited and unrelated communication received on the job. It is helpful for e-mails to have titles (subject lines) that easily enable readers to distinguish business from nonbusiness e-mails. Like memos, e-mails should begin with the point of the message and then state the case to support it. Efforts to move any forms of e-communication from informal social tools to effective business tools may be challenging.

Managers may be responsible for developing and implementing policies and procedures for e-mail and other emerging e-communication to control what may be an overwhelming work interference rather than a powerful communication tool. All managers and staff should be encouraged to be selective about initiating e-communication by asking, "Is it really necessary?" and "Is it the best means of communication?" They are valuable for distributing announcements and other important information quickly to large groups of people. However, the use of electronic mailing lists that reach many people at once may not be the most appropriate means for delivering complex or controversial information. Managers should develop a filing system for easy storage and retrieval (electronic or hard copy) of e-communication messages received and sent as documentation of communication to individuals and groups.

ACTIVITY 12.6
MEMOS AND LETTERS

Prepare a memo to advise a staff of changes in their work schedules with implementation of a new 7-day coverage model of providing care. Prepare a letter to offer a physical therapist a position that includes scheduling weekend work on a regular basis. Critique memos and letters provided for review.

Posted Announcements

Managers need to determine when the posting of hard-copy announcements complement or serve to replace other forms of communication. Strategic placement of bulletin boards in public areas for display of information or action to be taken by a group can be an efficient and powerful means of communication of official, general, non-sensitive information. Large organizations typically have policies and procedures for approval of content and appearance of announcements and time limits for their posting. This action keeps boards free from the clutter of outdated or irrelevant announcements. Legal requirements guide the public display of other mandatory information that commonly appear in separate designated spaces to meet legal requirements. Displaying professional licenses of staff is an example of such a requirement in some jurisdictions.

Managers must attend to the professional appearance of posted announcements because they reflect the organization's culture. Selecting a consistent color and format helps employees recognize announcements that require action. Providing a bulletin board out of the public eye for employees to post informal announcements and information helps managers control the content of official public announcement space.

Reports

Managers are frequently responsible for generating reports on a variety of topics, typically related to fiscal issues. Managers may generate some reports routinely while other reports are prepared in response to a particular request for information. Information is the key word. Reports are about data and their interpretation. The content of reports should not be subject to further interpretation.

Preparation of a report begins with determining its purpose and scope and to whom and how it will be distributed. The next step is identification of the data to be included, and their presentation. If the report includes graphs and charts, managers will need to determine their format. The text of the report should be arranged with bullets and other formatting to improve the chances that the facts presented are not misinterpreted or muddled. Reports prepared on an ongoing basis may follow standardized formats to ease communication. Managers should be concise in their preparation of reports so that only relevant information is included. See Activity 12.7.

Overcoming Communication Hurdles

Touchy Subjects

Particularly when the message may evoke strong emotions, managers need to review them from the point of view of the receiver(s) before they are sent or spoken. Timing and sensitivity may deflect negative reactions so that the message is actually received as intended rather than misinterpreted. Deferring a message or leaving it unsent may be a wise choice when the manager's emotions are high.

ACTIVITY 12.7
BEING IN TOUCH

The hospital's policy is that employees turn off their personal phones while at work. Enforcing this policy has been challenging. Some employees insist that they must have their phones on in case one of their children needs to reach them. Others think "at work" only means when they are with a patient. Others think that phones that are set on vibration modes are acceptable. Contingent workers seem to follow their own rules about phone calls.

Lisa Tyler, the rehab manager, has been lenient about this policy to keep her employees happy. Her failure to enforce the phones-off policy has had repercussions. Complaints from patients about therapists on phones were received by the nursing staff, who also resent the fact that the physical therapists use phones when they cannot. Lisa's boss happened to be on an elevator with a physical therapist who was on a personal phone call, and she is very angry about it. Lisa's boss gave her an informal warning to follow the procedure or else. Lisa said it was a flawed policy, explaining her staff's dissatisfaction with it. Her boss gave Lisa 1 week to prepare an alternative policy. What should Lisa recommend? Consider: What is the phone situation now? What does it need to be? What does Lisa have to work with? How will she get to where she wants it to be?

Lack of Clarity

When managers are not of the same discipline as the receiver(s) of oral and written messages, they should check for jargon and abbreviations that may be unfamiliar. A common language enhances communication, as does using the fewest number of words and syllables possible. Encouraging people to ask for further explanations when necessary promotes communication because the feedback allows senders to improve their future efforts.

Using action words (behaviors) may also result in a clearer message. For example, "great job everyone" may mean different things to different people. The message is clearer if stated as: "The team exceeded its goals by 10% this week. Each member of the team will be recognized in the next newsletter. Thank you all for your extraordinary efforts in this important project." Because it is often necessary to send the same message to all members of a team, sending it simultaneously may provide the opportunity for members of a team to seek clarification or confirmation from one another. This interaction may save time. It is likely that more than one person may have the same questions that can be posed by one person for the group. Of course, simultaneously sending a poorly prepared message may be problematic, particularly if it arouses anxiety or anger that is reinforced within the group.

Getting the Message Across

The more important a message is, the more directed it needs to be to a particular person. For example, an e-mail, phone call, or face-to-face meeting with the person who needs to make an important decision may be more effective than a hard-copy letter that may be delayed or handled by one or two other people before arriving in the decision maker's hands.

There are also challenges with making an important or sensitive announcement to a group of people. The news may be better received and understood by bringing everyone together in person for a meeting rather than sending a simultaneous e-mail to everyone. Other messages may be so important that managers introduce them in an e-mail, discuss them in a meeting, and follow them up in a memo. Changes in personnel benefits that require action or patient safety efforts are examples of this three-pronged approach. Non-critical, simple, clear information may be e-mailed or posted in a central location. For example, final plans for a holiday party or extended hours for building security are simple messages that require simple communication.

Teamwork

Another communication challenge is the formation of work teams for a particular purpose. Especially when a team is made up of people representing several different healthcare units, managers may need to make special efforts to facilitate its success. Establishing written guidelines that clarify expectations and timelines may increase a team's effectiveness, for example, sharing a teamwork document that includes:[2]

- The name, purpose, and goals of the team
- Deadline for meeting the purpose
- Number or frequency of meetings
- Names of team members and contact information
- Team member expectations:
  Attend all sessions prepared to work
  Be respectful, considerate, tactful, and concise
  Work collaboratively to reach consensus
  Actively participate with an open mind
- Submit assigned work on time (reports, recommendations, etc.)

Listening

Managers not only need to send messages but they also need to receive them. Listening is perhaps the most valuable and desirable skill in improving communications. Traditional hints for effective listening include the following:

- Ask, "What's in the message for me?"
- Do not jump to conclusions.
- Fight distractions.
- Focus on the message, not on the delivery.
- Hear tones of voice.
- Identify the central idea(s).
- Limit talking to "I see," "Uh huh," "Go on," etc.
- Make eye contact.

- Mentally summarize the message.
- Postpone judgment until the message is complete.
- Sort facts from opinions.
- Take notes to organize, not memorize, what is heard.

Encouraging others to listen can be just as difficult as listening for oneself. Modeling good listening may help. Asking, in a nonthreatening way, the receiver to summarize the message just sent may help him or her develop listening skills. It also allows managers to regroup and resend messages that need corrections or clarification. See Activity 12.8.

Grapevines and Rumor Mills

Informal communication channels and networks (grapevines and rumor mills) evolve from interpersonal relationships and social interaction patterns that occur in all work settings. They occur in parallel with the formal communication chains that are established by managers. Although grapevines may lead to difficulties if misused to spread rumors rather than facts, they can be the fastest way to get the word out—much faster than formal channels.

For instance, the fact that an organization was just named the best in the country in *U.S. News & World Report* is exciting news that would spread fast. That staff will be sent home because of a severe weather warning is another example of news that spreads through the grapevine before an e-mail can be typed. Rumors provide managers with information about communication networks and concerns of employees that are often valuable in decision-making but not directly available. See Activity 12.9.

Communication and Health Literacy

Managers may initiate and implement plans for communicating patient educational information as well. For instance, conducting a cost-benefit analysis of packaged computer programs for exercise instructions is a common responsibility. Reviewing the literacy level of materials purchased or developed to assure their value to the target patient populations may be another important responsibility.

In addition to basic literacy issues (the ability to read, write, and speak in English), healthcare managers must attend to the issue of health literacy. Health literacy is the ability to read and comprehend essential health-related materials (e.g., prescription bottles, appointment slips, discharge instructions) to function successfully as a patient, and to use information to promote and maintain good health. Health literacy[1] is context specific and can be a major barrier in communication with patients that managers must overcome. Many people do not understand the underlying biology of their symptoms and have

---

ACTIVITY 12.8
I'M LISTENING

Monique LaSalle is the manager of a large rehabilitation staff. She works very hard at communication and is proud that her efforts seem to be effective a great deal of the time. However, Charlie McGill is an annoyance. He just does not seem to get it—anything. Whether it is a memo, specific verbal directions, or participating in meetings, it is as if he is in his own world. Monique is beginning to wonder whether Charlie has some hearing or cognitive processing problem. She prefers not to think that he just chooses not to listen. When she confronts him or repeats information that he should already have, he always responds with, "I'm listening." What should she do? Consider: What is the situation now? What does it need to be? What does Monique have to work with? How will she get to where she wants it to be?

ACTIVITY 12.9
RUMOR HAS IT

Oliver Hendrix is regional rehabilitation manager for six All-American Rehab Services outpatient centers. One of his center managers has advised him that there is a rumor going around that two of the centers are closing and the staff is already looking for new positions. How might Oliver react to this news if it is true? If it is false?

unreasonable expectations about improvement in their conditions as a result, or they may not comply with treatments because they do not have the knowledge to understand their importance. More information on health literacy may be found at Web Resources.

Managers must determine whether the communication skills of staff improve patients' health and healthcare. Because so much information is available to people who are health literate, managers should direct their efforts to those who are not. For instance, the reading level of printed materials deserves attention. Using visuals and providing essential information only may help. Patients are often already intimidated or feeling anxious about their condition, which limits their ability to ask and respond to questions. Managers need to make staff aware of signs that may suggest that a patient has difficulty with basic literacy such as:[1]

- Taking a long time to sign forms
- Relying on others to complete paperwork for them
- Asking to take paperwork with them to complete later
- Saying their eyes are bad when given something to read
- Paying more attention to nonverbal cues than verbal messages

See Activity 12.10.

A Manager's Responsibility

Communication is the fundamental, underlying responsibility of managers that takes a surprisingly large amount of their time. Controlling that time can be challenging. Although, communicating effectively comes more naturally to some managers than it does to others, its importance demands that everyone make efforts to continue improving oral and written communication skills. There is no organization without communication. Managers must not only work on their own communication skills, but they must also guide others in their own skills so that the goals of the organization are conveyed and met.

ACTIVITY 12.10
A READABILITY TOOL

To determine the readability of a selected Microsoft Word document, enable the readability feature:
1. Click the File tab, and then click Options.
2. Click Proofing.
3. Under "When correcting spelling and grammar in Word," make sure the "Check grammar with spelling check" box is selected.
4. Select "Show readability statistics."

After you enable this feature, open a file that you want to check, and check the spelling (found at the review tab). When Word finishes checking the spelling and grammar, it displays information about the reading level of the document. NOTE: The Flesch Reading Ease test rates the text on a 100-point scale. The higher the score, the easier it is to understand the document. The score for this chapter is 40.3. For most standard texts, a score between 60 and 70 is desirable. The Flesch-Kincaid Grade Level test rates text on a U.S. school grade level. For example, a score of 8.0 signifies that an eighth grader can understand the document. For this chapter the grade level is 11.7. For most documents, aim for a score of approximately 7.0 to 8.0. Microsoft Office document readability levels available at http://office.microsoft.com/en-us/word-help/test-your-document-s-readability-HP010148506.aspx#BM13). Accessed November 22, 2013.

REFERENCES

1. Bernhardt JM. Accessing, understanding, and applying health communication messages: the challenge of health literacy. In: Thompson TL, ed. *Handbook of Health Communication*. Mahwah, NJ: Lawrence Erlbaum Associates; 2003.
2. Buchbinder SB, Shanks NH. *Introduction to Health Care Management*. 2nd ed. Burlington, MA: Jones & Bartlett; 2012.

WEB RESOURCES

Centers for Disease Control and Prevention (CDC). Health literacy information. http://www.cdc.gov/healthliteracy/. Accessed November 22, 2013.

National Network of Libraries of Medicine (NN/LM). Health literacy information. http://nnlm.gov/outreach/consumer/hlthlit.html. Accessed November 22, 2013.

MANAGEMENT IN SPECIFIC HEALTHCARE SETTINGS

This section provides the opportunity to take a more detailed look into the range of practice settings and the many managerial opportunities for physical therapists. Chapters include common issues managers in healthcare can address to influence quality patient care and positive business outcomes (Fig. S3.1). Each chapter in this section is devoted to management of physical therapy (or rehabilitation) services based in one of the major practice settings:

- Long-term care
- Outpatient centers
- Special education units of public schools
- Home health agencies
- Hospitals and healthcare systems

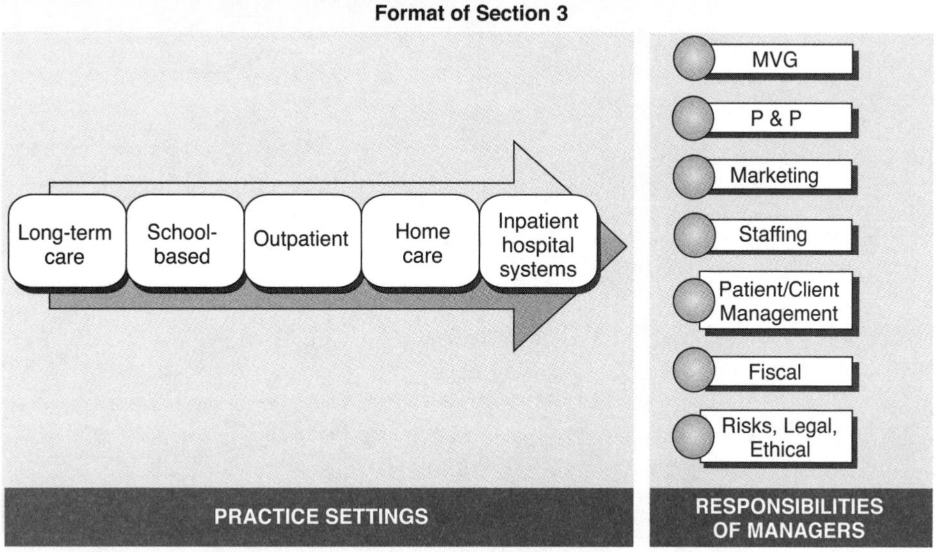

Format of Section 3

Figure S3.1 Practice settings and the responsibility of managers.

Each chapter in this section is divided into two parts. Part 1 of each chapter addresses contemporary characteristics and common issues in the setting that affect the work of physical therapists. Part 2 identifies the potential managerial roles in the setting and addresses the eight areas of managerial responsibility presented in Section 2 of the text—vision, mission, goals; policies and procedures; marketing; staffing; patient care; fiscal; risk management, legal, ethical; and communication. At the end of each chapter are activities that provide an opportunity to develop managerial decision-making skills in the context of each setting through the interweaving of all manager responsibilities.

CHAPTER 13

Management Issues in Long-Term Care

LEARNING OBJECTIVES

- Discuss components and characteristics of contemporary long-term care.
- Analyze key licensing, accreditation, and reimbursement requirements.
- Analyze the work of physical therapists in long-term care.
- Determine the role of the care team, particularly certified nursing assistants, in the accomplishment of patient rehabilitation goals.
- Determine the importance of family education in long-term care.
- Determine managerial roles and challenges to managerial responsibilities in long-term care.
- Analyze managerial decision-making in given situations.

PART **1**   The Contemporary Setting

Overview of Long-Term Care

The provision of social and medical services is intertwined tightly in long-term care to meet the needs of people with complex, multisystem problems across the life span. Only 53% of people who require long-term care are elderly. Many younger people who require long-term care have cognitive deficits and mental illnesses. The focus of long-term patient care shifts toward the ability of a person to function rather than on diagnoses and treatment of their diseases.[1]

Long-term care may be best represented as a continuum of care, which is anchored with skilled care and nonskilled on opposite ends as shown in Figure 13.1. Skilled care is defined as the provision of care by professionals (nursing and rehabilitation) who manage, observe, and evaluate patients. Care provided safely by nonprofessionals is considered nonskilled service. For example, staff or family members assisting patients with personal care and activities of daily living are nonskilled. Professionals play an important role in teaching nonskilled caregivers about these patient responsibilities.

Long-term care can occur in a variety of settings represented by the circles in Figure 13.1. Note that home care (provided in the patient's home) is a unique form of long-term care. It is discussed separately in Chapter 16. Because the need for skilled interdisciplinary care is a requirement for admission into skilled long-term care, most patients who qualify for admission are admitted directly from an acute care hospital.

Nonskilled residential care may be provided in many types of long-term care and assisted living facilities under a variety of names that may overlap and cause confusion. These facilities are inconsistently and variably regulated from one jurisdiction to another, but their services attend to the personal needs of their residents using nonskilled employees

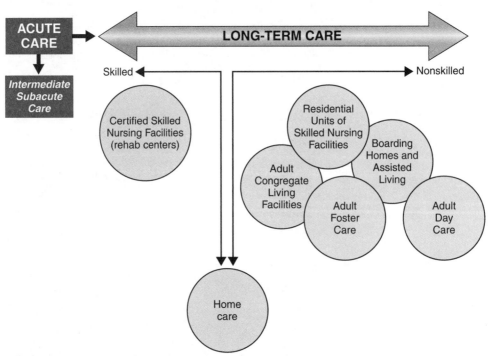

FIGURE 13.1 Healthcare continuum.

to help them with self-care. Some residential facilities may cater to particular populations, such as adults with mental retardation. Often there are restrictions for admission related to a required level of mobility. For example, patients may need to be, minimally, independent in wheelchair mobility to live in some centers.

A special type of residential care is the adult (congregate) living facility in which people maintain a private or semiprivate residence within a large building while sharing common areas for meals and activities. Transportation and housekeeping services are typically available. Nursing supervision 24 hours a day is available to monitor and assist with residents' medication and other healthcare needs. Typically, residents need to be ambulatory. They may receive intermittent physical therapy as outpatients or through home care services for short periods. Nonskilled care for assistance with activities of daily living or homemaking on a long-term basis may be provided.

A nursing home is another setting for residential care. Nursing homes may have two units. One unit is not Medicare certified, in which residential long-term care is provided. The other Medicare-certified unit provides skilled interdisciplinary care. Although they are in the same building, these units are treated as separate entities because they are regulated differently. As an example, a woman living in a residential unit may develop a new problem such as a hip fracture. Upon return from the hospital, instead of returning to her place in the residential unit, she is formally transferred to a "Medicare-certified bed" in the same building for skilled services. Conversely, patients admitted from a hospital to a nursing home for skilled rehabilitation services may be discharged to the residential care unit in the same building if they have not improved enough to warrant discharge to their homes. An example is a person admitted for stroke rehabilitation whose functional goals are limited or someone who lacks the family support needed to return home.

Individuals living in residential care units of a nursing home may qualify for outpatient Part B Medicare services or Medicaid skilled rehabilitation services as if they are living in their private homes, although they are residents in an inpatient facility. An example might be a residential-care patient with a rotator cuff tear who requires physical therapy three times a week. Another example is a patient who is transferred from the skilled care to the residential unit who continues rehabilitation or nursing services a few days a week under Medicare Part B services to reach new functional goals in the new living situation.

The level of assistance a person requires in the components of long-term care may range from general supervision for safety or administration of medications to maximum assistance for all activities of daily living. These needs may change over time. The concept of continuous long-term care bridges all of these needs. It typically takes the form of a campus-like retirement community with private homes, opportunities for many leisure activities, an assisted living facility, a skilled nursing facility (SNF), outpatient care, and a residential care home. Residents of the community buy or rent a private home or apartment and contract for lifelong care within the community that includes transfers among the continuum of the community's services as their medical and social needs change.

It is also important to note that an intermediate (subacute) level of care (between acute care and long-term care) is defined as a short period (normally about 6 weeks, but no more than 100 days) of intensive rehabilitation, treatment, or intensive care that may be provided in subunits of hospitals, skilled nursing facilities, or in patients' homes, typically after discharge from the hospital. Subacute care with hospitals is discussed in Chapter 17. It also may be used to deter admission to a more expensive hospital whenever possible. See Table 13.1 for the role of physical therapy in long-term settings. See Web Resources for more general information from the federal government on long-term care.

Skilled Nursing Facilities (SNFs)

The focus of this chapter is the most tightly regulated healthcare setting and the long-term care setting in which physical therapists play a major role—SNFs. These organizations, which may have "rehabilitation center" or "healthcare center" in their names, are clearly defined by certification requirements of Medicare and Medicaid. There are about 16,100 long-term care facilities with more than 1.4 million skilled nursing beds in the United States certified by Medicare and Medicaid that are 82% occupied.[2] Almost 20% of SNFs have

TABLE 13.1   Levels of long-term care and the role of physical therapy in them

TYPE OF LONG-TERM CARE	LEVELS OF SERVICE	ROLE OF PHYSICAL THERAPY
Skilled nursing facilities (rehabilitation centers)	Skilled nursing and rehabilitative services are an integral component of care. The length of stay may be shorter than the 100 days available for those needing intermediate levels of rehabilitation before transferring to a lesser level of care. Longer lengths of stay are common for people with complex chronic conditions.	Member of the interdisciplinary rehabilitation team to return people to the safest, optimal level of function. Establish restorative programs and functional maintenance programs to promote optimal quality of life and independence of residents in nonskilled units.
Residential care homes	Provide nonskilled personal care and supervision for people unable to meet their personal needs independently. The care may range from minimal to maximal assist for activities of daily living, medical management of chronic diseases, etc. There may be nonskilled units in SNFs.	When a residential care unit is in an SNF, physical therapists may treat residents as if they were Medicare B outpatients for brief periods, a few times a week (e.g., a resident receives physical therapy 3×/week for 3 weeks after hospitalization for viral infection). Establishing restorative programs and functional maintenance programs to promote optimal quality of life and independence of residents is another responsibility. Physical therapists may treat residents of boarding and foster homes as home-care patients in these settings.
Adult (congregate) living facilities	Provides meal services, organized activities, and supervision of medical status to residents who live independently in their own units. May also include lockdown units for patients with dementia to assure patient safety.	Physical therapists may provide home-care services to residents, residents may travel to outpatient centers for physical therapy, or there may be an on-site therapy clinic.
Continuing care communities	Provides services on a campus that may include apartments or homes where people live independently, an SNF, an adult congregate living facility, and a residential care home or unit. Residents buy into a program to meet their needs for the rest of their lives. They move from one type of care to another as their needs demand in a continuous manner.	Physical therapists may be employed by the community or contract their services through other agencies to provide inpatient services in the SNF, outpatient or home care to people who are living in their own homes on the campus or in the assisted living facility, and intermittent care to residents in the residential care units. They may have educational responsibilities for nursing staff development and resident educational programs. They may assist in the development of health and fitness programs for members of the community. It may be that different physical therapists or physical therapy companies provide services in different components of the community complex.
Adult day care	Provides assistance with personal care and social activities in a community-based center on a regular basis. Clients return to their own homes at the end of the day. May address the needs of particular groups such as patients with Alzheimer disease.	Physical therapists may serve as consultants to develop group exercise programs. They may treat individuals requiring skilled outpatient services in the centers although treatment resources may be limited.

physicians on staff and almost 69% use outside contract companies for therapy services.[2]

Because the acuity level of patients discharged from hospitals has increased, the number of people who require skilled nursing care at discharge has increased. This increase in demand has occurred at the same time that reimbursement reductions and financial constraints have been imposed. Many nursing homes closed or operate under bankruptcy protection. Frequent changes in ownership, management, and organizational structure have also resulted.[3] A trend toward large national chains that allow the shifting of resources among buildings may be one outgrowth of these healthcare policy and reimbursement decisions.

Nursing Home Regulations and Quality Management

Omnibus Budget Reconciliation Act (OBRA)

The 1987 Federal Nursing Home Reform Act, which included the Omnibus Budget Reconciliation Act (OBRA), was the primary catalyst for change in long-term care. It included the requirement that *each* resident "attain and maintain the highest practicable physical, mental, and psychosocial well-being" for the facility to receive Medicare and Medicaid funding. National standards of care and rights for residents were established that include:[4]

- Emphasis on a resident's quality of life and the quality of care
- New expectations that each resident's ability to walk, bathe, and perform other activities of daily living will be maintained or improved absent medical reasons
- A resident assessment process leading to development of an individualized care plan
- Rights to remain in the nursing home absent nonpayment, dangerous resident behaviors, or significant changes in a resident's medical condition
- A right to safely maintain or bank personal funds with the nursing home
- Rights to return to the nursing home after a hospital stay or an overnight visit with family and friends

- The right to choose a personal physician and to access medical records
- The right to organize and participate in a resident or family council
- The right to be free of unnecessary and inappropriate physical and chemical restraints
- Uniform certification standards for Medicare and Medicaid homes
- Prohibitions on turning to family members to pay for Medicare and Medicaid services
- New remedies for certified nursing homes that fail to meet minimum federal standards

The importance of rehabilitation services in meeting these standards becomes apparent. A shift has taken place from non-skilled care to skilled care to restore and maintain function at the maximal functional level. This move to skilled services became a major philosophical and managerial challenge for many nursing homes. The Omnibus Budget Reconciliation Act (OBRA) led to a focus on compliance with regulatory mandates on all aspects of the management of skilled nursing care. Staff/patient ratios, mixes of licensed and unlicensed personnel for the full 24 hours of care, and the development of the Minimum Data Set (MDS, discussed later) are the results of this legislation. Burdensome reporting requirements to demonstrate the efforts made to improve the quality of care and quality of life for residents continue to detract from the actual provision of that care.

Regulatory Surveys

Compliance with OBRA legislation is determined through an annual state survey and certification process established by the Centers for Medicare & Medicaid Services (CMS). The survey involves unannounced on-site audits of all nursing homes. It includes interviews of staff members, residents, and family members after a review of established quality indicators has been completed. The purpose of the survey is to assess whether the quality of care provided is in compliance with given standards and the needs of individual residents. Noncompliance with Medicare and/or Medicaid regulations and/or state certification laws may result in penalties, such as denial of payment for new admissions, fines, revocation of certification, and transfer of residents. To avoid these consequences, any identified deficiencies must be addressed within 30 days.

In addition to survey and other administrative data requirements, the CMS also monitors nursing homes through the MDS that is used to comprehensively report the status of each individual receiving care. The data are aggregated, analyzed, and then converted to specific indicators. These indicators cover all aspects of the quality of interdisciplinary care and compliance with residents' rights. They are presented in Nursing Home Compare, which is an important online resource that provides important information for families faced with decisions about placement for the care of their loved ones. See Web Resources for more information on Nursing Home Compare and other long-term care information from the Centers for Medicare & Medicaid.

Accreditation of Long-Term Care

Long-term care organizations have the opportunity to seek voluntary accreditation from two organizations. The Joint Commission expanded its accreditation activities to include healthcare organizations other than hospitals (see Web Resources for detailed accreditation information). This credential is probably more important to, and more feasible for, larger nursing homes or those that are part of a larger healthcare system. The Joint Commission's approval reflects a commitment to certain quality standards that may exceed those required in the SNF certification process.

The Commission on Accreditation of Rehabilitation Facilities (see Web Resources) recently acquired the Continuing Care Accreditation Commission (CCAC) and became the only accrediting body for continuing care retirement communities (CCRCs) and other types of aging services networks. Because government regulation of retirement communities and other aging services is not rigorous, CCRC accreditation may be important to set an organization apart in this competitive market.[5]

Unique Features of Physical Therapy Practice in Skilled Nursing Facilities

Regulatory mandates followed by physical therapists in SNFs are basically the same regardless of their differences. They may be for profit, nonprofit, or governmental organizations. Their organizational structures vary widely from small, freestanding, proprietary homes to large national nursing home corporations that include hundreds of nursing homes in many states. In those large multisite organizations, managers in each building meet their goals with the support provided by regional managers and corporate experts. This oversight also means demands for conformity that may limit a manager's ability to be flexible in daily decisions about operations and employees.

Managers need to consider those factors that make the work of physical therapists and other professionals fulfilling and rewarding in long-term care, a setting that presents unique challenges related to the clinical management of elderly residents with chronic diseases, residents' needs for sophisticated post–acute care, and complex regulatory demands. See Sidebar 13.1.

Skilled nursing care organizations provide upper-level management opportunities that may not be available in other healthcare organizations. Perhaps more than any other setting, career ladders for advancement of rehabilitation professionals present themselves frequently in long-term care. Opportunities to assume responsibility for interprofessional teams that extend beyond the typical rehabilitation team also are possibilities.

The Care Team in Skilled Nursing Facilities

Probably the most striking characteristic of SNFs is the shift in the major responsibility of resident care from a physician to the professional caregivers. SNFs hire a medical director (a part-time position in smaller facilities) who reports to a board of directors and has administrative and leadership responsibility for clinical services. Each resident has a physician of record (POR) who certifies the clinical decisions of the team. If a physician or physicians' group has a large number of patients in a particular nursing home, they may assign either a nurse practitioner or physician assistant to coordinate the care of all of their residents in the building on a regular, if not daily, basis. In other instances, physicians who have been conspicuously absent in the day-to-day management of their patients in nursing homes may now conduct weekly rounds in a building.

SIDEBAR 13.1

Characteristics of Work in Skilled Nursing Facilities

- Involvement with comprehensive care in inter-professional teams, which presents many opportunities for professional interaction and mentoring within and among disciplines
- Focus on residents' functional abilities and their independence to maintain quality of life
- Accomplishing significant outcomes with complex residents
- Focus on education and assistance for caregivers to establish specific programs for residents. Extended interactions often lead to a sense of being part of the family, particularly during discharge planning.
- Challenges of transferring resident care to family members who may be either unwilling or unable to assist with a person's complex conditions
- Ability to implement and follow through a comprehensive plan of care from beginning to end with a great deal of autonomous decision-making
- Opportunities to raise awareness of the importance of patient safety and optimal aging

- Many opportunities to expand clinical expertise with complex patients, develop new programs, and improve marketing skills
- Demanding paperwork and documentation of patient contact time
- Spurts of high activity and downtime over the course of a day because of difficulties in scheduling treatment sessions owing to the high demands placed on nursing staff to ready residents for therapy sessions and conflicts with other patient activities
- High-productivity demands while meeting multiple guidelines for compliance and reimbursement that may seem to conflict
- Dependence on certified nursing assistants (CNAs) and activity coordinators for carryover of rehabilitation programs into daily routines
- Challenges of caring for residents with dementia whose behavior may be disruptive
- Time required meeting strict regulatory demands to assure that the environment and care are in compliance
- High staff turnover across all disciplines

Managers of nursing and rehabilitation services use care plan meetings to represent their staffs in making interprofessional decisions about each resident's care. In larger centers, managers may monitor and evaluate the decisions of their staffs in this care planning. Despite the many regulations that are often restrictive and burdensome for the organization, physical therapists have high degrees of autonomy in their clinical decision-making with regard to the levels of care provided and the details of the daily management of residents—many of whom are acutely ill with complex problems.

Therapists also have increased responsibility, either independently or in consultation with nursing, for clinical decisions about immediate actions to be taken when unexpected responses to care occur or when there is an unexplained decline in a resident's medical status. Managers have a major responsibility for assuring that therapists are prepared for these higher expectations and demands for their expertise. Important decisions about residents' overall potential for rehabilitation as well as their safety are

at stake. Therapists in these settings are less likely to be able to rely on rapid decision-making of physicians when clinical concerns or medical emergencies arise. Instead, it is physicians who rely heavily on the expertise and daily contact that therapists and nurses have with residents as they make their medical decisions.

Managers also have an important role in evaluating information on applicants for potential admission to a facility. Making judgments about who gains admission to the SNF is probably a more important managerial responsibility than in any other type of healthcare setting. The people who are admitted influence all aspects of resource management. An accurate prediction about the residents' potential utilization of those resources is crucial in accomplishing positive clinical outcomes with the least financial impact on the organization.

Regardless of the organizational structure, nursing home operations rely heavily on dependable staff members who are flexible and responsive to regulatory changes, particularly because of the punitive nature of government regulations. Increased regulatory demands and limited reimbursement opportunities result in a lack of resources to pay competitive wages for the direct caregivers. Performing a difficult, demanding job for low compensation does not reflect the real, true value of these caregivers in healthcare. This workforce issue is one of the major management challenges of long-term care.[3]

Physical Therapists and Certified Nursing Assistants (CNAs)

Another important responsibility of rehabilitation service managers in skilled nursing facilities is establishing strong working relationships with certified nursing assistants (CNAs). Under the direction of licensed nursing personnel, CNAs interact with residents at a higher frequency and intensity than any other care provider.[6] Underestimating the important role that CNAs play in the management of the facility, and in the lives of the residents they care for, may result in major setbacks in meeting the goals of the rehabilitation services and achieving the optimum quality of life for residents.

The reported feelings of CNAs that they are undertrained, overworked, and underappreciated seem incongruent with their importance. This incongruence is likely to be reflected in job dissatisfaction and decreased efforts, not to mention the high turnover among this staff. A secondary effect is, of course, lack of continuity of care and dissatisfied residents and families that may have serious repercussions for the SNF.[6]

Particularly as the acuity level of residents in SNFs increases, rehabilitation managers may play an increased role in preparing CNAs for their expanded responsibilities. These responsibilities often involve increased emotional and physical work demands with residents who have more complex medical, emotional, and cognitive problems. Recommending and participating in programs that encourage increased involvement of CNAs in identifying barriers to their work and encouraging their recommendations should be considered. Having CNAs participate in discussions to solve problems rather than be given solutions to follow may be an effective strategy. The involvement of rehabilitation staff in collaboration agreements with local technical schools and the development of in-house training programs are other options for strengthening the care team.

Rehabilitation professionals are dependent on CNAs to reach their patient outcome goals in two important ways. Without the efforts of CNAs to assist them in bathing, dressing, and feeding, residents are not ready to participate in rehabilitation sessions. If residents are not attending therapy, the ability of therapists to reach their frequency and duration goals for reimbursement is compromised. Without the cooperation of CNAs, patient follow-through of exercise or activities to reinforce their rehabilitation progress is not accomplished and clinical outcomes are not achieved.

Realizing the physical effort required of CNAs to lift and bathe many residents who may be hostile, confused, and resistant to the care, physical therapists can establish a mutually beneficial relationship. Helping CNAs understand and redirect behaviors based on cognitive and functional ability may dramatically affect outcomes. Assisting CNAs to care for *specific* residents through demonstration and education enables them to contribute more effectively to the quality of care and rehabilitation of their assigned patients.

CNAs often face constant demands and even abuse from some residents with severe cognitive limitations. They may be so involved with behavior issues that, unsurprisingly, time and attention to established protocols or new interventions often are not available. Physical therapists can play a major role in making their jobs easier. Simply by asking their opinions and including them in decisions made about the people they care for can dramatically affect their difficult work.[6] This collaboration leads to CNAs who are able to work smarter, not harder, and physical therapists who have access to important information about residents that only CNAs know because of their intimate contact with them.

Physical Therapists and Family Education

Perhaps more important than in any other setting, family involvement is a critical component of rehabilitation in SNFs. Often the key determinant for whether the patient returns home or transfers to a residential care setting is the family. The following factors influence the effect family education may have on the achievement of reha-bilitation outcomes:[7]

- The family's knowledge, attitudes, and skills including physical capabilities
- The physical therapist's ability, willingness, and skills to involve family members
- The family's relationship with the patient before the injury or disability
- The availability and opportunity of family members to be involved
- The cognitive status of the patient (the more impaired, the more family involvement required)
- Multiple formal and informal avenues for family training (support groups, home visits, "open-door" policy visiting hours, and scheduling changes)

Although these factors are evident in any practice setting, rehabilitation managers in SNFs perhaps face the greatest challenges in family education because their patients rely on it the most. Residents in SNFs often have physical deficits, cognitive deficits, and/or complex medical problems requiring them to have more assistance from family members, whether they return to their homes or they are admitted to residential care. These family members, particularly spouses and adult children, may also be elderly with cognitive and/or physical challenges of their own that can limit their ability to assist. Convincing caregivers of the residents' limitations, as well as their own, is often the most important first step. Managers are responsible for assuring that the abilities and limitations of family members are accurately assessed to ensure a safe discharge and reduce the exposure to lawsuits because of inappropriate discharge planning.

If family members have the cognitive and physical ability to assist, they are often available and likely to be involved in family education and the direct care of residents in SNFs. Managers need to be aggressively proactive in creatively establishing a variety of means for including family members in the rehabilitation process at every opportunity and advocating for the inclusion of rehabilitation staff in educational programs in other services. The starting point may be staff development to improve the skills of therapists so they effectively include families in their interventions and goal setting for residents. In return, therapists may feel gratified by the effect they have had on a family's ability to care for a loved one. Focusing on this aspect of long-term care may provide managers with an important recruitment tool.

PART **2**   Management Issues

Overview of Management in Long-Term Care

More than any other factor, the size of the nursing home and the number of beds certified by Medicare and Medicaid determine the model for rehabilitation services in an SNF. The number of SNFs with fewer than 50 Medicare-certified beds is about the same as the number with 200 beds or more.[2] (Note: *Bed* is the term used to identify the space available for a patient who will be admitted for Medicare services under Part A.) Because of the increased need for skilled care for the elderly and other complex patients, it is now more common for a nursing home to have all patient beds certified as Medicare beds.

These size and organizational differences mean that managerial responsibilities in SNFs vary widely. They may include responsibility not only for clinical outcomes but also for budgets, quality control, marketing, and customer satisfaction in one or more buildings. The availability of managers and their contact with the staffs they supervise may range from constant and predictable to long-distance and intermittent. Their level of involvement with direct patient care also contributes to the extent of their managerial role. Managers in long-term care may be heavily imbedded in patient care, which may reduce the time they have to spend on managerial responsibilities.

At the other extreme, managers may be so far removed from observing or participating in direct patient care that their managerial role becomes top-down rather than bottom-up; that is, they focus on profitability, the oversight of budgets, and the development of managers in their assigned buildings rather than direct patient care. Striking a balance between these two extremes is often a challenge for SNF managers in their responsibilities for high-quality rehabilitation services that comply with all regulatory demands.

Some examples of managerial roles for physical therapists in SNFs include:

- Traditional director of physical therapy services in a larger SNF (rarely seen because the number of discipline-specific managers has decreased).
- Interprofessional director with responsibility for all disciplines in a rehabilitation service of an SNF. The director may be a physical therapist assistant or occupational therapy assistant in efforts to reduce costs or because therapists are simply unavailable.
- Area manager for rehabilitation services with responsibilities for several staffs and patient care in multiple facilities (5–10) of a national chain of SNFs. Regional managers may have similar duties as area managers but for more buildings (15–20). As part of the management team, a manager may also have responsibilities that include making contributions to decisions related to the organization as a whole and interpreting outcomes and other data. They may report to a vice president who is the manager for several states. Clinical specialists for each rehabilitation profession at the corporate level may advise and consult with area and regional managers about clinical issues.
- Solo physical therapist, employed in a smaller SNF with all patient care and managerial responsibilities.
- The director of rehabilitation in a large teaching hospital who is responsible for all aspects of physical therapy services provided in the hospital's SNF and all other inpatient and outpatient units. The larger the organization, the more likely it will be that unit supervisors will manage the day-to-day operations of these units. They may have some flexibility in shifting staff among units, as staffing needs demand.
- Owner of a private practice who contracts with nursing homes to provide services and coordinate assignments of physical therapists who may have a mix of outpatient and SNF care duties.
- Manager of contract therapy service company whose responsibilities may include negotiating contracts for assignment of physical therapists in any of the above settings.
- Physical therapist who is a consultant to groups of SNFs to monitor physical therapy or rehabilitation services, train staff in interprofessional models, and advise administrators.

Management Responsibilities

Mission, Vision, and Goals

Rehabilitation managers need to participate in the creation or regular review of the mission and vision of SNFs so that the role of contemporary rehabilitation practices is soundly incorporated. As healthcare policy changes, opportunities for identifying and clarifying the role of rehabilitation in the goals of SNFs lie with managers. They must collaborate with nursing home administrators and directors of nursing as SNFs take on these regulatory and philosophical challenges.

Managers may need to identify a variety of means for transforming the mission and vision into action and for demonstrating the link between the goals of the organization and the day-to-day responsibilities of rehabilitation professionals. Particularly at times of organizational change, managers need to be particularly diligent in transitioning changes in mission and goals into the behaviors of staff. Reconciling potential conflicts between professional responsibilities and the demands that set the culture of the organization may be of particular importance to managers in SNFs, particularly for those in for-profit corporations.

In a typical scenario, a large national corporation purchases a small independent nursing home that is providing private residential care. All of the beds are converted to Medicare-certified beds, which immediately places higher demands on all of the staff for documentation and a high level of quality of care demanded by Medicare regulations.

A rehabilitation manager in this situation needs strategies for transitioning from the former philosophy of care (nurses taking care of people) to a rehabilitation philosophy of setting care plan goals for the highest level of function for each resident. Insurers also expect a focus on functional improvement as a basis for reimbursement. Managers need to take the initiative to identify regulatory changes and modify policies and procedures just as other implemented changes are taking place. As visions and missions are revised, resolving potential conflicts between corporate directives and professional practice guidelines also may require close monitoring by managers.

Policies and Procedures

Policies and procedures that clarify roles and responsibilities become especially important when care is interdisciplinary. Implementing regulations rather than establishing policies and procedures is more of the role of managers in SNFs. Again, being held accountable for regulations and rules for which they had no input during development can lead to managerial frustrations.

If the SNF contracts with an outside agency to provide rehabilitation services rather than hiring its own staff, those contract managers may have additional burdens in sorting out competing or contradictory priorities of the contracting agency and the SNF. Employees of agencies are bound to the agency's policies and procedures as they move from SNF to SNF in their assignments. These policies and procedures must be reconciled with those of the SNF. Identifying where loyalties lie, and should lie, may be difficult for some employees.

Marketing

Rehabilitation managers may have many opportunities to contribute to program development in SNFs that are part of large corporations, or they may have to take the initiative in program development in smaller SNFs. Identifying niche markets to target particular groups of patients for systematic, well-defined programs to meet their specific needs is one commonly used marketing strategy. The group of patients with memory deficits is one example of a target market. SNFs may also focus on marketing their home-like environments with attention to meeting individual needs. These

marketing strategies are also driven by surveys in some states that encourage strategies that promote privacy and care with dignity in a more home-like atmosphere including restaurant-style dining in a hospitable environment. Rehabilitation managers are usually considered part of the marketing team. They need to be prepared to market rehabilitation services and their centers aggressively because of the competition with other SNFs and other types of long-term care services.

Even if driven primarily by healthcare policy changes at first, nursing home administrators increasingly rely on rehabilitation managers. They assist the SNF in attracting appropriate patients for skilled care through promoting strong relationships with referral sources, optimizing patient outcomes, and identifying niche markets. Managers need to advocate for appropriate utilization of rehabilitation services and, as important, identify new services that may be offered.

Nursing personnel have traditionally dominated long-term care (as would be expected in skilled *nursing* facilities), so managers of other services need to take every opportunity to consider nursing staff as a target market as well. Shifting skilled nursing care for patients with all diagnoses to a focus on improving patients' function becomes critical. Rehabilitation managers are better positioned as key players in skilled nursing care as a result as they assist nursing staff to transition from their comfort with the medical model of care with its focus on treatment of disease to a rehabilitation way of thinking and decision-making.

Staffing

Staff turnover is probably the biggest issue for SNF managers. The cost of recruiting, selecting, interviewing, checking credentials, and orienting a new employee may far exceed the monthly salary of an employee. Therefore, managers are compelled to retain employees as much as they need to hire additional employees. Retention becomes increasingly important during growth periods. When competition for qualified employees is high, workforce demands and turnover increase simultaneously.

Avoiding turnover is especially crucial in long-term care because of its effect on elderly residents who come to rely heavily on their caregivers and who do not tolerate changes in personnel very well. New employees face the additional challenges of attempting to adhere to the routine of the usual, consistent care that many people depend on to function at their optimal levels.

Meeting workforce needs with temporary workers may be more problematic than helpful in long-term care because these employees lack the history of care and knowledge of the complex conditions and idiosyncrasies of residents. Temporary or prn (as needed) staff may not have a strong commitment to the rehabilitation because of negative biases or stereotypes about the elderly. This lack of history and interest places the SNF at a higher risk for errors in judgment in caring for residents. A vicious cycle of losing personnel because of the errors that occur, followed by more errors made by their replacements, can be difficult to break.

Rehabilitation professionals accepting positions as traveling therapists is common during times of workforce shortages. They are offered short-term assignments (e.g., 6 to 13 weeks) that offer high salaries and the opportunities for a wide range of experiences. Because managers know that the end of the short-term assignment is always near, any professional and behavioral performance issues may not be addressed effectively. The added expense of fees paid to agencies to provide these services may be high but unavoidable. The alternative—recruitment costs for full-time, permanent staff—is another important financial consideration for nursing homes as they seek to provide the quality of care and the quality of life that the residents deserve.

Supportive Personnel

State statutes guide administrative rules about the role of licensed physical therapist assistants and other supportive personnel in SNFs. In some states, physical therapist assistants may work in an SNF without a requirement that a physical therapist be on site. Although this level of direction and supervision may be legal, managers need to determine the roles of assistants by considering the levels of complexity and acuity of patients' conditions in addition to the expertise of particular assistants. The more unstable and unpredictable a patient's condition is, the less appropriate it may be for physical therapists to direct others to perform interventions independently. Having responsibility for decisions about each resident at any point in time, physical therapists must know and trust the skills and knowledge of physical

therapist assistants whom they direct and supervise, particularly when not on site.

At the same time, to remain efficient and control costs, determining the appropriate utilization of physical therapist assistants, and hiring them, is critical to managing physical therapy services. Clarification of the duties and responsibilities for provision of care and reporting that care to the physical therapist of record is necessary to reduce the risk of adverse physiological responses of patients with complex conditions. The strengths and weaknesses of physical therapist assistants should not be assumed any more than the strengths and weaknesses of physical therapists should be assumed.

Because of the risks inherent in the SNF population, the direction of personnel other than the physical therapist assistant should be limited to non-treatment responsibilities such as maintenance of the environment, transporting patients, running errands, filing, and assisting with other managerial requirements. Should other personnel be considered for direct patient care, considering them as an extra set of hands to assist during treatment sessions is probably the most appropriate view of these tasks. However, if rehab aides or techs are also CNAs, they may be very helpful in performing CNA tasks while patients are in their therapy sessions. Conversely, their experience in rehab enhances the skills they take to the nursing service. This crossover training provides CNAs with additional work opportunities.

Managers should consider how valuable the physical therapist assistant might be in family education and teaching CNAs and other caregivers. Providing one-on-one instruction and classroom instruction may be a vital role for assistants. These assignments result in the ability of therapists to attend to the complex clinical decisions that need to be made in one-on-one direct patient care.

Perhaps more than any other setting, SNFs provide physical therapist assistants a wide range of upward career opportunities as they engage in other administrative duties, and the opportunity to develop strong clinical skills with complex patients in what may be considered a specialty practice for them. For instance, because of workforce shortages, assistants may become the managers of rehabilitation services because of their administrative skills and expertise. Perhaps they may be the most senior person on staff because of the turnover of therapists or the percentage of staff who are temporary or traveling therapists.

As managers, physical therapist assistants may have the administrative expertise, but lack the clinical expertise and responsibility to make the difficult decisions regarding direct care of patients. Assistants in managerial positions need to verify for themselves that they are not practicing physical therapy without a license while performing both managerial and patient care responsibilities. The assistants must shift to their supervisory roles to manage the performance and duties of the licensed physical therapist. Confusion may arise between managerial assistants and licensed physical therapists when trying to differentiate between the direction and supervision of a licensed physical therapist while performing patient care duties. These daily interactions require a clear mutual understanding of these dual roles. Further, managers who are assistants may also need to clarify their positions with patients. Patients need to be aware that physical therapists and other therapists are responsible for *all* of the important *clinical* decisions about their care, although responsibility for administrative decisions lies with the manager.

This unusual dynamic may be another reflection of the change for healthcare managers who are expected to deal with finances and staffing rather than clinical practice issues. Managers in positions that include supervision of staff from many professions are required to be healthcare-discipline neutral in their managerial decision-making. It may be helpful for physical therapist assistants to remain neutral as well in physical therapy clinical decisions. The potential for gaps in the need for professionals to have role models and mentors in their clinical decision-making is at risk in these models.

Patient Care

Reimbursement is tightly intertwined in patient care in SNFs, resulting in patient care decisions that have a direct impact on tight financial circumstances. In addition to this complicated financial factor, managers have to be certain that therapists are well prepared for evaluating the physiological effects of their direct interventions on the complex conditions of their patients. Close monitoring during treatment sessions is essential to reduce the risk of harm to patients. Therapists in SNFs also must be cognizant of the impact of their choice of interventions on

the psychosocial needs of patients who may find it difficult to learn new motor tasks, or who may be struggling with the losses they experience because of a serious illness. Further information on the role of rehabilitation in long-term care can be found in the Cochrane Database of Systematic Reviews; see Web Resources. The American Physical Therapy Association webpages on Payment and Practice and Patient Care should be checked regularly to remain abreast of current issues; see Web Resources.

Prospective Payment in Skilled Nursing Facilities

Assuring that evidence-based interventions are used to achieve patient goals efficiently within a discipline or among disciplines that provide care to a resident is paramount because of the prospective payment system imposed on SNFs. Complying with established plans of care and projecting the number of minutes/day that patients must receive skilled therapy services are required for payment of services. Plans of care are based on standardized assessments of patients using the MDS tracking forms (see Web Resources for Medicare MDS forms). The skill involved in compliance with regulations in this process is as important as the delivery of appropriate, effective interventions themselves. Additional information on this complex payment system can be found at the Centers for Medicare & Medicaid: Nursing Home Quality Initiative (NHQI) and MDS Data Set Public Reports webpages listed in Web Resources. They should be referred to frequently because of ongoing modifications that require new action. Current highlights of this complex payment system are presented here:[8]

- The Medicare Part A prospective payment for care provided by SNFs is based on a per diem rate/patient admitted. This base rate bundles the payment for all services. The rates are established and reviewed regularly by the federal government to cover *all* costs of the nursing home, not just patient care. There are different rates for urban and rural nursing homes.

- The base per diem rates are adjusted for each patient based on the results of the Resident Assessment Instrument (RAI) that includes the MDS triggers, Resident Assessment Protocols (RAPs), and utilization (treatment time) guidelines. The RAI is intended to be completed by an interprofessional team (i.e., dieticians, therapists, nurses, pharmacists). The RAI scores determine the case mix for each patient and the wages for providers at the level of skilled care (time) required to provide the care a particular patient needs.

- The case mix and time adjustment is based on a classification system, the Resource Utilization Groups III (RUGs). Each patient's RUG is determined by the data generated by each member of the care team as entered into the standardized MDS that must be signed by a nurse—typically with the title of MDS coordinator. The MDS data may trigger one or more of the 18 RAPs that lead to more assessment of potential problem areas. Typically, different sections of the MDS are assigned to different members of the team.

- This MDS reimbursement requirement also affects the quality of care by requiring a thorough evaluation of each patient (resident) with this standardized, comprehensive, and reproducible assessment. It improves communication within the facility and among facilities because everyone is speaking the same language. This reimbursement/quality approach is designed to prevent the avoidable decline of patients and build on their current strengths to improve their quality of life through high-quality care.

- Assuring that there are no inconsistencies or contradictions in the MDS among the data generated by different team members is critical for accurate determination of each patient's case mix RUG group. Rehabilitation managers are included in this decision-making for each patient admitted to a nursing home. Identifying all factors that may qualify patients at the highest RUG level is important to the financial stability of the nursing home. The nursing home cannot afford to provide more care than it will be reimbursed for, so the determination of the level of care that will be required must be accurate. The skill and knowledge to contribute to this process are important for managers to develop.

- The 53 RUG III classifications (expected to increase to 66 RUG IV classifications) that are most important to the nursing home because of their higher levels of per diem

rates of reimbursement just happen to be those that involve the patient's need for rehabilitation services. See Table 13.2 for examples of RUGs.

- To which of the 53 levels of the RUG classifications a patient is assigned determines, for example, the services a patient will receive and the number of minutes that must be met for each therapy service. This assignment has serious implications for rehabilitation managers who are responsible for staff compliance to these reimbursement requirements.

- The data from individual patient MDSs are transmitted to centralized databanks in each state and then forwarded to a national database at the CMS. There they are analyzed and used in the measurement of outcome-based quality improvement criteria.

Nursing Rehabilitation

At the other end of the spectrum of long-term care is the managerial responsibility for nursing rehabilitation (restorative care services) that is provided to individual patients in residential care. The rehabilitation manager has responsibility for assuring that all patients in residential care are walking and exercising to maintain their maximal level of performance for as long as possible with the establishment of individualized programs for all residents. Educating CNAs to perform these activities as part of their routine care of patients and reinforcing the need for group physical activity as part of the center's activity programs are other ways that rehabilitation managers have a major impact on positive patient outcomes. As the medical management of chronic diseases increases in importance, the sophistication and consistency of restorative care must improve accordingly.

Fiscal

Historically, reimbursement policies have shaped the delivery of therapy services in all practice settings. SNFs may face some unique challenges in assuring that documentation of care matches the billing for that care, all of which are electronically transmitted for reimbursement. The care is interdisciplinary, yet the documentation and billing are discipline unique. Regulatory surveys include

TABLE 13.2 Resource Utilization Groups III (RUGs) examples

RUG LEVEL REHABILITATION NURSING	PATIENT REQUIREMENT	REHABILITATION MINUTES AND DISCIPLINES	TYPICAL PATIENT	ACTIVITIES OF DAILY LIVING (ADLS) INDEX AND RUG CODES FROM MDS*
Ultrahigh/ Extensive	IV, tracheotomy, ventilator, or suctioning in past 14 days. Feeding tube, nil per os (NPO) orders, parenteral fluids in past 7 days.	720 minutes or more of rehabilitation/ week. One rehabilitation discipline 5 days/ week and another 3 days/week.	People with neurological diagnoses who were independent with excellent rehabilitation potential to return home or to lower level of care.	16–18 RUX 7–15 RUL *If ultrahigh without extensive nursing then:* *16–18 RUC* *9–15 RUB* *4–8 RUA*
Very High/ Extensive	Same	500 or more minutes. At least one rehabilitation discipline for at least 5 days.	People with cerebral vascular accident, joint replacement, new condition that required limited assistance with very good rehabilitation potential to return home or lesser level of care.	16–18 RVX 7–15 RVL *If very high without extensive nursing then:* *16–18 RVC* *9–15 RVB* *4–8 RVA*
High/ Extensive	Same	325 or more minutes of rehabilitation/ week. At least one rehabilitation discipline 5 days/ week.	People with cerebral vascular accident, hip fracture, elective surgery who will likely be discharged to long-term care.	16–18 RVX 7–15 RVL *If very high without extensive nursing then:* *13–18 RHC* *6–12 RHB* *4–7 RHA*

*Go to http://www.cms.hhs.gov/SNFPPS/downloads/RUGDesSch.pdf for definitions of RUG codes.

review of billing documentation that leads to review of clinical documentation to support the claims for reimbursement.

In addition, *actual* time spent in treatment *must* be accurately reflected in the documentation because billing is based on time to meet current Medicare requirements. Requirements include guidelines for treating patients one-on-one and for treating more than one person at a time. The group or concurrent charge is one-half the one-on-one charge, so the mix of the two types of treatments sessions becomes a major factor in staff mix and case mix decisions.

To assure consistency and accuracy, decreasing the number of different providers who work with any particular patient increases the likelihood that there will be agreement among treatment notes, weekly progress notes, and billing sheets, as well as better coordination of care among disciplines. Management accountability for accurate reporting may require ongoing audits of documentation and billing. This important responsibility reduces the risks of payment denials and provides the opportunity to identify treatment activities that may not be assigned easily to a particular billing category. Avoiding documentation of activities that overlap with that of other professions is another possible area of concern that calls for clarification so that records and billing forms are both accurate. Therapists expect, rightfully so, that managers will assist in these important responsibilities because accountability for documenting and billing stops with the individual providing the care.[9]

Their fiscal responsibilities require that rehabilitation managers remain current in their understanding of Medicare and Medicaid rules and the frequent changes that occur. They must share this information not only with their staffs for implementation, but also with upper management to advise them of potential areas of risk—fraud, abuse, underutilization or overutilization of services.

Rehabilitation managers may not have responsibility for financial planning, but they do have input into budgeting decisions, particularly about capital equipment (typically for the expansion of services) and space allocation. They are often more accountable for implementing a budget than they are for developing it, and most frequently face decisions calling for a reduction in resources that have been allocated. Controlling costs, particularly workforce costs, becomes a focus of managerial efforts. Finding the resources to cover important patient care–related functions that are directly billable also causes pressure, particularly in for-profit corporations, to maintain certain profit levels.

Legal, Ethical, and Risk

Long-term care is a high-risk environment because patients often have both cognitive deficits and complex medical conditions that require extended periods of care during which many variables impact their well-being or recovery. Attention to the rights and dignity of patients is paramount regardless of their ability to participate in their own care and decisions. This demand is the basis of the high level of responsibility that the staff in SNFs often holds for the care of the most vulnerable people in society. From the use of restraints to control patient mobility to living wills, the staffs in SNFs face major legal and ethical issues on a daily basis. Managers have a responsibility to question and understand the values of the people they supervise. The potential for a failure to respect the dignity of or to violate the rights of the individuals they care for can thereby be avoided.

Delegation of skilled care to family members and other non-skilled paid helpers increases safety risks. The ramping down of therapy intervention toward discharge to a safe environment presents a variety of opportunities and legal challenges for managers. Managers are responsible for representing the rehabilitation perspective in comprehensive, interprofessional discharge planning, which is needed for a smooth, **safe** transition to the next living environment. Identifying the potential risk factors and assuring that safety requirements can be met are major responsibilities.

Remaining rational and objective about safety when patients and family bear pressure because of their strong desire to return to their prior living situations often takes courage and understanding. The physical and cognitive needs for skilled services has to be distinguished from services that people may prefer to have to meet their social needs. Creative planning and the desire to help people overcome many barriers to go home again make rehabilitation in SNFs rewarding and exciting. Managers who are able to convey the importance of this role and the satisfaction of these accomplishments may have one of the most powerful recruitment tools.

Communication

Because of the fast pace of the work in SNFs, opportunities for informal conversation among staff may seem to occur rarely. Formal communication about patient care, however, is often mandated and documented in detail. Depending on the size of the SNF, staff may be grouped into teams that work in particular units with the same residents throughout the entire length of their care. This team model is effective in improving formal and informal communication. Because of the individualized, long-term needs of most residents, it is more effective for everyone taking care of a patient to meet about that particular patient than to gather caregivers together to discuss global, generic issues about patient care. These team or utilization meetings for resident-based care are formalized so that each discipline is represented as interprofessional decisions are made and documented about each patient's care.

Managers often feel that all they do is attend meetings. With the MDS coordinator, social worker, business office manager, admissions coordinator, and perhaps others, rehabilitation managers attend daily, brief, stand-up meetings. The topics for discussion typically include a review and updates of the census in the building (admissions and discharges), 24-hour nursing reports to report any patient incidents or problems, review of RUG classifications, and reminders of days remaining in patient benefit periods. These meetings demonstrate the importance and urgency associated with controlling those factors that affect the finances of SNFs. Other meetings are necessary to assure accurate interprofessional completion and revision of the MDS for each patient.

Rehabilitation managers may have a great deal of interaction with the director of nursing (DON) in SNFs. They face many of the same responsibilities and jointly arrive at many decisions. For instance, both are responsible for efficient utilization of staff and management of financial resources to provide care and the day-to-day staffing and overall operations of their services. Shared responsibilities include developing and implementing plans of care for each patient. Assuring nursing and rehab documentation that presents consistent clinical pictures of patients is also a partnership. The directors of nursing are often depended on the most by the nursing home administrators, who may defer a great deal of decision-making to them. Rehabilitation managers who establish a strong professional relationship with DONs may find that they are part of a powerful managerial team, particularly when the clinical problems are many and common to both disciplines.

Rehabilitation managers also may meet formally every day with the nursing home administrator. This frequency may vary depending on the role of the DON and the presence of assistant administrators in certain centers. Managers should not assume they would have the same direct working relationships with each nursing home administrator as they move from one building to another. These meetings typically include review of Medicare statistics, authorization for care of indigent patients or others with special needs, budgeting, marketing plans, and patient census building. Rather than direct responsibility for individuals in a nursing home, the administrator typically has the broad legal responsibility for the patient outcomes and finances of the nursing home as a whole.

As the size of SNFs continues to grow, managers need more opportunities to interact with larger staffs to monitor their performance both formally and informally. With the increased number of therapists in a building, new therapists can also receive a higher degree of mentoring and assistance with clinical decision-making. Although inter-professional teams are paramount in long-term care, managers have more opportunity to facilitate the development of discipline-specific teams who are able to apply and contribute to the evidence in each of their professions for the care of patients with complex conditions and for chronic disease management. For example, developing new physical therapy approaches for the care of people with cognitive and psychological disorders presents opportunities for brainstorming and program proposals. Promoting these professional interactions (e.g., journal clubs) either within a building or within an area in which there are several facilities may be an important management tool. These activities may lead professionals to pursue board certification in geriatrics, assist in recruitment efforts, and reduce staff turnover.

Conclusions

Long-term care, more than any other component of healthcare, provides many management opportunities for physical therapists because of the breadth of services provided and the anticipated growth for high-quality services to manage chronic diseases among the elderly. The management of skilled nursing care today is similar to the management of acute care hospitals of the past in terms of the variety of clinical learning experiences and opportunities for upward career mobility. Managers may need to focus on the transfer of these exciting characteristics to the long-term care setting to improve the recruitment of therapists who often have negative preconceived notions to overcome.

Either through internal corporate-management programs or self-directed professional development, physical therapists and assistants may prepare themselves for careers in long-term care at a variety of levels of care and management. They may anticipate new approaches in aging services that will continue to broaden the scope of physical therapy services. Such approaches are limited only by the imagination and initiative of managers. Activities 13.1 through 13.17 present scenarios for working through some long-term care management challenges.

ACTIVITY 13.1
MORE INFORMATION

Determine 10 key aspects of Medicare requirements that are most important to managers in SNFs based on the following resources:

1. Go to the CMS's Guidance to Surveyors for Long-Term Care Facilities at http://www.cms .gov/Medicare/Provider-Enrollment-and-Certification/GuidanceforLawsAndRegulations/Downloads/som107ap_pp_guidelines_ltcf.pdf,

especially §483.45, Specialized Rehabilitation Services.
2. Review Medicare requirements for reimbursement of rehabilitation services at http://www.cms.gov/Research-Statistics-Data-and-Systems/Monitoring-Programs/Medical-Review/Downloads/TherapyCapSlidesv10_09052012.pdf.

ACTIVITY 13.2
THE SKILLED NURSING FACILITY MANAGEMENT TEAM

Pleasant Valley Care Center is a 200-bed skilled nursing facility with one wing of 30 beds for nonskilled residential care. Sam Simmons, administrator, Rebecca Romano, Director of Nursing, and Louise Lopez, Director of Rehabilitation, meet every Monday for 1 hour to brainstorm and solve one selected problem.

The issue that continues to be unresolved is the decline in the quality of care on weekends. Despite efforts to provide consistent weekend staff from their per diem pool and to improve in the transfer of information from the weekday to the weekend staff,

they have not been very successful. Resident, family, and staff complaints continue about what seems to be every aspect of care delivered on Saturdays and Sundays.

Sam is very concerned that these complaints will lead to noncompliance in several areas during the next state survey.

What should the team do? Consider: Where are they now? Where do they want to be? What do they have to work with? How will they get there?

ACTIVITY 13.3
THE NEW PHYSICAL THERAPIST

Latosha Wilkes is the new rehabilitation director at Still River Nursing and Rehabilitation Center. After years of using contract rehab services, the center was able to recruit her as a full-time employee. Latosha was very excited about this opportunity to improve the rehab services because of her love for geriatric patients. However, she is not as far along as she would like to be in her plans. A stumbling block is the administrator, Cynthia Carruthers. Although Cynthia has been effective in many areas,

she prefers to focus on marketing. In their weekly meetings, Latosha finds it difficult to get Cynthia to discuss specific rehab questions and issues. She believes this is because Cynthia relied on the contract company's regional manager to handle rehab and never really devoted much attention to it. What should Latosha do? Consider: Where are they now? Where does Latosha want them to be? What does she have to work with? How will she get there?

ACTIVITY 13.4
EQUALS

Latosha Wilkes is the new rehab director at Still River Nursing and Rehabilitation Center. She has been successful in staffing the department with employees rather than contract therapists. Rehab Services is becoming the most valued department in the nursing home. This has created a little problem for Latosha in her working relationship with George Johnson, the Director of Nursing. When rehab services were contracted, the staff reported to George who became accustomed to telling them what to do. He has not fully accepted that he does not supervise Latosha who has equal managerial status. What should Latosha do? Consider: Where are they now? Where does Latosha want them to be? What does she have to work with? How will she get there?

ACTIVITY 13.5
THE WORK OF PHYSICAL THERAPY IN SKILLED NURSING FACILITIES

Louisa Lopez, the Director of Rehabilitation at Pleasant Valley Care Center, faces the challenge of high turnover among the rehabilitation staff, with an average stay of only 6 months. Applicants often tell her that they would like to work in nursing homes because they like old people. However, she finds that they just do not understand the complexity of their patients' conditions and of the regulatory demands on their care. What should she do? Consider: What is the current status of staffing efforts? Where should the result of staffing efforts be? What does Louisa have to work with? How will she get there?

ACTIVITY 13.6
PHYSICAL THERAPY RUSH HOUR

Louisa Lopez does not know what to do. Although her staff is scheduled to work 8-hour days, it seems that all the patients receiving therapy are treated between 10 a.m. and 2 p.m. The therapy areas are crowded and noisy during these hours and empty otherwise. Both patients and therapists feel rushed, and the therapy rooms look like therapy mills rather than therapeutic settings. Her staff reports that patients are not ready to come to therapy any earlier and they are scheduled for other social activities in the afternoons. What should she do? Consider: What is the current status of patient scheduling? Where should it be? What does Louisa have to work with? How will she get there?

ACTIVITY 13.7
FAMILY EDUCATION

Louisa Lopez, Director of Rehabilitation at Pleasant Valley Care Center, has another issue to resolve. Although she sees many family members in the therapy rooms during treatment sessions, they seem to be observing rather than participating. She believes this contributes to the low rate of discharges to home. She is trying to decide whether to focus her energy on intensifying one-on-one family education or on developing family education classes in light of the Health Insurance Portability and Accountability Act (HIPAA) privacy rules. Which should she do? Why? Consider: What is the current status of family education? What should it be? What does Louisa have to work with? How will she get there?

ACTIVITY 13.8
OWNERSHIP CHANGE

Robert O'Reilly has been the manager of rehabilitation services at Mountain Top Nursing Center, a rural SNF with 20 skilled and 30 residential beds, for 3 years. As the only physical therapist in the SNF, he has been responsible for all physical therapy services with the help of a full-time physical therapist assistant. He is also responsible for hiring and evaluating the occupational therapist and speech-language pathologist who work on a per diem basis. He places great pride on his achievements in the development and incorporation of rehabilitation services in the SNF and on his strong work relationships with the nursing staff. Things could not be better.

The administrator/owner of Mountain Top calls a general staff meeting to announce that he has sold Mountain Top to All Nation Care, a nursing home corporation. Effective the first of the month, All Nation Care's transitional team will be at Mountain Top to facilitate the transition to new ownership. He assures the staff that all changes will be for the better including across-the-board salary increases in anticipation of doubling the size of the facility. After the shock wears off, what questions should Robert prepare for his meeting with All Nation Care's corporate coordinator of rehabilitation?

ACTIVITY 13.9
A PATIENT FALLS

Robert O'Reilly receives a call at home on Sunday morning from the licensed practical (LPN) charge nurse on the north wing. She reports that while the physical therapist assistant and CNA were performing a transfer of Mrs. Langdon, requiring the maximum

assist of two people from bed to chair, the patient fell. The LPN thinks that Mrs. Langdon's hip is fractured and wants to know what she should do. Fill in the blanks: Robert should_____immediately. He should also_____to prevent a similar incident in the future.

ACTIVITY 13.10
DUPLICATION OF SERVICES

When conducting his monthly audit of rehabilitation records, Robert O'Reilly notices that physical therapy and occupational therapy goals, interventions, and billing for several patients appear to be overlapped.

How should he resolve this duplication of services? Why does it need to be resolved? Consider: What is the current status of billing and coding? What should it be? What does Robert have to work with? How will he get there?

ACTIVITY 13.11
A NEW OPPORTUNITY

Seashore Pavilion is a 200-bed SNF that is completely Medicare/Medicaid certified. Tina Tirelli has just begun her position as Director of Physical Therapy with a staff of five physical therapists and 10 physical therapist assistants. One of her challenges is the 16-bed, state-funded pediatric unit for children with complex medical needs. None of the current staff is qualified or even willing to learn how to provide services to children,

and there is a hold on new hires. State funding of the unit is at risk if they do not comply with regulations regarding the provision of rehabilitation services to these children.

What should she do? Consider: Where are the pediatric staff members now? Where do they want to be? What does Tina have to work with? How will she get there?

ACTIVITY 13.12
A FULL RANGE OF SERVICES

Moonlight Bay is a large retirement community with a full range of social and medical services for its residents. Rehabilitation services are of concern to Janet Blackstone, the administrator. Although the staff in the SNF are employees of Moonlight Bay and residents of the community can receive outpatient rehabilitation services there, they often choose to go to other outpatient centers in the nearby town. Residents of the adult congregate living facility receive home care rehabilitation services through City Home Health, although home nursing care is provided by Moonlight Bay nursing staff. Concerned about the promise of continuity of care to the residents, she asks Robin Blessing, the Director of Rehabilitation at the SNF, to explain how they reached this state of affairs and to propose a plan for keeping all rehabilitation services within the community.

What should Robin do? Consider: Where is the range of therapy services now? Where do they want them to be? What do they have to work with? How will they get there?

ACTIVITY 13.13
PATIENT PROGRESSION

Inez Roberts, PT, is very upset as she meets with Robin Blessing, Rehabilitation Director. Inez reports that Karl Smith, the Physical Therapist Assistant, is impossible to work with. Despite her warnings to Karl, he has often progressed a patient's exercise or weight-bearing without consulting with Inez first. None of the other therapists seems to have a problem with Karl.

Today was the last in a series of problematic issues with Karl. Inez just received a call from an orthopedic surgeon who is outraged that his patient has been instructed to walk with more weight-bearing than he ordered. As a result, the patient will require surgery to revise her total hip replacement. Karl has provided all of the patient's care in the past 2 weeks and only reported to Inez that the patient was doing well. Inez says she has had enough and plans to submit her resignation.

What should Robin do? Consider: Where are they now? Where do they want to be? What does Robin have to work with? How will she get there?

ACTIVITY 13.14
PATIENT DIGNITY

Joanna Barnes is a physical therapist assistant with 6 years of experience in a large medical center where she rotated among inpatient and outpatient care. She accepted a position at Moonlight Bay Nursing and Rehabilitation Center. Robin Blessing, Rehabilitation Manager, has been very pleased with her clinical skills but is concerned, however, because Joanna, not in a malicious or hurtful way, often makes fun of patients with cognitive problems or who appear or behave oddly. The remarks and mimicking are funny, and her presence has lightened the mood of the rehabilitation department. Everyone really likes Joanna. Robin, though, is concerned that Joanna often crosses the line with some of her comments, which may be perceived as disrespectful with a disregard for a patient's dignity. She does not want to lose Joanna.

What should she do? Consider: Where are they now? Where do they want to be? What does Robin have to work with? How will she get there?

ACTIVITY 13.15
TRAVELING THERAPISTS

Robin Blessing has been promoted to area manager for six nursing homes in Manatino County Nursing and Rehabilitation Corporation (MCNRC). She feels fortunate to have been able to establish a good relationship with USA Rehabilitation Travelers. They have been providing a steady stream of competent therapists who typically work 6- or 13-week assignments in one of the nursing homes and then move out of the area. A few of the traveling therapists have been a very good match with MCNRC, and they have expressed an interest in continuing to work in any of their centers.

What should she do? Consider: Where is the staffing now? Where do they want staffing to be? What does Robin have to work with? How will she get there?

ACTIVITY 13.16
A CLINCAL AND FINANCIAL CHALLENGE

Belinda Gentry, Director of Rehabilitation at Seashore Health and Rehabilitation Center, receives a call on Monday morning from the Executive Director, William Winters, requesting to meet today about a patient. During their meeting he asks Belinda whether she had the opportunity to see the new patient, Mr. Beasley, who was admitted over the weekend. Belinda reports that she had and that Mr. Beasley is a 66-year-old man who has had a left total hip replacement. He was admitted on Saturday with orders for physical therapy and occupational therapy. Mr. Beasley was evaluated by a physical therapist on Saturday, and an occupational therapist is in the process of completing her evaluation today.

William is pleased and asks Belinda for assurance that they will not miss the opportunity to capture the reimbursement for Mr. Beasley at a RUG-level of Rehabilitation Ultrahigh. He has reviewed the monthly report and shares with Belinda the fact that utilization for the higher RUG levels of reimbursement has dropped by 25% and the average patient length of stay has declined by 4 days. He attributes these unfavorable numbers to the new therapy staff. He believes they are not seeking to treat patients aggressively enough, and they fail to strongly encourage patients to come to therapy. The result, he tells Belinda, is that the therapy department is losing the nursing home money and he wants to know what she will do about it.

How should Belinda respond? Does William have a valid concern? What action does Belinda need to take? Consider: Where are they now? Where do they want to be? What do they have to work with? How will they get there?

ACTIVITY 13.17
HELPING THE HELP

Keisha Williams has been a CNA at Seashore Health and Rehabilitation Center for about 1 year. She has been surprised at how much she enjoys her work and the people she is assigned to care for in the residential unit. She is very pleased that Belinda Gentry, the Rehabilitation Director, has asked the Director of Nursing that Keisha be assigned to the rehabilitation wing because she is so efficient and works so well with her patients.

Keisha tells Belinda that she is flattered and appreciates that her work has been recognized, but she is also concerned about the transfer. She feels her work will be harder physically and she doesn't know whether she likes the idea that there is so much patient turnover on the rehabilitation wing.

What should Belinda do? Consider: Where are they now? Where do they want to be? What does Belinda have to work with? How will she get there?

REFERENCES

1. Pratt JR. *Long-Term Care: Managing Across the Continuum.* 2nd ed. Sudbury, MA: Jones and Bartlett; 2004.
2. National Center for Health Statistics. *Health, United States, 2006, With Chart Book on Trends in the Health of Americans.* Hyattsville, MD: Centers for Disease Control; 2006. http://www.cdc.gov/nchs/fastats/nursingh.htm. Accessed May 15, 2013.
3. McCarthy J, Friedman LH. The significance of autonomy in the nursing home administrator profession: a qualitative study. *Health Care Management Review.* 2006;31:55-63.
4. National Long-Term Ombudsman Resource Center. OBRA '87 summary. http://www.ltcombudsman. org/ombpublic/49_346_1023.cfm. Accessed September 12, 2007.
5. Commission on Accreditation of Rehabilitation Facilities. Who we are. http://www.carf.org/consumer. aspx?content=content/About/News/boilerplate.htm. Accessed November 1, 2007.
6. Hill RD. *Geriatric Residential Care.* Mahwah, NJ: Lawrence Erlbaum Associates; 2002.
7. Ryan NP, Wade JC, Nice A, et al. Physical therapists' perceptions of family involvement in the rehabilitation process. *Physiotherapy Research International.* 1996;1(3):157-179.
8. Department of Health and Human Services. Prospective payment system and consolidated billing for skilled nursing facilities-update-notice. http://www.cms.hhs. gov/snfpps/downloads/cms-1530-n-display.pdf. Accessed November 16, 2007.
9. Erhart A, Delehanty LM, Morley NE, et al. Consistency between documented occupational therapy services and billing in a skilled nursing facility: a pilot study. *Physical & Occupational Therapy in Geriatrics.* 2005;24(2):53-62.

WEB RESOURCES

American Health Care Association. http://www.ahcancal.org/about_ahca/Pages/default.aspx. Accessed November 29, 2013.

American Physical Therapy Association. Practice and Patient Care. http://www.apta.org/Practice/. Accessed November 29, 2013.

Centers for Medicare and Medicaid Services, Long-term Care Facilities. http://www.cms.gov/Regulations-and-Guidance/Legislation/CFCsAndCoPs/LTC.html. Accessed November 29, 2013.

Centers for Medicare and Medicaid Services. Nursing Home Compare. http://www.medicare.gov/nursinghomecompare/?version=default&browser=IE%257C6%257CWinXP&language=English&defaultstatus=0&pagelist=Home&CookiesEnabledStatus=True&AspxAutoDetectCookieSupport=1. Accessed June 11, 2014.

Centers for Medicare & Medicaid Services. Nursing Home Quality Initiative (NHQI) website provides consumer and provider information regarding the quality of care in nursing homes. http://www.cms.gov/Medicare/Quality-Initiatives-Patient-Assessment-Instruments/NursingHomeQualityInits/index.html?redirect=/nursinghomequalityinits/. Accessed November 29, 2013.

Cochrane Database of Systematic Reviews. http://www.ncbi.nlm.nih.gov/pubmedhealth/PMH0012677/. Accessed November 29, 2013.

The Commission on Accreditation of Rehabilitation Facilities (CARF). http://www.carf.org/ and http://www.carf.org/aging/. Accessed November 29, 2013.

The Joint Commission. Long-Term Care Accreditation. http://www.jointcommission.org/accreditation/long_term_care_accreditation_requirements.aspx. Accessed November 29, 2013.

LongtermCare.gov. http://longtermcare.gov/the-basics/. Accessed November 29, 2013.

Medicare and Medicaid-certified nursing home compare. http://www.medicare.gov/nursinghomecompare/search.html?AspxAutoDetectCookieSupport=1.

Medicare Minimum Data Set (MDS) basic assessment tracking forms. http://www.cms.gov/Medicare/Quality-Initiatives-Patient-Assessment-Instruments/NursingHomeQualityInits/downloads/MDS20MDSAllforms.pdf. Accessed November 29, 2013.

Minimum Data Set (MDS, 3.0 Public Reports) is part of the federally mandated process for clinical assessment of all residents in Medicare and Medicaid certified nursing homes. http://www.cms.gov/Research-Statistics-Data-and-Systems/Computer-Data-and-Systems/Minimum-Data-Set-3-0-Public-Reports/index.html. Accessed November 29, 2013.

National Institutes of Health, Senior Health. http://nihseniorhealth.gov/longtermcare/whatislongtermcare/01.html. Accessed November 29, 2013.

CHAPTER 14

Management Issues in Outpatient Centers

LEARNING OBJECTIVES

- Discuss components, characteristics, and types of contemporary outpatient care.
- Analyze key licensing, accreditation, and reimbursement requirements.
- Discuss contemporary outpatient practice issues (i.e., referrals, kickbacks, use of the term *physical therapy*, reimbursement limits).
- Analyze the work of physical therapists in outpatient centers.
- Determine the managerial roles and challenges to managerial responsibilities.
- Analyze managerial decision-making in given outpatient situations.

PART 1   The Contemporary Setting

Overview of Outpatient Physical Therapy

Physical therapy was typically based in hospitals or physicians' offices in the early years of the profession. However, the emergence of nationwide rehabilitation corporations with the inception of the Medicare program in the 1960s and 1970s provided many additional outpatient employment opportunities for physical therapists. The advent of the Medicare program also led to another important outpatient development—private practices owned and managed by physical therapists as reimbursement policies made these opportunities attractive and lucrative.

Interest in outpatient physical therapy continues today. In 2010, 33.6% of the American Physical Therapy Association (APTA) physical therapist members reported private outpatient or group practices as their place of employment. Others working in healthcare systems may be assigned to outpatient centers.[1]

A shift from inpatient to outpatient care at all levels of healthcare also contributes to the self-employment of professionals. The more important factor, however, is that many physical therapists often find caring for outpatients with subacute and chronic musculoskeletal disorders more preferable than caring for patients with more acute, complex conditions found in all other practice settings. Based on a 2010 survey, about 82.6% of patients in outpatient settings receive physical therapy services for musculoskeletal conditions.[2] This focus on outpatient care is supported by the fact that more than 16,000 physical therapists belong to the orthopedic section of the APTA,[3] and in 2012 the 12,937 APTA-board-certified specialists were overwhelmingly certified in orthopedics (7,655), and sports (1,094).[4] Medicare reimbursement policies also skew the patients to those with acute musculoskeletal problems or those who have had orthopedic surgery. People with other diagnoses associated with chronic musculoskeletal or other complex medical conditions are less likely to receive outpatient services because of reimbursement policies. Therapists may also find it more difficult to develop goals for patients with chronic conditions if their potential for improvement is limited. These complex patients also tend to be sicker, which makes it more difficult for them to make their way to an outpatient center on a regular basis.

Licensure, Certification, Regulation, and Accreditation

Regardless of the type of center, all outpatient physical therapy providers must be certified as individuals or as a group practice to be reimbursed for their services. Provider organizations are certified by agencies in each state to be either rehabilitation agencies or certified outpatient rehabilitation facilities (CORFs). These certification processes are complex. Simply stated, the difference between the two types of certifications is in the services provided. A CORF must provide physician services, physical therapy, and psychological/vocational counseling. Typically, occupational therapy and speech/language pathology are also included. A rehabilitation agency (or outpatient physical therapy facility) must provide services in an office, although it also may provide services in a patient's home. A rehabilitation agency must provide at least physical therapy or speech/language pathology and social or vocational counseling. Occupational therapy may be included.

The certification process involves an on-site survey and ongoing attention to recertification. In all cases, either the group or individuals also must seek approval of the appropriate Medicare carrier to obtain a provider number to bill Medicare for their services. See Web Resources for more information on the State Operations Manual that guides each state's regulation of outpatient services. Readers may wish to explore the webpages of a particular state for more information on these outpatient regulations. Certification does not mean accreditation, however. The Joint Commission accredits many types of healthcare organizations including rehabilitation and outpatient physical therapy in its list of ambulatory care centers. The Commission on Accreditation of Rehabilitation Facilities (CARF) also accredits outpatient centers. Seeking accreditation of outpatient centers is voluntary. Managers may see accreditation as a tool to formally review their processes and outcomes. Achieving accreditation status may also give a practice a marketing edge. See Web Resources for more information on Centers for Medicare & Medicaid Services (CMS), The Joint Commission, and CARF.

Contemporary Outpatient Issues

Turbulent changes in Medicare reimbursement policies have presented many hurdles for managers in all outpatient settings and for independent practitioners in physical therapy. These policies also influence the professional relationships between physical therapists and physicians. These relationships are generally and usually collaborative, ethical, and legal, resulting in positive outcomes for many, many patients. However, four important issues may negatively affect this professional relationship and demand the attention of managers. These issues are direct access of patients to the services of a physical therapist, practice without referral, self-referral, and kickbacks. Other issues related to reimbursement are also addressed in this chapter. Chapters 3, 4, and 10 present outpatient issues related to the Affordable Care Act of 2010, such as accountable care organizations (ACOs) and bundling payment models.

Direct Access

Efforts led by the APTA to influence state legislators to permit consumers direct access to physical therapists without physician referral through each state's practice act rules have been very successful. These efforts have resulted in a variety of access models that legally permit patients to seek care directly from therapists. However, the association continues its lobbying efforts to convince members of Congress that Medicare payment for physical therapy services without physician referral should be allowed. Continued negotiations by the APTA with other private third-party payers about physician referral requirements for payment are equally difficult.

The inability of some patients to directly access physical therapy services without the referral from a physician may deny them the care they require to meet their functional needs. The need for a physician referral also places many independent outpatient practitioners at a competitive disadvantage with physician-based physical therapy services. Without the resources available in large corporations, solo practitioners may also have more difficulty establishing referral relationships with physicians who are willing to refer therapy patients to practices outside of their own offices.

Practice Without Referral

Despite the legal ability to treat patients without physician referral, many physical therapists choose not to do so. One reason is reimbursement requirements discussed above. Another reason is their reluctance to give up the valued interactions they have with physicians in their clinical decision-making. For instance, in a hospital-based outpatient practice, doctor–therapist interactions may be frequent and expected, because this communication is a strong part of an organizational culture that is often physician centered. Managers may need to be aware of financial arrangements that hospitals have with physicians who have a referral relationship with its outpatient centers.

Identifying expectations for relationships with staff physicians and developing strong relationships with them facilitates the transition of patients from one setting to the next within the hospital or healthcare system. This communication responsibility is important for hospital-based managers just as developing a strong referral base is for managers in other outpatient settings.

Other outpatient therapists may feel that they lack the competence and skills for the independent decision-making involved in the examination and evaluation of patients who have not seen a physician. There is some comfort in receiving physician referrals that includes important patient information, particularly when there is a need for diagnostic testing that is beyond physical therapists' scope of practice to order or interpret. The ability to call a referring physician for more information is routine.

Physical therapists in outpatient settings need to have relationships with physicians to initiate important conversations about patient care. For example, patients with direct access to physical therapists may have suspicious findings discovered during their examinations that require further medical testing. It may be more difficult and time consuming for physical therapists to make referrals to patients' physicians or to the most appropriate physician if a patient does not have a physician of record. To avoid delays in the continuity of therapy services, managers may establish policies and procedures to standardize referrals to physicians and patient follow-ups.

Self-Referral

Professional opposition to both referrals for profit and physician ownership of physical therapy services has been a long-standing legislative agenda item for the APTA. Such business relationships present a potential conflict of interest for physicians that may not be in the patient's best interest. They also may negatively affect the autonomy of physical therapists in their clinical decision-making and in their fiduciary responsibilities to patients. Although the negative impact of self-referral on physical therapy autonomy and fiduciary responsibility may occur in *any* setting, the focus of the efforts of the APTA has been the provision of outpatient physical therapy Medicare services. The competitive disadvantage for private practice physical therapists that results from self-referral is difficult to overcome.

Physicians are in the position of "cherry-picking" patients who have the highest potential for the greatest reimbursement for their own practices. They also can exhaust a patient's benefits for outpatient rehabilitation services in their practices before referring them to another provider to continue service in order for patients to meet their therapeutic goals. Moreover, they may refer to other professionals only those patients who are the most difficult—financially or because of conditions that demand more treatment time. These financial and ethical issues fueled the development of federal legislation regarding self-referral.

Concern about the potential for the fraud and abuse inherent in self-referral, federal legislation, generally referred to as the "Stark Law," now prohibits a physician from referring a Medicare patient to any organization for certain designated health services (i.e., laboratory services, radiology, physical therapy) if that physician holds a financial interest in that organization. The Stark Law has been in effect in one phase or another for about 20 years with the inevitable development of exceptions to the prohibition of self-referral. The final Phase III of the Stark Law continues to refine this law to close loopholes and clarify financial relationship rules.

Probably the most important part of the complex and confusing Stark legislation for physical therapy managers has been the exceptions to self-referral related to the provision of ancillary services in a physician's office. The resultant "rules" have evolved to include several conditions that must be met for physicians to bill Medicare for physical therapy services provided in their offices. Essentially, the rule is that physicians are permitted to order and to provide physical therapy in their offices if it is ancillary to the medical services that they provide. In other words, the patient receiving physical therapy must also be a patient of the physician for medical services. Other criteria are that the services must be provided in the same building as the physicians' offices, and physicians no longer need to provide direct supervision of those services to be reimbursed. (For more information on physician self-referrals see Web Resources.)

For physicians to bill for physical therapy under Medicare provider numbers, only those personnel who are identified by Medicare as providers of physical therapy (i.e., physical therapists and therapist assistants) can provide services. They must comply with state statutes regarding direction and supervision.

These employment arrangements raise several important concerns for physical therapy managers in physicians' offices. Establishing strong professional relationships with physicians in a practice is a key responsibility for a manager, who must clarify and assure that the expertise of the physical therapists is respected. It is crucial so that the therapists' clinical decision-making about specific patients is preserved. Simply following the specific, standard orders of the physicians must be avoided to assure autonomous decision-making.

Because the physician's Medicare provider number and business office are used for processing physical therapy bills, physical therapy managers may have a higher responsibility for assuring the accuracy of claims submitted for reimbursement. Educating the business office staff about legal and ethical concerns that may override either contract agreements with Medicare carriers or office policies and procedures may be an ongoing primary managerial responsibility. Managers in this type of setting may need to be even more cautious about productivity goals and physician-established protocols for care that may be in the best interest of the practice rather than in the best interest of a particular patient.

Kickbacks

The Stark Law should not be confused with the Medicare and Medicaid Patient Protection Act of 1987, commonly called the "Anti-Kickback Statute," which was passed to address compensation arrangements that had the potential to adversely affect clinical decision-making and lead to unfair competition. This law prohibits the *offer or receipt* of any kickback, bribe, or rebate directly or indirectly in the form of cash or in kind for referrals by physicians (or their recommendations to purchase or lease supplies and services) of patients insured under Medicare and Medicaid.

Violation of the Anti-Kickback Statute is a criminal offense, and it has been enforced to a greater degree than the Stark Law, a civil statute, which relies more on whistle-blowing than criminal investigations to identify violators. Like exceptions in the Stark Law, there have been revisions of the Anti-Kickback Statute that identify safe harbors that exempt certain forms of kickbacks. Managers seeking to widen their referral base must be careful to comply not only with these federal statutes related to Medicare and Medicaid patients but also anti-kickback statutes in their states, which may apply more generally to all types of patient referrals.

Despite these legislative solutions to serious problems, the current reimbursement system continues to support the positions that physicians hold in healthcare decision-making, and reflects their ability to lobby Congress for policies that favor their practices financially. Physicians also have the advantage of their positions of power and influence over patients. Although many people are more interested and skillful in gathering and analyzing information about their healthcare choices, the impression is that most people continue to rely on and trust the recommendations of their physicians, although these recommendations may be influenced by factors other than the best interest of the patient. See Web Resources for more information from the Office of the Inspector General.

Changing this patient dependence on physicians requires not only managerial strategies but also strategies for the physical therapy profession as a whole. Managers are faced with almost daily decisions about how much of their efforts should focus on "working the system" rather than changing it to achieve some of their most important business goals.

Use of the Term *Physical Therapy*

It is possible that physicians may bill other non-Medicare healthcare insurance companies for "physical therapy" that they either provide themselves, hire a physical therapist or physical therapist assistant to deliver, or direct nonlicensed staff to perform the services. Because any healthcare providers who are licensed to do so may bill Medicare using any current procedural terminology (CPT-4) code, they may treat patients using the interventions of heat, ultrasound, massage, exercise, and the like. They often tell patients that they are receiving "physical therapy" although a physical therapist is not providing the care.

Using the term *physical therapy* exclusively to denote only those services that physical therapists perform is another dilemma for the profession. Many Medicare policies limiting access and reimbursement for outpatient services are linked to the high incidence of fraud and abuse in outpatient billing for the CPT codes most commonly used in treatment of musculoskeletal conditions— primarily the 97000 series. The problem continues to be that Medicare establishes the value of each CPT code in the Physician Fee Schedule but does not control or determine which health professionals bill for the services they provide using these codes. Medicare has assumed that all providers licensed to provide interventions that fall in the 97000 series are equally qualified to do so.

This Medicare assumption means that physical therapists in private practice not only compete with other physical therapy outpatient providers in corporations and healthcare systems, but they also compete with chiropractors, physicians, and any other provider who may directly bill for 97000 interventions. Sorting out which of these practitioners may be responsible for the fraud and abuse associated with the billing for CPT codes in the 97000 series remains elusive. The initiation of the National Provider Identification Standard may help to clarify this situation by identifying who is actually providing the care billed for and to allow comparisons of different types of practitioners.[5]

Reimbursement Limitations

Lobbying efforts also have been directed to reversing the implementation of an annual financial limitation (capitation) on Medicare Part B payments for physical and speech therapy combined and for occupational therapy. Until recently, hospital-based outpatient services have been exempt from this capitation to ensure that access to therapy services is not denied to Medicare beneficiaries because of the limits imposed by this capitation. Outpatient managers must develop processes to assure that patients are not moving from one therapy provider to another within 1 year ("therapy hopping") to attempt to overcome these caps on the coverage of their outpatient rehabilitation services.

Identifying which patients may have already reached their annual capitation amount in one setting before initiating services in another setting can be time consuming. For example, a patient may receive physical therapy in a physician's, chiropractor-based, or corporate practice setting and exhaust his or allowable charges or reach his or her capitation amount. The patient's physician may make another referral and direct the patient to a private practice or hospital-based practice to continue therapy. The risk of denials of claims may be high if a patient's goals were documented as met in the prior setting. Private practitioners who continue any patient's care in this situation may risk denial of the claim for reimbursement if the annual cap has been reached even without their knowledge.

Authorizations

Managers also must be certain that approvals necessary to initiate and continue services are consistently and accurately followed by members of their professional and business office staff members for both Medicare and non-Medicare patients. The aim is to avoid denials of payment for services rendered because they were not preauthorized or rules for continuing care were not followed. This required communication with insurers is another means of ensuring that payment for patient care is not intentionally, or unknowingly, denied.

Authorizations for the care of patients who receive services as part of their workers' compensation benefits or through personal injury protection (PIP) insurance (auto accident insurance) is determined by state rather than federal statutes. Managers also must track these state statutes and rules for ongoing policy changes. Because many of the patients receiving workers' compensation benefits have been injured while working for large corporations, it is not unusual that attorneys also attempt to become involved in medical discussions as they champion benefits for their clients. Interactions with attorneys related to their clients' rehabilitation can be time consuming for managers. More information to compare workers' compensation in different states may be found through the Workers Compensation Research Institute (WCRI) Benchmarks Study found in Web Resources.

Insurance Coverage for Rehabilitation Services

Congress continually acts to cut Medicare payments for rehabilitation services, regulate payment fees though annual adjustments of CPT code values, and adjust annual capitation on fees for rehabilitation services. This perpetual legislative activity keeps many outpatient physical therapy managers on an unpredictable course as they not only manage the current financing of physical therapy practice but also attempt to predict the growth of their organizations.

For private insurers, controlling costs has often meant limiting or eliminating coverage of "ancillary" health services, such as rehabilitation. However, rehabilitation and habilitation services are among the 10 essential benefits required by the Affordable Care Act for insurance policies offered in 2014 as discussed in Chapter 4. Frequently, only organizations with extensive resources are able to support business offices prepared to deal effectively with Medicare, workers' compensation, personal injury, and other types of insurance concurrently. The complexity of any one of them can be overwhelming. Further, it may be important to contract with different types of insurers because changes in any one of their policies may make one type of insurance more attractive than another at any point in time.

Alternative Income Sources

Physical therapists who wish to be truly autonomous may decide not to contract with insurance payers at all and rely on a strictly cash business with patients who are able to directly access their services. The introduction of health savings accounts may allow more people to select and pay out of pocket for particular services they need. In any type of outpatient physical therapy setting, becoming the provider of choice is a major responsibility of the physical therapy manager.

Turf wars with chiropractors for patients with spinal disorders, with occupational therapists for patients with hand injuries, and with other providers who are on the fringes of formal healthcare (i.e., acupuncturists, Rolfers, massage therapists) often raise the concern of rehabilitation managers. Personal trainers are also eager to meet the needs of people who may have exhausted their insurance benefits and are willing to pay cash for individualized, private exercise sessions to continue their "therapy." Deciding when to align with other professionals to enhance a physical therapy practice, or when to clearly differentiate physical therapy from them, is not an obvious decision.

A recent managerial response to declining reimbursement for rehabilitation services has been diversification of physical therapy practices. Efforts to provide related services, such as spa services, health-club memberships, or wellness programs, that are paid for in cash rather than health insurance reimbursement are becoming more common. Managers of physical therapy practices may need to consider, however, the image these business decisions may project. It is their responsibility to clarify and solidify the role of the profession while promoting exclusivity of the use of the term *physical therapy*.

Unique Features of Physical Therapy Practice in Outpatient Settings

The focus of most physical therapy practices or rehabilitation outpatient centers is the care of people with musculoskeletal conditions. Sports-related injuries are often identified as a special set of conditions treated within these centers. Outpatient practices also may care exclusively for children, or they may focus on particular conditions, such as the management of patients with lymphedema, women's health, wound care, or work-related injuries. Other general practices provide a broad range of services

to meet the needs of patients with diverse movement disorders.

Sometimes, the specialization of a practice evolves from the specialty of the physicians who refer to that practice. For instance, if an orthopedic surgeon specializes in the treatment of shoulder impairments and refers the majority of his patients to one particular physical therapy center, that center will likely, by default, "specialize" in rehabilitation of disorders of the shoulder. Other centers establish themselves as a sports medicine center, for instance, and then build referrals to develop that specialty practice. It may be that the unexpected opportunity to hire a board-certified specialist (e.g., women's health) drives the specialization of a clinic. Another management strategy for developing a niche practice may be the deliberate recruitment of only a certain type of board-certified clinical specialist (e.g., geriatric).

Types of Practices

The use of the term *outpatient* demands further definition more often than any other healthcare setting because of the range of organizational possibilities. Outpatient settings are found in large healthcare systems, comprehensive long-term care campuses, the workplace, physician offices, national rehabilitation corporations, and private practices. However, there are commonalities within this variation that are presented in Sidebar 14.1.

Patient Outpatient Choices

Physician referrals for outpatient rehabilitation may be based on locations convenient for patients. They may be dependent on a center having a contract with a patient's insurer. Regardless of the preference of the physician to refer to a particular center, the third-party payer may limit where a person receives outpatient therapy to facilities that are within their provider network, with extra cost to the patient who chooses a center outside the network. The reality is that patients are most likely to do what their physicians recommend whenever possible, and physicians try to honor referrals to providers within patients' networks.

The most defining feature of outpatient physical therapy is that, unlike all other settings, the therapists do not have a captive audience. Because they are dependent on people voluntarily coming for treatment sessions managers must, above all,

---

SIDEBAR 14.1

Characteristics of Work in Outpatient Centers

- Typically, provide highly specialized services, but may be general practices meeting the needs of patients across the life span
- Identification of niche markets that are primarily related to patients with musculoskeletal conditions, but opportunities for formally achieving orthopedic or other clinical specializations
- Establishment of a referral base a major challenge
- Negotiation of reimbursement contracts a key factor
- May include services of other professionals, but typically *not* interdisciplinary care (e.g., an occupational therapist may treat a patient who is not concurrently receiving physical therapy services)

- May be one unit of larger organization with a great deal of autonomy in clinical and business decisions, but relies on centralized support for contract negotiations and other aspects of billing, marketing, and quality care, etc.
- Opportunities for upward career mobility in multi-center outpatient organizations or healthcare systems
- Risk of professional isolation in solo practices, or more collaboration in larger outpatient centers because of the physical environment
- Close working relationships with physicians
- Typically large caseloads with high productivity demands
- Stockholders may be important stakeholders in settings other than private practice

---

get patients in the door. An important first step in this responsibility is arranging as many contracts with insurance carriers as possible so that the organization is a potential provider for as many patients as possible. It is difficult for managers when people who seek to come to their centers cannot pass through the doors because they are "out of network." Many potential patients cannot afford the additional costs of going to a provider they prefer rather than one that is "in network."

Competition within a third-party-payer network for the same patients, particularly for those deemed most desirable for a variety of reasons, becomes fierce. To be competitive and profitable, physical therapy managers in any outpatient practice setting must focus on the quality of services provided and payments for their services. Communication by word of mouth about the successes and efforts of the staff in a practice may be the most valuable marketing tool a manager has. Perhaps the only way to tip the power and influence of physicians on patient choices about their physical therapy is to have more patients who are empowered to say that they prefer to go to a particular practice because of the reputation it has. At the same time, it is important for referring physicians to have confidence in the quality of the services that their patients receive.

Quality of Care

Physical therapists who are considering management positions in different types of outpatient centers need to consider accountability expectations for assuring the quality of care as well as the profits. A discussion with potential employers about the amount of time a manager is expected to devote to these two broad categories of responsibilities may be revealing. The business side of these managerial responsibilities may be complemented or supplemented by other staff, but the professional ability to assure the quality of care cannot be delegated effectively to nonprofessionals, or even professionals from another discipline. The strength of a practice may lie with a quality emphasis, or approach, to management decisions.

Unlike other healthcare settings in which Medicare has linked required electronic data collection for each patient to quality outcomes and costs, there is no standardized, formal documentation at this time for physical therapy outpatient centers.[6,7] Because documentation is required of any outpatient rehabilitation setting from any payer, there are documentation and billing systems available for purchase. Large organizations may develop their own. The use of a variety of systems makes it difficult to compare the quality of care and cost-effectiveness of outpatient organizations. Unlike other healthcare settings, this important information is not as available for public comparisons of outpatient rehabilitation centers at this time.

Recent initiatives by the APTA may provide the ability of centers to participate in a national outpatient database. This effort faces challenges because of the diverse setting in which outpatient services are provided—hospitals, private practices, physicians' offices. Because there is no requirement to share data on the services they provide, outpatient centers may prefer to avoid comparisons with other centers. Larger organizations such as rehabilitation chains or PT networks may already have national, standardized outpatient documentation and outcome measurement systems in place.

Patient Satisfaction

Surveys to determine patient satisfaction with physical therapy outcomes and care also may be useful in studying the quality of outpatient care, particularly because hands-on orthopedic treatments may be threatening or painful, and patients are expected to be active participants in their therapy.[8] One study of survey results suggests that outpatient satisfaction with physical therapy is most associated with a high-quality interaction with the therapist (e.g., time spent with patients, adequate explanations and instructions to patients, less use of supportive personnel) rather than environmental factors such as clinic location, parking, time spent waiting for the therapist, and type of equipment.[9] See Chapter 9 for more discussion of patient satisfaction.

PART 2   Management Issues

Overview of Management in Outpatient Centers

Management opportunities in outpatient physical therapy are numerous and can be found in a variety of organizations and models that are attractive to entrepreneurs and employees who seek career ladders within large organizations. These managerial opportunities include:

- **A solo practice, typically one office, in which the physical therapist provides all of the patient care and manages the practice with limited support personnel.** This practice may also include provision of home-care or contract services for other organizations. It is often a highly specialized service, or it may be a general practice meeting needs of patients across the life span. Solo practices provide the greatest opportunity for autonomy in clinical and business decisions, but it may be more difficult to negotiate contracts with third-party payers. Solo practitioners may need to make a special effort to avoid

professional isolation and to remain current with both clinical evidence and reimbursement policies.

- **A large private physical therapy practice with either a single office that employs several other professional and support staff or multiple locations.** Private practice provides the greatest opportunity for unlimited business growth and the development of niche markets. Business responsibilities of managers often override direct attention to patient care because the livelihoods of employees are based on responding to unpredictable reimbursement policies and contract negotiations. Cash flow and capital resources are common management concerns.

- **Solo or private practices that are part of physical therapy networks with centralized support for many aspects of the practices.** Members participate through flat payments to the network or profit-sharing arrangements. Depending on the nature of the agreements, the practices in the network commonly operate with relatively independent decision-making. A manager of a network provides centralized support for contract negotiations and other aspects of billing, marketing, and quality care.

● **Solo or private practices that lease space and pay for support services in a physician practice.** This arrangement allows the establishment of strong professional ties with physicians while clearly maintaining professional and business autonomy.

● **A workplace-based practice.** These are contracted services with a large employer(s) to provide all physical therapy services to employees, typically including job analysis and injury prevention services. They are frequently located at the business location, and involve a per capita payment model that eliminates third-party payer challenges. The other advantages of this type of practice are development of specialization in work-related injuries, reduction in or elimination of space and equipment costs, convenient location for employees to keep appointments, and opportunities to consult in the development of on-site prevention and wellness programs.

● **Outpatient services provided in long-term care centers or retirement communities.** Outpatients may be residents in the center who are eligible for Medicare Part B outpatient rehabilitation, or patients who have been discharged from the facility and return from their homes to continue rehabilitation. Managers typically have responsibility for inpatient services in the same long-term care organization that may extend to people living in assistive living or congregate living units in the same organization. Managers supervise the care of a higher percentage of patients with complex, chronic medical conditions that provide professionals the opportunity to pursue geriatric specialization opportunities.

● **Physician-owned (single or group) physical therapy services.** These are services that are offered in-house only to patients of that particular physician or physician group. The role of managers may be more limited because of the financial interests of physicians in the physical therapy practice. Managers monitor the close working relationships of physical therapists and physicians to assure that professionals are making autonomous clinical decisions. These are physician practices with large numbers of patients, so staff members maintain larger caseloads with high productivity demands. Because of these factors, managers are compelled to closely monitor the physical therapy practice for potential ethical and financial conflicts.

● **A national corporation that owns a chain of outpatient centers.** Upward career mobility opportunities are presented in these organizations from manager of one center, to regional management of several centers, or upper-level executive positions at the corporate level. Managers at any level rely on central corporate control of resources for development, marketing, and staff recruitment. Managers may need to address the potential risk of a corporation's focus on quantity rather than quality of care to please shareholders.

Within any of these outpatient settings, there may be board-certified specialists and niche target markets. Practices may focus on particular diagnoses or age groups, or they may be broad generalist practices that address a wide target market in a small community. In any outpatient setting, managers assume similar responsibilities that are addressed in the following sections. But first, some unique aspects of hospital-based outpatient services are explored.

Hospital-Based Outpatient Services

Hospital-based outpatient rehabilitation services may address a wide range of specialty services. The range depends on the type and number of physician-owned or private practices in the community. For example, orthopedic surgeons who perform surgery in the hospital may refer those patients to their own practices or other outpatient centers rather than the hospital's outpatient rehabilitation services. The hospital's specialization, therefore, may, by default, be anything other than postsurgical orthopedics. This self-referral leaves hospital-based outpatient centers dependent on referrals from other medical specialists. Hospitals are frequently the only provider of services to people who are underinsured or uninsured.

A recent trend for hospitals and health systems to develop outpatient centers separate from the hospital itself that are more conveniently located and accessible for patients is a response to the competition for outpatients. The more centers one organization has in an area, the fewer contracts a third-party payer requires to meet the needs of the people it insures. This is good for insurers who are able to reduce their administrative costs with fewer contracts, but it often presents difficulties for independent practitioners in those communities who also seek contracts with the same insurers.

Managers in hospital-based outpatient practices are part of a larger organization that meets a wider range of community needs. Their staffs may more likely be involved in staff meetings, clinical instruction, and institutional activities related to accreditation. Finding the means to address the needs of a broad patient base rather than a niche market may be a management responsibility that is not found in other settings.

Deciding how much to meld the inpatient and outpatient staffs into one unit may be an important decision in hospital-based practices, particularly if staff shortages are a major concern. Ideally, having staff who are willing and able to float from inpatient to outpatient services and vice versa allows managers flexibility in staffing assignments. More often, the two staffs are either unwilling or unable to transition easily from one setting to the other as needed. The skill set, pace of work, and clinical specialties may be very different in these subgroups of therapists.

These factors contribute to a manager's decision to deliberately treat the two groups as separate entities, particularly when the inpatient and outpatient services are physically isolated from each other. Other managers may insist that staff maintain their skills in both areas. The ability of a physical therapist to remain a broad generalist to meet these job demands may only be possible in less complex hospital settings with a limited range of patient problems to be addressed.

Upward career mobility opportunities for managers in healthcare systems may range from supervisory responsibilities in one of several satellite outpatient offices to management of all inpatient and outpatient rehabilitation services in one hospital, or all units within an entire healthcare system across a large geographic area. Managers may be more engaged in decisions related to continuity of care as patients transition from one part of the system to another (especially if the healthcare system is an ACO). Facilitation of communication and face-to-face interaction of staff may make these organizations attractive to many professionals. The ability to move among several different types of practices within one organization may also be an important recruitment factor. Managers often have better resources for state-of-the-art facilities and equipment to meet the needs of staff and patients in large organizations. They may also be challenged by the development of both general and specialty practices within one organization.

Managerial Responsibilities

Mission, Vision, and Goals

There may be more variation in mission, vision, and goals among outpatient settings than any other healthcare settings because of the range of possibilities of ownership and size. Hospital-based outpatient units are linked to the larger organization's goals and outcomes to meet the mission and vision of the organization as a whole. Outpatient managers in those settings may contribute to the development of the hospital mission, vision, and goals; they will certainly be accountable for their unit's contributions to achieving them.

Managers in corporate-based outpatient centers also are likely to be handed the mission and vision of the corporation with minimal input into their development unless it is part of a special assignment to review or modify them. Private physical therapy practitioners have to consider the creation of a vision, a mission, and goals as the starting point for setting their practices apart from others.

Managers in all types of outpatient settings work a little harder to differentiate themselves through their visions and missions because the competition for patients is different from that in other practice settings such as home care or hospitals. For example, if compared, the visions and missions of home-care agencies would be similar, but the visions and missions of outpatient practices vary widely. Clearly differentiating the strengths of a practice through vision and mission statements may also be a powerful tool for recruitment of personnel and for development of a referral base, provided they are effectively communicated to stakeholders.

Policies and Procedures

Outpatient managers' responsibilities for policies and procedures also vary according to the size and type of organization. Managers may receive policies and procedures manuals developed at higher organizational levels for implementation, or they may assume total responsibility for development and implementation in independent practices or in physicians' offices. The larger and more complex the organization is, the more complex policies and procedures become. In addition to the required policies and procedures that are needed to become a Medicare-certified provider organization, larger organizations may expand their policies and procedures to reflect the more complex interactions and management of resources that are the result of their size. Independent practitioners may feel less urgency for policies and procedures because the running of the business is more automatic and reflexive with less staff and simpler physical space.

Professional Courtesies

A policy and procedure that may be unique to outpatient settings is one that addresses extending the professional courtesy of free or discounted fees for treatment of physicians, other health professionals, and/or family members of employees. Although professional courtesy may be an effective marketing strategy, there are inherent issues related to unfairness (unintentional or deliberate) or a potential violation of anti-kickback legislation. The Stark Law also addresses professional courtesy but only in hospitals. It does, however, address issues to be considered in any setting. The Stark Law requirements for professional courtesy include the following:[10]

- The policy for professional courtesy must be in writing and approved by the governing body responsible for the organization. It must not violate state or federal anti-kickback legislation
- The services offered are routine and typical and offered to all physicians regardless of the volume or value of their referrals
- The physician or family member cannot be a federal health beneficiary unless there is a financial need

Establishing limits on the percentage of the annual visits that can be devoted to professional courtesy may be necessary, particularly for the private practitioner. Determining the number of courtesy visits per physician and their extended families also may need to be set. Balancing professional courtesy and pro bono services may need to be considered in some practices.

Although managers cannot afford to give away their services, they also cannot afford to jeopardize the goodwill that may be accumulated through these actions. Establishing written guidelines for scheduling of these patients will avoid disruptions of services to clients who are paying for their services. Policies should assure that *all* patients are receiving the same level of service whether they are paying for it or not.

A similar policy may be necessary for the treatment of coworkers who require physical therapy services when there is an expectation that they also receive a professional courtesy. Professionals who treat family members may want to consider the ramifications of that decision. Managers should have a policy to address how professional courtesy extends to staff who treat family members directly and family members who are treated by other people on staff.

Pro Bono Services

Similar policy and procedures questions often arise in relation to the delivery of pro bono services. *Pro bono publico* is derived from the Latin and means "for the public good." It is used to describe professional services that are voluntarily provided without payment to people who are unable to afford them. With a basis in the legal profession, pro bono services commonly are offered by professionals in all fields. Some professions require their members to provide pro bono services to meet legal and ethical responsibilities, while others believe that pro bono is the voluntary choice of each individual.

Organizations do not have pro bono obligations, but they often provide services to people who are unable or unwilling to pay. This loss of revenue is a bad debt, not pro bono service. Because the reduction of bad debt losses can be difficult, it is unlikely that managers are willing to encourage staff to provide pro bono services that they do not charge for when they should be generating billable units of care. However, they may establish guidelines for staff to engage in pro bono services on their own time in community-based organizations.

Typically, the use of its own facilities, even after hours, to provide pro bono services is discouraged because of liability concerns. Because professionals can often meet their pro bono responsibilities through a variety of means other than the direct provision of free services (e.g., financial donations to charitable groups), employers typically expect professional employees to meet their required or voluntary obligations on non-work time.

Marketing

The managerial duties for marketing vary widely from one type of setting to another. Typically, large healthcare organizations and corporations have full-time marketing staff who generate materials and plans for implementation by managers among the units of the organization. Because of the expenses involved, independent practitioners may be at a disadvantage in their marketing responsibilities. The time needed for inbound- and outbound-marketing activities intended to set a practice apart from others may be limited because the bulk of the manager's time is devoted to direct patient care and the management of finances. Moreover, the costs of a strong outbound-marketing program may be prohibitive, forcing these practitioners to rely on word of mouth to develop a strong, professional reputation for the services they provide.

A priority target of marketing efforts for the private practitioner may be insurers. Overcoming their reluctance to enter into contracts with private practice physical therapists is a major managerial challenge. Although the prices set by private practices are commonly competitive, insurers often are not interested in negotiating a contract for their services. Perhaps the reason for this lack of interest is that one business priority of insurers is minimizing their administrative costs, which are typically fixed regardless of the size of an organization they contract with. If a managed care corporation already has a contract with a hospital in the community, it has little incentive to also contract with several small private practices. Each new provider that is added to their panel of providers increases their administrative costs.

Provider Networks

These third-party-payer contract difficulties led to the development of physical therapy provider networks that allow multiple private practices to negotiate collectively with insurers. This model increases the possibility of gaining a contract that includes all centers because the network has enabled the insurance company to reduce their administrative costs. Their combined ability to develop a broader diversification of populations to be served or to address the unmet needs of particular populations also improves their ability to negotiate as a single entity with third-party payers. The capability to present quality assurance, utilization review, and outcome studies across several practices also makes the idea of private practices more attractive to third-party payers, particularly if a group of practices can be flexible about the different types of reimbursement models insurers may offer. These network business opportunities also present professional opportunities for providers to share ideas and improve clinical practice. This may be an attractive opportunity for managers of solo practices willing to sacrifice some of their independence and control to continue operating a private practice.

Staffing

Because outpatient services are enticing and appealing to many physical therapists, managers may have a little less difficulty in recruiting staff than they do in other healthcare settings. However, they may face hurdles recruiting particular therapists with specialized skills for program development in niche markets. For instance, managers in different types of outpatient centers are more likely competing with each other than they are with other types of healthcare settings in the recruitment of musculoskeletal specialists.

Salary and benefits are likely the big negotiating factors because of the number of outpatient opportunities in any location. Managers need to be insightful interviewers who can spot an applicant who has the strong interpersonal skills requisite to establish trusting relationships that lead to high levels of patient care satisfaction and strong professional relationships with referring physicians.

Personnel decisions often are directed to the development of specialized services. Supporting specialist certification or advanced degrees in exchange for a long-term employment commitment to the organization is often good management strategy. Identifying both physical therapist and physical therapist assistant staff who have the potential to assume more administrative responsibilities is important as well. Programs that nurture that potential have many advantages. Having the means to grow one's own staff with career ladder plans may be the most important decision about the utilization of human resources in outpatient practices.

Support Staff

Because services must meet the definition of *skilled* for Medicare reimbursement, the use of supportive personnel, other than physical therapist assistants, for direct patient care provided to Medicare recipients is typically not a management option. However, the use of other physical therapy extenders may be tempting, particularly in times of workforce shortages and reduced reimbursement. The direction and supervision of others who are not physical therapist assistants, and careful delineation of the duties that they may perform, must receive the close attention of managers.

Even if these extenders (i.e., aides, technicians) are licensed in other disciplines, such as athletic training or massage therapy, or have education and credentials as exercise physiologists or personal trainers, they are not licensed to practice physical therapy. Although the skills they bring to a position in an outpatient practice may be very attractive, what they can be legally assigned to do and whether the services they perform can be billed for must be weighed against the value of their contributions to patient care.

In some practices, there may be a reluctance even to hire physical therapist assistants. A practice that relies heavily on manual therapy is an example. The manager may decide that this staffing model is not conducive to a practice that is committed to consistent, one-on-one, high-touch therapy. Therapists directing others to deliver patient care are not part of this model. However, because staffing costs are so high, managers may have no choice but to hire physical therapist assistants. If not delivering direct patient care in this type of practice because it is so specialized, physical therapist assistants may be able to contribute effectively to other types of interventions and assume more administrative roles.

Supervision of Students

Small private outpatient practices, in particular, may show reluctance to engage in clinical education programs. Because outpatient practices have less difficulty recruiting staff, and their marketing commitment is to provide patients with highly skilled specialists, they may hesitate to incorporate students into their practices. Other outpatient centers may be reluctant because of high productivity expectations that may not be met because of additional duties placed on clinical instructors. Conversely, other outpatient centers may be very eager to have students because of the extra hands that students bring to heavy caseloads with no additional personnel expenses, and the ability to use the clinical learning experiences as the opportunity to screen a potential employee.

Outpatient managers in *all types* of physical therapy practices have an obligation to ensure that the learning goals of students take precedence over maximizing billable units generated in those situations. Preparing staff to meet their important professional responsibilities as clinical faculty is key to meeting this obligation. Other managerial issues related to clinical education include:

- Integration of clinical education in the vision, mission, and goals of the organization
- Criteria for establishing contracts with physical therapy and physical therapist assistant programs
- Determination of which and how many staff are committed to the supervision of students at any time
- Integration of clinical teaching into career ladders
- Modification of staff assignments and productivity goals that reflect a commitment to students' learning goals
- Evaluation of both teaching and clinical performance

Patient Care

Managers must develop strong orientation sessions and establish monitoring systems (peer-review audits of documentation, for instance) to ensure not only the quality of services, but also compliance with the accurate and timely completion of documentation to meet legal and reimbursement requirements. There are challenges in meeting these requirements. For example, the goal-setting component of documentation for reimbursement of outpatient services demands a functional focus that requires therapists to adjust their thinking about patients. Outpatients who require physical therapy must be well enough to get dressed and travel to therapy, which are high-level functional activities. Yet they must be "sick" enough to require the skilled services of physical therapists.

Although the need to report functional status of patients has always been important, CMS linked reporting functional limitations to reimbursement in 2013. Claims for payment of services depends on submitting G codes and modifiers that reflect the functional limitations of patients initially, at least at 10 days and at discharge. Managers should follow the monitoring of these new requirements by the APTA at its webpage in Web Resources.

Because no standardized measurement of function has been adopted for this reporting, managers may refer to the APTA for guidance in selecting these tools. The premorbid functional level of many outpatients is often high. Pain or impairments rather than functional limitations are typically the basis of their need for physical therapy. Physical therapists must be diligent in linking their patients' concerns to functional goals. Other patients may have chronic conditions in which improving long-standing functional limitations is not a reasonable goal, although therapy certainly may significantly influence their quality of life. It is often difficult to determine what is "reasonable and necessary" that "requires the skill of a physical therapist" for many patients with chronic conditions. Managers should also frequently access CMS Web pages for therapy services found in Web Resources.

Documentation

A primary patient care responsibility is that accurate documentation of the high-quality services that were provided comply with requirements for reimbursement established by Medicare and other insurance companies. The link in Web Resources provides details on these requirements in the CMS *Outpatient Rehabilitation Fact Sheet*. Generally, for each insurer, managers should determine:

- Which staff members are recognized as certified providers responsible for clinical judgments and supervision of other personnel

- The level of care required for reimbursement as a skilled service
- Documentation requirements (Level of skill? Justification for care? Goals? Patient response?)
- Content to be included in standardized forms to be submitted during the episode of care
- Data needed for reauthorization or modification of plans of care
- Required content in encounter (treatment) notes and progress notes
- Discharge and discontinuance requirements

An increased interest in medical necessity and outcomes is expected to be the federal government's next focus on Medicare rules about rehabilitation services. Pay for performance is expected to be the next major reimbursement initiative. Managers will need to evaluate the usefulness of new instruments and databases designed to address these issues, such as the Activity Measure-Post Acute Care Computer-based Format (AMPAC-CAT),[11] Focus On Therapeutic Outcomes (FOTO),[12] and the Outpatient Physical Therapy Improvement in Movement Assessment Log (OPTIMAL).[7]

Fiscal

A major financial concern, once contracts with insurers have been negotiated, is meeting the requirements for a clean claim (i.e., 100% complete, clear, no errors, no questions) that is reimbursable on its first submission. Being paid for services provided often seems to be based on capricious and arbitrary, if not silly, rules set by carriers. Outpatient managers must check that carriers are consistent with federal legislation regarding Medicare coverage policies. Keeping abreast of current decisions about reimbursement policies is also critical. Breaking the rules because they were unknown can have a very serious impact on cash flow and profits of an outpatient practice. The Medicare Coverage Database (MCD) contains all National Coverage Determinations (NCDs) and Local Coverage Determinations (LCDs), local articles, and proposed NCD decisions. See Web Resources for more information on coverage. Managers of outpatient services should refer to this resource frequently.

In addition to the coverage rules, the high deductibles and co-payments in some benefit packages may deter many people from choosing to attend physical therapy sessions at all, or to reduce their attendance (i.e., no-shows and cancellations) to levels that they can afford. This type of insurance plan may be ideal for major catastrophic illnesses or injuries, but they may have a negative effect on services such as physical therapy that have a co-payment due at the time of each treatment session. The Medicare co-payment for outpatient services also may be prohibitive for many senior citizens on limited retirement incomes.

Managers need to be prepared to have open discussions with patients about their ability to pay and the potential negative effects of ignoring problems that may be relieved with physical therapy intervention. Payment plans and other creative strategies may be necessary within the scope of what is legal and permissible. Offering certain discounts and waiving fees may be illegal.

Legal, Ethical, and Risk

A broad ethical issue for the profession is the potential disparity in patients who are able to access services. A recent study summarized some factors that determine utilization of physical therapy services. Generally, participants in this study were more likely to receive physical therapy if they had more than one musculoskeletal condition, had some limitation in function, had seven or more diagnostic codes, had a college degree, and resided in an urban area. People who were not as likely to receive physical therapy were older than 65 years of age, had no high school degree, were of Hispanic ethnicity or African American, had public or no insurance, and were living anywhere except the northeastern United States.[13] Patients with musculoskeletal disorders were more likely to be referred by an orthopedic surgeon or an osteopathic physician than primary care physicians, particularly if they also had workers' compensation insurance.[13]

Although overutilization of services is the focus of third-party payers, this study suggests that outpatient managers may find an urgent need to address underutilization. To do so, managers may develop business goals that address social and cultural norms along with programs to educate groups about physical therapy.

Overcoming language barriers may be a powerful way to counteract underutilization. Many patients with the need for physical therapy and the insurance to pay for it may not seek it because of these communication barriers. Other patients may face cultural barriers because their physicians have been educated in other countries and lack an understanding of contemporary physical therapy practice in this country. Managers also need to advocate for patients who need rehabilitation in Medicaid programs that may be very restrictive and vary from state to state.

The salient legal and ethical issues in outpatient settings lie with fraud and abuse in Medicare billing. *Fraud* is knowingly and willfully scheming to defraud a benefit program by false or fraudulent pretenses to obtain money or property from a health benefit program. *Abuse* is obtaining payment that results in unnecessary costs to Medicare through payment for services that fail to meet professionally recognized standards of care, are billed inappropriately, or that are medically *unnecessary*.

Federal investigations have directed a great deal of attention to fraud and abuse in the Medicare system with physical therapy (or more accurately, the use of physical medicine CPT codes) at the heart of this investigation. For more information see Web Resources for Operation Restore and Trust, CMS CERT program, Office of the Inspector General, and CMS's Medicare Fraud and Abuse.

Federal and state agencies have cooperated in these investigative programs to reduce fraud and abuse. These programs have also enabled public citizens to use hotlines to directly report suspected Medicare fraud and abuse to the proper authorities. These initiatives have been very successful in recovering millions of dollars and have resulted in the prosecution of many healthcare providers. Some examples of fraud and abuse are fraudulent diagnoses, billing for services that were not provided, duplicate billing, and claims for medically unnecessary services.

Monitoring efforts that include the statistical analysis of claims and on-site reviews of Medicare providers with high reimbursement rates continue to reduce inappropriate payment of Medicare claims. Utilization management programs assure that payments are made only when it is clear that beneficiaries actually received the services that were billed. Incomplete or inaccurate documentation about patients' diagnoses and conditions, extent of services provided, and lack of medical necessity underlie suspicions of fraud and abuse. Managers can expect continued initiatives to address Medicare payments, which forces them to be diligent about documentation requirements and the skills of therapists to meet them.

Many problems with the reimbursement of rehabilitation services relate to the fact that data on a particular diagnosis are more difficult to pinpoint when the need for therapy is often the result of multiple diagnoses. It is also difficult for outsiders to understand why there is a wide range in the length of time the same condition may be treated. The wide variation in the quality and outcomes of those services does not seem to be in direct relationship to the amount of therapy received. Defining the amount or mix of services needed for specific patients or categories of patients remains elusive. See Chapter 10 for the latest APTA efforts on an alternative payment model for CPT codes. All of these initiatives make it important for managers to be aware of their organization's inclusion in these data collection and analysis efforts by federal agencies and to remain current about actions taken in response to these analyses.

Communication

Most outpatient physical therapists rely on phone and fax in their communications with physicians regarding the care of particular patients. The opportunities to communicate about patient data or problems may be most important in outpatient centers because the source of information is often limited to what a patient reports. Access to diagnostic test reports and other information from medical records is not always available. Each communication with a physician also becomes important as an opportunity to strengthen a referral base and establish goodwill and professional relationships. Outpatient practices that are components of ACOs may have less difficulty because medical records are electronically linked among all providers. Physical therapists directly employed by physicians have the advantage of more immediate physical access for direct conversations and access to medical records.

Managers need to constantly remind staff of the importance of these communications. Calls to physicians for clarifications of referrals or additional diagnostic information also are opportunities to demonstrate the knowledge and expertise of staff and to determine the preferences and needs of the referring physicians.

Establishing strong communication patterns with the staff members in a physician's office alleviates the need for repeated attempts to speak directly to a physician. By developing a rapport with the people who answer the phones in physicians' offices, physical therapists make it known that they would not be calling unless it were something that demanded attention to meet a patient's needs or a concern. Managers must instill the importance of establishing this trust in all staff in a practice.

Verbal Orders

Managers need to assure that all requirements are being met for receiving verbal orders from physicians or physician extenders. State statutes or third-party payer rules may determine who may refer a patient to physical therapy. For instance, in an exchange of phone calls about modifying a patient's plan of care, the result may be that a physician assistant returns the call to the physical therapy clinic approving the change request. The only person available to accept the call is a physical therapist assistant who may or may not be involved in that patient's care.

Whether or not the phone conversation between the physician assistant and physical therapist assistant is acceptable may depend on several factors. For instance, whether the physician assistant is speaking for the physician who is engaged in other activities at a particular moment, or whether the physician assistant is independently making the decision on the revised plan of care must be made clear if physical therapy statutes specify from whom physical therapists may accept orders or referrals.

At the same time, it may be acceptable in some jurisdictions for the physical therapist assistant to take the call while the physical therapist is engaged in other activities as long as it is not perceived as though the physical therapist assistant is modifying the plan of care rather than simply taking a message. Documentation of all of these communications must be clear and detailed to reduce legal and reimbursement risks. Managers should encourage their staffs to avoid assumptions and blanket rules about these communications related to patient care decisions.

Peer Support

The outpatient setting is conducive to opportunities for professional interaction and mentoring in all but the solo practitioner setting. This may be another factor that makes the setting attractive for many physical therapists. Interdisciplinary teamwork is not a driver of most outpatient practices, but interactions among therapists of the same discipline in larger centers is much higher than other practice settings in which they may be more isolated in their daily work.

There is more opportunity for professionals to consult with each other and share their expertise because the more open, common "gym" area in outpatient centers permits more ongoing interaction among staff. Managers have more opportunity to observe work performance as well. This environment strengthens communication about clinical decision-making, which may contribute to improving the quality of care. Outpatient managers may more easily identify common clinical issues that can be addressed in staff meeting or journal clubs because of the large number of patients with similar conditions.

Caseload Models

Managers in larger outpatient settings also need to consider the impact of their caseload model. Does the same therapist follow assigned patients from admission to discharge? Are daily patient assignments made based on a generated master schedule, which means that any available therapist or physical therapist assistant may see a patient at any point? As an efficiency issue, managers may prefer that each therapist's schedule be filled regardless of who initially treated the patient. From a patient satisfaction perspective, there may be a risk in frequently changing the providers who see the patient. If this is the case, establishing timely, written documentation requirements may be necessary to avoid the need for staff to make and take time to discuss patients with the providers who saw

them at the last visit. These models also require managers to assure the patients' rights to confidentiality and privacy. The more people there are involved in a patient's care, the greater the risk will be of inadvertently violating these rights.

Direction

Perhaps more than any other setting, outpatient clinics also provide the best opportunity for unquestionable direction and supervision of physical therapist assistants and other supportive staff, again because of the open, yet contained environment that facilitates interaction among the staff. Communication about patients may become an issue depending on the ratio of physical therapists to physical therapist assistants. Situations in which there are many physical therapist assistants and one physical therapist may require managers to identify communication methods that are very different from those required when there are many physical therapists and one physical therapist assistant.

Conclusions

As new technology, new healthcare business models, and new opportunities for specialized practice continue to develop in a system shifting to outpatient care, managers will find, and create, many opportunities. As the most popular work setting of physical therapists, outpatient physical therapy services provide many professional opportunities for managers who are willing to carefully attend to the complexities of billing and payment for the services provided. Managing professionals who are often specialized and highly skilled can be very rewarding. Activities 14.1 to 14.15 address many of the decisions facing managers in outpatient settings.

ACTIVITY 14.1
A CHANCE MEETING

Benny Landers is a physical therapist at the Carter City office of Nationwide Rehabilitation Services. He asked Mary Driscoll, his area manager, whether he could see his niece as a professional courtesy. His niece could visit during his lunch hour for advice about her ankle injury. Mary gave permission and wished his niece a speedy recovery. A few weeks

later, Mary happened to be driving through Carter City and noticed the lights on in the office after hours. Concerned, she stopped to investigate. She found Benny treating a patient who turned out to be his injured niece. Benny said he was providing pro bono care for his uninsured niece. He was surprised that Mary objected. Should she have objections? Why?

ACTIVITY 14.2
DIVERSIFYING OUTPATIENT SERVICES

Patrick Peterson is manager of the 5th Avenue Physical Therapy Center that is one of 123 centers owned by U.S. Rehabilitation Corporation. At the last regional meeting, all eight managers including Patrick were assigned to devise a plan for expanding services in their centers. All of these centers are solo practitioner centers with limited floor space.

What might Patrick recommend to the group? Consider: Where are they now? Where do they want to be? What does Patrick have to work with? How will he get there?

ACTIVITY 14.3
PERSONNEL RECRUITMENT

Jack Steuben is Manager of Outpatient Services for the Great Plains Healthcare System. His responsibilities include staffing the six outpatient centers that are 30 to 40 miles from each other in the rural area around the county seat. Currently, he has an open position in each center because of population growth in the county and marketing efforts that have increased the visibility of rehabilitation services in the system. He has asked for another meeting with Linda Lopez, who is his contact in the Great Plains Human Resources Department. Although there have been three applications from physical therapists submitted over the past few months, Jack has been reluctant to hire any of them because they are board-certified specialists who want to limit their assignments to their specialty areas.

What can Jack and Linda do? Consider: Where are they now? Where do they want to be? What do they have to work with? How will they get there?

ACTIVITY 14.4
EXPANSION OF A PRACTICE

Michael Moriarity has been a successful solo practice physical therapist for 7 years in Greendale, a suburban community. He feels that he is ready to take on more responsibilities. Recently he has been approached by U.S. Rehabilitation Services, which is interested in buying his practice and having him stay on staff as the manager of his clinic and two others. He has also identified a possible location for another office in his practice, in Whitehurst, another suburb, which is growing rapidly. Finally, Westshore Village, the largest retirement community in the area, has approached him with a contract to provide rehabilitation services in their nursing home and outpatient center.

How should Michael decide which professional opportunity is most attractive? Consider: Where is Michael now? Where does he want to be? What does he have to work with? How will he get there?

ACTIVITY 14.5
STAFF RETENTION

Joslyn Robertson has owned and managed Robertson and Associates, Physical Therapists, for 10 years and currently has a staff of three physical therapists and three physical therapist assistants. Her most senior therapist, Annabelle Walsh, tells Joslyn that she has been offered another position with U.S. Rehabilitation Services that is opening a clinic about 3 miles away. Although she likes her current position, the opportunity to move up within the U.S. Rehabilitation Services is very attractive.

What should Joslyn do? Consider: Where is Robertson and Associates now? Where do they want to be? What does Joslyn have to work with? How will she get there?

ACTIVITY 14.6
NONLICENSED PERSONNEL

Tony Massino is the new manager of Citywide Rehabilitation. Although he knew when he accepted the position that there were two athletic trainers and a massage therapist on staff, it was not until he got into the position that he became concerned. The athletic trainers and the massage therapist have been assuming a great deal of responsibility for patient care. They even have their own caseloads and they complete charge slips for the patients whom they treat. When he asks the other physical therapists about this, they report that they turn patients over to them once they have stabilized. They are not sure why he is concerned. Should he be?

ACTIVITY 14.7
PHYSICIAN RELATIONSHIP

Dr. Ramirez has called Susan Wishart, manager of Rehab Action, to voice his concerns. He has been receiving complaints from his patients in the past few months about the therapy they have been receiving at Rehab Action. The complaints include patients who say they are ignored for long periods of time, another who says the therapy made her injury worse and increased her pain, and others who have asked whether they can go somewhere else for their therapy because the clinic is so busy.

He wants Susan to resolve her problems or he will call Americare, the primary insurance carrier for these patients to find another provider. Susan is very upset because she had no idea patients were so unhappy. She has relied on Dr. Ramirez as her primary referral source for the past several years and her business is at financial risk without his patients. She also wants to avoid any problems with Americare.

What should she do? Consider: Where is Rehab Action now? Where do they want to be? What does Susan have to work with? How will she get there?

ACTIVITY 14.8
A BILLING ISSUE

Daniel Devereau is one of the six staff physical therapists who work in the physical therapy department of Northern Orthopedic Associates. He tells Polly Alberts, Rehabilitation Manager, that he believes the billing department is not posting charges as he has submitted them. Although he and the other therapists are not involved with billing, he happened to see a former patient at the market last night who was very upset with him because the bill she received for therapy did not match the therapy she received. Daniel was embarrassed and promised to look into it and get back to her.

What should Polly do? Consider: Where are they now? Where do they want to be? What does Polly have to work with? How will she get there?

ACTIVITY 14.9
DOCUMENTATION

Despite the several warnings that Burt Duncan, the manager of the outpatient rehabilitation services at St. Anthony's Hospital, has given Tamara Berkman, she has gotten several days behind on her patient documentation again. Although she is a very effective physical therapist who is admired by her patients and coworkers, she just seems unable to manage the paperwork. When pushed, she stays after hours to catch up but reverts to her old patterns very easily.

What should Burt Duncan do? Consider: Where are they now? Where do they want to be? What do they have to work with? How will they get there?

ACTIVITY 14.10
GIFTS

Getting signatures on the plans of care from the physicians in Northern Orthopedic Associates has been very difficult and frustrating for Karen Larson, the manager of a small private practice. About 20% of her patients are referred from Northern Orthopedic yet she seems to spend 80% of her time resolving issues with them. At a meeting with her staff, they brainstorm some ideas to solve their issues with Northern Orthopedic. One of the staff suggests that they offer an in-service on rehabilitation of the shoulder to the physicians and provide a nice dinner to encourage them to come. Another therapist says that is a kickback and it's illegal to do that.

Is she right? What are other ideas for resolving the plans of care issue? Consider: Where are they now? Where do they want to be? What does Karen have to work with? How will she get there?

ACTIVITY 14.11
SCHEDULING

Marla McCormick has been the receptionist and scheduler in the Sandy Shores Physical Therapy practice for several years. She really likes her job but feels overwhelmed with the recent expansion that includes four physical therapists. She seems to make one of the physical therapists angry every day because of some scheduling decision that she made. Discussing these problems with them makes her very nervous. She tells them that she is just trying to

accommodate the patients, no matter what. This has been what she has always done with scheduling, and has been encouraged to do by Burt Evans, the owner of Sandy Shores.

What needs to be done? Consider: Where are they now? Where do they want to be? What do they have to work with? How will they get there?

ACTIVITY 14.12
WORKERS' COMPENSATION

Cynthia McLean, the manager of the Rehabilitation Care at Southside, overhears one of her staff therapists, Kitty Salmonson, on the phone. Kitty is discussing a patient's care and condition in detail.

When Cynthia asks Kitty whom she is speaking with, she says it is Mr. Caan's workers' compensation attorney. What should Cynthia do?

ACTIVITY 14.13
SERVICE EXPANSION

Eleanor Prentiss is the new regional manager for U.S. Rehabilitation Services. She has been asked to develop a clinic in a predominantly Hispanic, middle-class neighborhood where most of the people are employed by a nearby assembly plant. This is the first effort of U.S. Rehabilitation Services to break into this underserved market.

What should Eleanor do to make this a successful venture? Consider: Where are they now? Where do they want to be? What does Eleanor have to work with? How will she get there?

ACTIVITY 14.14
SURVEY RESULTS

Tonya Montes is very surprised. She has reviewed the results of the patient satisfaction surveys completed in the past 3 months and 30% of the patients rated their experience in her outpatient clinic as "somewhat dissatisfied" or "very dissatisfied." The only change that has been made is the hire of two physical therapist assistants

about 4 months ago, but they seemed to be doing very well and handle their assigned caseloads without difficulty.

What does Tonya need to do? Consider: Where are they now? Where do they want to be? What does Tonya have to work with? How will she get there?

ACTIVITY 14.15
A DILEMMA

Jerome Fielding has a problem. One of his patients reported receiving physical therapy at a U.S. Rehabilitation Services clinic a few months ago but only for three visits. Jerome treated the patient in one of his All County centers and received a denial because the patient had reached the cap for treatments for this year.

What should Jerome do? He believes the patient received only the services she reported.

REFERENCES

1. American Physical Therapy Association. Physical therapist member demographic profile 2010. Available to members only. Accessed on May 16, 2013.
2. American Physical Therapy Association. Patient types and time management by facility. Available to members only. Accessed May 16, 2013.
3. American Physical Therapy Association. Chapters and sections: orthopedic section. http://apps.apta.org/custom/wstemplate.cfm?cfmltitle=Chapters%20and%20Sections&cfml=componentsonline/index.cfm&processForm=1&componentType=Sections&specChoice=J&convertList2Form=yes. Accessed May 17, 2013.
4. American Board of Physical Therapy Specialties. ABPTS certified specialists statistics. http://www.abpts.org/About/Statistics/. Accessed May 16, 2013.
5. Centers for Medicare & Medicaid Services. National Provider Identifier Standard (NPI). http://www.cms.hhs.gov/NationalProvIdentStand/. Accessed May 16, 2013.
6. American Physical Therapy Association. APTA CONNECT. http://www.apta.org/CONNECT/. Accessed May 16, 2013.
7. Guccione AA, Mielenz TJ, DeVellis RF, et al. Development and testing of a self-report instrument to measure actions: outpatient physical therapy improvement in movement assessment log (OPTIMAL). *Physical Therapy.* 2005;85:515.
8. Monnin D, Perneger TV. Scale to measure patient satisfaction with physical therapy. *Physical Therapy.* 2002;82:682-691.
9. Beattie PF, Pinto MB, Nelson MK, et al. Patient satisfaction with outpatient physical therapy: instrument validation. *Physical Therapy.* 2002;82:557-565.
10. Justia US Law. 42 C.F.R. § 411.357. Exceptions to the referral prohibition related to compensation arrangements. Title 42-Public Health. See Professional courtesy § 411.357 (s). http://law.justia.com/cfr/title42/42-2.0.1.2.11.10.35.8.html. Accessed May 16, 2013.
11. Jette AM, Haley SM, Tao W, et al. Prospective evaluation of the AMPAC-CAT in outpatient rehabilitation settings. *Physical Therapy.* 2007;87:385-398.
12. Resnik L, Hart DL. Using clinical outcomes to identify expert physical therapists. *Physical Therapy.* 2003;83:990-1002.
13. Carter SK, Rizzo JA. Use of outpatient physical therapy services by people with musculoskeletal conditions. *Physical Therapy.* 2007;87:497-512.

WEB RESOURCES

American Physical Therapy Association. Functional limitation reporting under Medicare. http://www.apta.org/Payment/Medicare/CodingBilling/FunctionalLimitation/. Accessed November 29, 2013.

Centers for Medicare & Medicaid Services. Comprehensive Error Rate Testing (CERT) Program. http://www.cms.gov/Research-Statistics-Data-and-Systems/Monitoring-Programs/CERT/index.html?redirect=/cert/. Accessed November 29, 2013.

Centers for Medicare and Medicaid Services. Fact Sheet: Outpatient Rehabilitation Therapy Services: Complying with Documentation Requirements. https://www.cms.gov/Outreach-and-Education/Medicare-Learning-Network-MLN/MLNProducts/downloads/Outpatient_Rehabilitation_Fact_Sheet_ICN905365.pdf Accessed June 12, 2014.

Centers for Medicare & Medicaid Services. Fraud & abuse: prevention, detection, and reporting. http://www.cms.gov/Outreach-and-Education/Medicare-Learning-Network-MLN/MLNProducts/downloads/Fraud_and_Abuse.pdf. Accessed November 29, 2013.

Centers for Medicare & Medicaid Services. Medicare coverage database. http://www.cms.gov/medicare-coverage-datbase/overview-and-quick-search.aspx?from2=index_lmrp_bystate.asp&. Accessed November 29, 2013.

Centers for Medicare & Medicaid Services. Part B National Summary Data File (previously known as BESS). http://www.cms.gov/Research-Statistics-Data-and-Systems/Files-for-Order/NonIdentifiableDataFiles/PartBNationalSummaryDataFile.html. Accessed November 29, 2013.

Centers for Medicare & Medicaid Services. Physician self-referral information. http://www.cms.gov/Medicare/Fraud-and-abuse/PhysicianSelfReferral/index.html?redirect=/physicianselfreferral/. Accessed November 29, 2013.

Centers for Medicare & Medicaid Services. *State Operations Manual, Appendix K–Guidance to Surveyors: Comprehensive Outpatient Rehabilitation Facilities.* http://www.cms.hhs.gov/manuals/downloads/som107ap_k_corf.pdf. Accessed November 29, 2013.

Centers for Medicare & Medicaid Services. Therapy services. http://www.cms.gov/Medicare/Billing/TherapyServices/index.html?redirect=/therapyservices. Accessed November 29, 2013.

Commission on Accreditation of Rehabilitation Facilities—International (CARF): providers information. http://www.carf.org/Providers/. Accessed November 29, 2013.

The Joint Commission. http://www.jointcommission.org/assets/1/18/Ambulatorycare_1_112.pdf. Accessed November 29, 2013.

Office of the Inspector General (OIG). The Department of Health and Human Services and OIG work plan for fiscal year 2012. http://oig.hhs.gov/reports-and-publications/archives/workplan/2012/. Accessed November 29, 2013.

Office of the Inspector General (OIG). A roadmap for new physicians: avoiding Medicare and Medicaid fraud and abuse. http://oig.hhs.gov/compliance/physician-education/index.asp. Accessed November 29, 2013.

Workers Compensation Research Institute (WCRI). Detailed benchmark/evaluation (DBE) database. http://www.wcrinet.org/benchmarks.html. Accessed November 29, 2013.

CHAPTER 15

Management Issues in School-Based Services

LEARNING OBJECTIVES

● Discuss the characteristics of contemporary school-based services.
● Analyze key legislation impacting the delivery of school-based services.
● Discuss contemporary school-based practice management issues.
● Analyze the work of physical therapists in public schools.
● Determine the managerial roles and challenges to managerial responsibilities.
● Analyze managerial decision-making in given school-based situations.

PART 1 The Contemporary Setting

Overview of School-Based Rehabilitation Services

Although school systems are not part of the health-care system, many of the 6.5 million people ages 3 to 21 in special (sometimes labeled *exceptional*) education receive interdisciplinary rehabilitation services in the schools they attend.[1] In addition, almost 300,000 infants from birth through age 2 receive early intervention services through local school systems or other approved agencies to improve their opportunity for success when they enter school.[2] These special education and related services are provided by each state through federal legislation mandates, primarily the Individuals With Disabilities Act (IDEA).

The Individuals With Disabilities Education Act (IDEA) and the Individuals With Disabilities Education Improvement Act (IDEIA)

Initiated in 1975 with subsequent revisions—IDEA was reenacted and revised in 2004 as the Individuals With Disabilities Education Improvement Act (IDEIA) to align with the No Child Left Behind Act (NCLB) in 2001. The IDEIA has four parts: Part A deals with the administrative components of the Office of Special Education Programs, Part B lays out the educational requirements of the act, Part C creates guidelines for children with special needs who are under 2 years of age, and Part D creates national grants and resources for implementation of the act.[3]

Of these parts, Part B is of particular interest to managers in school systems. Part B of IDEIA defines children with disabilities as individuals between the ages of 3 and 21 who have one or more of the following conditions that adversely affect their educational performance:[3]

- Mental retardation
- Hearing impairment (including deafness)
- Speech or language impairment

- Visual impairment (including blindness)
- Serious emotional disturbance
- Orthopedic impairment
- Autism
- Traumatic brain injury
- Specific learning disability
- Attention deficit disorder (ADD)
- Attention-deficit hyperactivity disorder (ADHD)
- Other health impairment

School systems are required to provide a *free and appropriate* education, although what that is has not been clearly defined, and the support or related services necessary for each student in the least restrictive environment to achieve his or her educational goals. These related services include:[4]

- Speech-language pathology and audiology services
- Psychological services
- Physical and occupational therapy
- Recreation, including therapeutic recreation
- Social work services
- Orientation and mobility services
- Medical services for diagnostic and evaluation purposes
- Interpreting services
- Psychotherapy
- One-to-one instructional aide
- Transportation
- Art therapy
- Technological devices
- School nurse services

Least Restrictive Environment

A key element of IDEIA is that special needs students receive an education in the least restrictive environment, which requires that any child with a disability, to the extent possible, be educated with children who are not disabled. Only when the disability of a child is so severe that he or she is unable to participate in regular classes, even with supplementary aids present and services available, should the child be educated separately.[3] This requirement means that a child with a disability may be "mainstreamed" into some regular classes while taking other classes in special learning environments.

The Individualized Education Plan

School districts are held accountable for ensuring that every student with special needs is identified and evaluated through Child Find, which is another program mandated by IDEIA. After students are identified, the determination of a free and appropriate education in the least restrictive learning environment is made through a detailed process conducted by interdisciplinary teams of professionals to develop an individualized education plan (IEP). School districts assume the final responsibility for assuring that an IEP is established and implemented for every student identified with special needs.

Each student's IEP must be reviewed annually. Typically, a meeting with parents (legal guardians and others who assume the roles of parents) as equal partners is held to discuss the student's current status and annual educational goals through the proposed IEP. Parents have the right to accept or reject an IEP. Whenever possible, students are included in this planning process. Unique to students in special education, school districts are responsible for ensuring that each special child's right to an evaluation of learning needs, an appropriate education in the least restrictive environment, an IEP, and notice of changes in the IEP are met and documented as part of the formal school record. Students, through their parents, may dispute that schools have met their responsibilities for ensuring these rights. These disputes may be resolved through mediation or formal administrative hearing processes that each school district must have in place.

The IEP is essentially a binding agreement and the school district provides for the specifics outlined within each plan. Because this is typically completed toward the end of the school year, any necessary changes in an IEP because of unanticipated changes in the student during the summer, or as the school year progresses, must be agreed on in writing.[5] The IEPs include descriptions of:[6]

- Specific educational goals for the next school year
- The effect of a student's disability on involvement in and progress toward the goals for the general curriculum used in the regular classroom
- The means for meeting the student's need to be involved in general curriculum
- The special education and related services that will help a student reach annual educational goals (involvement in general curriculum, extracurricular, and nonacademic activities and participation with students with and without disabilities)
- Related services to meet the developmental, corrective, and other needs for the student to meet individualized educational goals
- The frequency, duration, and length of treatment sessions, provider qualifications, and ratio of providers to students
- Necessary program modifications or support for school personnel
- Plans to regularly inform parents of a student's progress
- The student's participation in any district or statewide assessment of student achievement used for the general education population and required modifications or accommodations that will be necessary

Other Parts of the Individuals With Disabilities Education Improvement Act (IDEIA)

Physical therapists and other members of the rehabilitation team may also be involved in state-approved early intervention programs that operate under IDEIA Part C's Early Intervention Program for Infants and Toddlers With Disabilities. The program guidelines encourage the most natural environment possible for interventions, and many of them are offered through school systems. There is much less consistency from state to state in these programs than there is in the implementation of Part B of IDEIA. For instance, in some states these programs may fall under the U.S. Department of Health rather than the U.S. Department of Education. A lead state agency typically coordinates and supports the services of all early intervention providers.

The target population of the Program for Infants and Toddlers is that of children who already have, or who are at risk for, developmental delays that may impede their education. In some states, this Part C of IDEIA, which includes children from birth through 2 years of age, may be extended to cover children until they reach age 6. These early interventions may decrease referrals to special education because they assist a wider range of students who are struggling with language or learning as they develop, but the major goal is successful *transition* of the young child with an actual or potential disability into the least restrictive school environment.

The required Part C Individualized Family Service Plan (IFSP), which is comparable with the IEP required in Part B, reflects the mandate that Part C of IDEIA is family focused rather than child focused. Recognizing the emphasis on providing care in the context of the family system requires the physical therapist to develop strong collaboration skills and to develop more respect for the priorities of the family than might be expected in healthcare settings.

At the other end of the educational spectrum is another transition point. Beginning at age 16, IDEIA demands that IEPs address a transition plan for how the student will proceed after high school. Whether it is the development of skills to live independently as an adult or preparation for college or a training program, the plan must have measurable postsecondary education goals and a plan to meet them.

Assistive Technology

Another component of IDEIA sets regulations related to the provision of assistive technology and the associated services related to these assistive devices and equipment. The IEP team determines that assistive technology is necessary to support the right to access the general curriculum, special education, or related services. Assistive technology may range from eyeglasses to complex, specially designed communication systems. The equipment may be used at home if it supports education but it remains the property of the school. For many students assistive technology may be the only way for them to access a general curriculum.

Some school systems may collaborate with community agencies to exchange, recycle, and refurbish assistive equipment that students no longer need or have outgrown. Payment for assistive technology may come from a variety of resources beyond the funds in the school system's budget, such as grants, third-party payers, and private donations. It is not unusual for school districts to have centralized assistive technology services that coordinate the provision of equipment and devices recommended by the IEP teams throughout the system.

Other Legislation Affecting Special Education

Several other pieces of legislation are related to the rights of people with disabilities. Those most important to schools include the Americans With Disabilities Act (ADA), Section 504 of the Rehabilitation Act, and No Child Left Behind (NCLB) education legislation. NCLB resulted in revisions of the original IDEA.[7] The 2009 American Recovery and Reinvestment Act included additional grant funding for states to support special education.[8]

The ADA Title II addresses *all* activities of state and local governments and requires that people with disabilities receive an equal opportunity to benefit from all of their programs and services, which includes public education. Accomplishment of this equal opportunity goal may take two forms. Specific architectural standards in the new construction and alteration of buildings must be met or programs may need to be relocated to more accessible locations. Standards include alternative means of communicating with people with hearing, vision, or speech disabilities so that they may maneuver within the buildings (i.e., floor announcements in elevators and Braille signage). The other component of ADA requirements is for reasonable modifications to policies, practices, and procedures where necessary to avoid discrimination of people with disabilities.

The ADA is a broader application of older legislation—Section 504 of the Rehabilitation Act. Section 504 must be followed by any program or agency that receives any federal funding. Section 504 and ADA are similar but not the same. Section 504 requires that those funded entities do not discriminate against or deny benefits to qualified individuals with a disability. Each federal department and agency has its own set of Section 504 regulations that applies to its own programs. They all include the requirement that reasonable accommodations are to be made, which is similar to the accommodations required in ADA. Because Section 504 does not come with funding to meet its requirements as does IDEIA, school systems may find it more difficult to comply with these regulations.[9] Children receiving services under Section 504 are required to have a plan in place similar to the IEP required for IDEIA.

Section 504 is broader in scope than IDEIA because IDEIA addresses only the rights of children with specific diagnoses. Section 504 requires the elimination of any barriers for *anyone* with a physical or mental impairment that substantially limits one or more major life activities. The ability to learn in school is considered a life activity. This broad scope includes all students eligible for IDEIA services, but it may also include children who may have temporary or intermittent disabilities, such as asthmatic episodes or self-limiting infectious diseases. To compare another way, IDEIA is often considered an affirmative action rather than an antidiscrimination act because children who qualify for IDEIA receive additional services and protections, which go beyond the equal protection assured by Section 504.[9]

The newer NCLB Act imposed standards for teacher qualifications and core academic subjects that were included in the amendments to IDEIA in 2004. States imposed educational standards for reading and math, demanding school districts show annual improvements in scores. Corrective actions and opportunities for students to transfer from schools that are not meeting the standards or to seek supplemental services to meet standards are part of this act. Although too soon to tell, the potential negative financial impact on special education is a possible concern as funding is directed to meeting standards for all students.

Unique Features of School-Based Physical Therapy Practice

The most obvious feature of school-based physical therapy is that services are provided in schools rather than in a healthcare setting. *Collaboration* may be the best word to describe the effort required by physical therapists to work with members of the related services team and with general and special education teachers to evaluate, plan, and support instruction. Without an understanding of instruction and curriculum, physical therapists may find it difficult to contribute to decisions about the least restrictive environment for students.

For the students with gross motor deficits, the physical therapists' collaboration with adaptive physical education teachers becomes very important in the development and implementation of IEPs. Adaptive physical education is part of the federal special education mandate so it must be provided to all qualified students. If physical therapy is no longer needed for a student to benefit from instruction, adaptive physical education may be a powerful means to continue to work on goals related to movement and physical activity. It provides an opportunity for physical therapy and adaptive physical education programs to complement each other when resources are limited.

The needs of students during a school year and their needs as they advance in grade levels make school-based positions the only positions in which physical therapists establish such long-term relationships with patients (students). Although it may not be typical, it is possible that a school-based physical therapist could work with the same child from ages 3 to 21. Participating in IEP meetings and the other, less formal contact with parents over the years leads to establishing lasting professional relationships with families that are unknown in healthcare settings. These collaborations place parents on equal footing with teachers and related service providers in the care of their children.

Funding Sources

Federal funds do not cover all of the costs of special education. School districts must find the rest of their funding from state and local taxes that may fluctuate widely from year to year. As a result, managers at all levels of school administration may need to make a point of following federal and legislative action closely. Some states permit Medicaid reimbursement to school systems for children who are eligible and require related services. The shifting of state and local resources from education to other public demands is common. Expectations to do more with less funding continues to be a challenge in special education, particularly in terms of salaries, which are often established through collective bargaining negotiations.

Salaries

Teachers are usually represented by the National Education Association's bargaining units in each state. Although physical therapists may not be members of these units, they may be bound by the pay scales and merit pay raises negotiated for teachers. These pay structures may make it difficult to recruit physical therapists because school-based salaries often are not competitive with the health-care sector. Some school districts may choose to contract for related services through community-based organizations that provide pediatric rehabilitation services. These practices can offer higher salaries to their employees because they receive reimbursement from other sources in addition to school system contracts.

This contracting of services may solve the need for more competitive salaries, but it presents other challenges for physical therapists. Many therapists who are employed by school districts may be perceived as "related to" rather than strongly integrated into some schools. If they are employed by an outside agency, there is a risk that overcoming the perceived or actual distances between teachers and therapists may be even more challenging.

Collective bargaining may also lead to strict rules about teaching assignments and the time devoted to specific assignments. Because school systems tend to be tightly regulated bureaucracies anyway, these two factors may make the integration of related services challenging. The daily scheduling of classes, lunch breaks, transportation, and other activities may be made down to one-half minute intervals with very little room for deviation. Physical therapists who are more accustomed to the freedom of scheduling their own patients and control of their workdays may find schools very restrictive. This type of environment may conflict with their approach to addressing students' needs and goals.

Concurrent Community Services

Another challenge for physical therapists new to school systems may be the required limitation of therapy goals to those related only to the accomplishment of educational goals in the least restrictive environment. The hours a child spends in school are, after all, only a small proportion of time compared with the challenges faced by a child with disabilities. For instance, independent bed-to-chair transfers or elimination of environmental barriers in the home may be important goals for a child with disabilities and are not related to the child's learning and ability to function in school. As a result, some students concurrently receive community-based therapy services. If so, school-based physical therapists may need to extend their collaboration networks to include other professionals who are providing services to students outside of school.

Collaboration is also important to managers who rely on a special, centralized, countywide team for acquisition of any item, equipment, or system needed to improve the functional abilities of particular students. Assistive technology may be purchased, fabricated, or leased. In addition to training students and others in the use of the technology, the responsibility for fitting, repairing, and maintaining the devices or technology lies with the rehabilitation team. Remaining current in new technology becomes an important professional responsibility for school-based therapists in collaboration with their colleagues in community-based practices and pediatric hospitals.

Sidebar 15.1 summarizes the factors that managers may present as components of the fulfilling and rewarding world of school-based physical therapy. As a member of the education team, physical therapists have an important role in assuring the achievement of educational goals of children.

SIDEBAR 15.1

Characteristics of School-Based Physical Therapy

- Establish long-term relationships with students, families, and interdisciplinary education team
- Services integrated into a tightly controlled schedule

- Need for creative approaches to focus only on the educational needs of students rather than more general patient goals

Continued

- Detailed collaboration with education professionals and other members of the rehabilitation team
- The role of physical therapy may be poorly understood by education professionals
- Coordination and collaboration with community-based providers offering concurrent care
- Highly individualized planning for meeting yearly education goals
- Outcomes of therapeutic efforts may be long term rather than immediate and more difficult to determine
- Shift focus of care to educational rather than therapeutic goals for students

- Competition for limited resources (often including space) available to school systems leading to financial and administrative constraints on services
- Shorter workdays because of public school schedules and potential for extended time off during the summer months
- Isolated from other physical therapists because of distances among schools in a system
- May involve travel among several schools in a school district

PART 2   Overview of Management in Public Schools

Management of School-Based Physical Therapy

Each school district may have a central coordinator of special education services who is based at the county's board of education. There may or may not be another person who coordinates the related services in special education for the entire district. Depending on the number of students in special education and the need for related services, supervisors for each of the related disciplines may be assigned to regions within a district. This makes school-based management a field operation similar to management of rehabilitation services in home care.

Because most IEPs are completed for each child before the beginning of the school year, districtwide needs for related services can be somewhat predicted. Because the needs of each child may vary from year to year, new students transfer into the system, and others graduate, the assignment of therapists among schools each school year remains a major challenge.

Depending on the number of students in each level of educational placement, physical therapy staff may be assigned to:

- One special school where there are many students with multiple disabilities and many related needs. They may provide actual, direct physical therapy interventions in therapy rooms in the schools and devote more attention to assistive technology in special education classes.
- Travel among several schools at all levels of education where students may be in both general education and special education classes. Their role may be more consultative (indirect) and intermittent to assure inclusion in these least restrictive environments.
- Programs for infants and toddlers who are at risk. Physical therapists may provide direct services with an emphasis on family education in early intervention centers.
- Some combination of the above models.

School district coordinators meet these needs by hiring therapists who are employees of the school district or by contracting the services of private companies or independently practicing physical therapists. Assuring that these contracts allow time for participation as an active team member beyond the provision of direct services is important so that contracting physical therapists are prepared to meet all of the responsibilities of school-based therapists.

The needs of students in special education cover a broad range of diagnoses and levels of disabilities, and a particular child's needs change over time. Physical therapists must have a broad range of skills to address a wide variety of conditions complemented by a strong understanding of teaching and learning for these special populations. Coordinators of related services in larger school districts may assign physical therapists the responsibility for interdisciplinary rehabilitation teams providing services in a cluster of schools in a particular location.

Management Responsibilities

Mission, Vision, and Goals

Perhaps the most important challenge to the mission, vision, and goals is orienting new staff not only to the philosophy and mission of IDEIA, but also to an educational rather than healthcare approach to the provision of services. Managers may need to clarify each particular school's philosophy and commitment to the "idea" of IDEIA and compliance with its rules and regulations. Although the interdisciplinary focus may have become second nature to many physical therapists, the heightened role of parents and teachers in decision-making may be something that managers need to convey to the people they supervise. Limiting goals to those related to education in the least restrictive environment may be another important component of orientation for new employees.

Policies and Procedures

To meet the letter and intent of the laws governing special education services, policies and procedures are developed in the offices of the school board. They are distributed throughout school districts for consistent implementation by managers. Clarification of the roles of the members of the IEP team may be the most important policy and procedure. Perhaps more than any other practice setting, the integration of services is critical. Avoiding overlap and identifying gaps in related rehab services not only assures educational outcomes, but also demonstrates compliance with legal requirements.

In addition to IEP mandates, policies and procedures may need to be in place to clarify the responsibilities of members of the team and to establish stopgap measures in the provision of services. For instance, it may be helpful to develop a list of assessments and interventions commonly used by physical and occupational therapists and to create a chart to delineate which discipline is primarily responsible for each. A similar clarification of the roles of supportive personnel in the related services and instructional paraeducators becomes important to ensure compliance with professional licensure regulations. Managers must establish clear lines of responsibility and communication.

Managers may also be responsible for determining which standardized developmental and functional scales should be used across the district and which should be used at the discretion of individual therapists. Investigating the evidence to support these decisions may be a new role for managers as their accountability for the outcomes of services provided becomes dependent on standardized measurements.

Unlike their role in healthcare decisions, physicians may never be involved in actual IEP processes and decisions. Whether or not school-based therapists must have physicians' orders to "treat" children in school systems may vary from state to state. Managers may have to assure that policies and procedures address the expected relationships with physicians and compliance with legal requirements for the provision of service, particularly if Medicaid funding of services is a consideration. Assisting staff in a major shift of responsibility for clinical decisions without the medical support that is more common in healthcare settings is another role of managers.

Marketing

Because related services in special education are so dependent on federal and state legislation, new programs may be limited to those that are mandated with little opportunity for creating other new programs. However, some managers may have the opportunity to identify funding sources and prepare grant proposals for alternative funding from other public and private sources. The support services available for preparation of proposals may vary widely from one school district to another, so grant-writing workshops and in-services may be valuable to managers who either are assigned or take the initiative to pursue outside funding.

Networking may be a more appropriate function than marketing for school-based managers. Because of IDEIA requirements for referral of students to identify their potential need for related services, managers may not need to internally market related services in most schools. Internal networking may be more important to managers to identify and establish working relationships with all of the key players in each school. Beginning with the principal and continuing with teachers and other service providers, it may be critical for managers to clarify the roles of the physical therapists and other members of the rehabilitation team to confirm that the goals for services are incorporated in the plans and mission for each school on an ongoing basis.

Formal and informal community networking is also important for the identification of support groups for caregivers and other community resources important to special education in general, and to meet the goals of specific IEPs. For example, managers may need to take the initiative to establish professional relationships with durable medical equipment suppliers, orthotists, and prosthetists.

Getting to know the family physicians, orthopedic surgeons, and other doctors who care for children receiving related services may be critical. Their understanding of the services provided in schools may be limited. Managers may make opportunities to educate physicians in face-to-face encounters to broaden the service network that supports the requirements of children with special needs while opening doors for better interdisciplinary communication between school-based and community-based providers of care.

Perhaps most important, managers need to be the face and voice of the school-based team to other providers of pediatric rehabilitation services. Not only are these services important as potential sources of providers in the school, but also managers may need to open these doors so that school-based staff are able to effectively coordinate all of the care a child receives.

Staffing

Determination of a full-time caseload presents challenges to school-based managers. Three major factors to be considered in school-based caseloads have been identified:[10]

- The students to be served: type and amount of services provided to each student, geographic area to be covered, number of schools, and distances between them.
- The therapists' other responsibilities: documentation, meetings, consultation with teachers and parents, outcomes studies, and supervision of support personnel.
- Other factors: consultation with other classroom staff and parents, support available, number of one-on-one sessions, community contacts required, and continuing education requirements.

Taking these identified tasks, managers may analyze staff caseloads by creating a log to determine the percentage of time in a 37.5-hour week that each full-time equivalent (FTE) employee devotes to various activities. Possible activities in a time log may include direct student contact, paperwork, IEP and other meetings, travel time, assessments, consultation, lunchtime, and other union contract work conditions (e.g., breaks, preparation time).[10] Managers may ask staff members to complete the time logs consistently or they may select certain weeks for data collection with time logs. Data analysis may assist managers to adjust work assignments on an ongoing basis, redistribute staff, compare the work of full-time and part-time staff, or establish productivity goals for each staff member.

Recruitment

Recruitment of full-time staff to be employees of the school board may be challenging because salaries tend to be less than competitive with those offered in other work settings. Juggling the needs of students in all schools with the needs and preferences of contract service providers or independent per diem contractors and aligning them with the expectations of full-time school board employees makes assignment decisions and scheduling, particularly in large school districts (i.e., either population or geographically large), very time consuming. For instance, contracting with a community-based pediatric practice may mean it provides services to the school district only on Tuesdays and Thursdays because they have outpatient visits in their offices scheduled on other days, although IEPs call for related services to be delivered three times per week. Independent contractors may work only in one particular school that is convenient for them or choose not to work into extended year programs during the summers. Full-time employees may become resentful if they are always representing other per diem or contract therapists in IEP meetings because the full-time therapists are more available.

School-based managers may face more pressure than managers in healthcare settings to avoid staff turnover because the services provided in schools are long-term and complex. The time required for new people to establish rapport with children may delay or interfere with the progress toward goals. Consistency of personnel is more likely to result in better collaboration among members of the IEP team as well, particularly in field operations where a physical therapist may be a part of numerous teams in several schools.

As in other field operations, therapists who travel among schools may spend as much time commuting between schools as they do delivering services. Often the staff are available but unevenly distributed because some locations are more desirable than others. This preference for a particular location presents another management challenge if there are no resources to offer incentives that make less attractive assignments more attractive. Hiring physical therapist assistants at lower pay scales may be one management solution, particularly if more assistants than therapists are available for hire. Because physical therapist assistants may be more tightly tied to a particular community, turnover of staff may be reduced, but managers should be cautious about other potential problems that may arise.

Physical Therapist Assistants

The roles of physical therapist assistants may be limited to the provision of direct care and providing instructions to teachers and support staff because consultation and the development of IEPs may be beyond their scope of practice. Evaluation, treatment planning, and supervision of others are typically the responsibilities of physical therapists that cannot be delegated to assistants. This delineation of roles further limits the distribution of the potential workforce. Utilization and supervision of physical therapist assistants is determined by state statutes, which may mean that physical therapists do not need to provide direct or on-site supervision to physical therapist assistants in schools. Depending on those practice rules, supervision of assistants by the physical therapist of record may mean that the therapist has supervisory responsibility for several assistants who are assigned to different schools. When a physical therapist assistant is assigned to only one school serviced by an itinerant physical therapist, managers may need to pay particular attention to assure compliance with practice acts.

For instance, if the physical therapist assistant is more readily available in a particular school than the physical therapist is, care needs to be taken that practice acts are not violated. There may be unintentional, well-meaning decision-making and problem-solving by the physical therapist assistant that occurs because of the day-to-day questions that arise about the care of a child, which are actually the responsibility of the physical therapist. Managers may find it necessary to spend more efforts distinguishing the legal responsibilities of physical therapists and physical therapist assistants for parents and education professionals. Orientation of therapists and assistants in school-based practices may need to include communication strategies for dealing with these potential issues about decision-making to avoid potential practice act violations.

Patient Care

Even for physical therapists with pediatric experience in other settings, distinguishing only those goals that are related to the achievement of school-based goals may require a careful analysis of a child's ability to function. Moving from a "medically necessary" model of thinking to a "learning relevant" model may not be as easy as it sounds for some therapists, particularly if the therapists are also working in community-based pediatric services where the emphasis is on one-on-one interventions. Changes may not happen without significant effort.

Managers' monitoring of this critical component of school-based services and their assurance of staff expertise to address a wide range of diagnoses and learning needs may be their primary roles in the actual delivery of services. Managers should not be hesitant to hire therapists who seek new opportunities in school systems even though their prior work experience may be with adults. It may be somewhat easier to start with a clean pediatric record than it is to modify strong, long-held opinions about the care of children with disabilities.

Classroom Integration

Another management concern in school systems is to make certain that direct interventions are provided *only* when necessary, and consulting (indirect) services are *always* provided when necessary. Clarification of these two roles of therapists is useful in determining the appropriate type and level of integration of therapy services into the classroom. Deciding when to shift services from isolated therapy rooms to integrated services in the classrooms remains controversial as therapists balance the child's need for practice to learn new skills with the need to function in the most natural environment—the classroom. It follows that determining the frequency of treatment interventions also becomes challenging because the effectiveness of interventions is muddied by many external factors—positive and negative, including the actual implementation of recommendations made to teachers and caregivers.[11]

Managers may need to encourage their staffs to be creative in identifying resources and in collaborating to meet the needs of students. Increased collaboration may require having the tools to resolve potential conflicts among the rehabilitation team, teachers, and family members. School-based managers may need to offer more assistance to their staffs in reaching more compromises than are expected in healthcare practices. Teachers become vested in students that they have known for years, and parents' opinions are taken very seriously.

The negotiation skills of managers also may be more important in school-based practice because resolving conflicts at one level of management may create additional problems at others. For instance, if upper-level district managers of special education and related services do not come from the same professional disciplines as the people they supervise, or if members of one IEP team report to different supervisors in a district, additional management issues can arise. School districts are complex, bureaucratic organizations in which the chains of command are not always clear, particularly as limited resources demand frequent organizational changes.

Performance Evaluation

Because school-based services are a field operation, evaluation of performance of staff may be difficult. There may be only one annual opportunity to observe treatment sessions to determine the therapist's clinical expertise and ability to manage the behavior of children. Managers often rely on input from other members of the IEP team, including parents and students to complement these direct observations. Tweezing out the contribution of each discipline in student outcomes may not always be straightforward or clear, and the outcomes of education are often long term, with many intervening variables along the way. Having staff self-report on their activities and their contributions to IEPs may be an important management tool. For instance, in addition to the direct provision of services, evaluation of performance may include:

- Compliance with the IDEIA, Section 504, and ADA
- Knowledge of the general education curriculum as it relates to therapy
- Effective use and analysis of assessment tools
- Consultation and collaboration skills

Fiscal

Although managers in healthcare settings may face many budgeting and cash-flow challenges, they seem to be compounded in school systems. Through complex federal and state funding, which is typically driven by legislative budgeting processes, school-based managers may have a minimal role in any financial decision-making, but a great deal of accountability for controlling costs.

School districts may enroll as providers of Medicaid services, which allows them to be reimbursed for services provided under IDEIA Parts B and C to eligible students. This Medicaid Certified School Match Program includes reimbursement for direct services, such as all of the rehabilitation services, counseling, nursing, and transportation. Administrative activities, such as referrals to determine Medicaid eligibility and for the coordination of services, also are reimbursed.

The intent of these Medicaid match programs is to improve students' access to medical care and to promote a better understanding of care available to families, which will improve students' health. It is also a source of income for school districts that helps to meet their costs for delivery of these mandated services, with some remaining funds available to reinvest in the expansion of services and to purchase supplies and equipment for special education programs. Managers may need to develop the means to prevent duplication of Medicaid services when children are concurrently receiving therapy in community-based agencies.

Legal, Ethical, and Risk

Because special education is so tightly linked to legislation, failure to meet these mandates presents potential legal issues. There are numerous legal cases surrounding special education and IDEIA that have been taken to the U.S. Supreme Court. For instance, courts have been asked to determine what constitutes a related service versus a medical service. The determination of the adequacy of physical therapy services for a particular child also has been addressed by the courts.[10]

Role Release

In addition to the legal issues surrounding the supervision and direction of physical therapist assistants, the delegation of care to paraeducators (also called paraprofessionals or instructional aides), teachers, and parents may be equally risky, although necessary. These professional decisions about who does what are about directing and instructing rather than delegation. They require careful consideration because it is more the rule than the exception that physical therapists and other health professionals in the related services "release" their roles to others in the schools and to parents for students to meet their IEP goals.[12]

Therapists are often less available for the daily carry through of interventions that students need to practice because they are spread thin among schools to meet the demands for services when workforce and other resources are limited. It is important that physical therapists understand that role release does not mean abdication of responsibility. Documentation of the training of others to perform assigned tasks and supervising that performance with a particular student is critical especially in this transdisciplinary, educational model of care.[12]

These role-release decisions are even more complex because IEPs are discipline neutral. This transdisciplinary nature of therapeutic services in schools may cause physical therapists to struggle with reinforcing what is and what is not physical therapy. Because physical therapy is defined as only what a physical therapist does or directs a physical therapist assistant to do, it may be helpful to clarify that others who are following the instructions of the physical therapist in the classroom or at home are not legally "doing physical therapy."

Managers also must understand that their legal responsibility for patient/client instruction and the education of other caregivers are also professional responsibilities. They may take on greater significance in complex school settings in which many people are involved in students' IEPs, particularly when the therapist is intermittently on the premises. The fact that all care providers are adequately trained for their global responsibilities and for particular tasks assigned for each student must be confirmed and documented by the physical therapist and other providers of related services.

Confidentiality

Another legal and ethical concern is maintaining the confidentiality of student records, which is as important as maintaining the confidentiality of medical records. Therapists may need to be reminded that all statutes regulating practice, professional codes of ethics, and standards of practice apply to healthcare and school-based settings.

As in many healthcare settings, inadequate or lack of resources in school systems often leads to ethical dilemmas. Pressure from principals or school board members to standardize policies and procedures about the frequency and duration of related services for children with particular diagnoses, or to establish productivity goals that negatively impact IEP outcomes, requires managers to be prepared to present the legal and ethical dilemmas that such actions place on therapists.

Communication

Managers of any field operations often take a variety of means to communicate with staffs that are scattered over a large geographic area following different work schedules. E-mail, phone conferences, cell phones, access to electronic databases, and other forms of communication have facilitated efforts to communicate and track services provided.

School-based managers may find the need to spend much time in the field to determine the effectiveness of services provided under their supervision in each school.

Managers may need to confirm that physical therapists who supervise physical therapist assistants have established the importance of scheduling ongoing communication and supervisory sessions. Physical therapist assistants must have accurate contact information so that the physical therapist is readily available should student emergencies arise. Whether or not the level and frequency of supervision of supportive personnel in school-based practice are defined in state statutes, supervisory responsibility and the documentation of communication are essential. This is particularly important if the physical therapist and the physical therapist assistant are not in the same place at the same time—which may be a more common staffing model in school-based practice than it is in healthcare settings. Similarly, instructions and follow-up of care provided by nonlicensed school aides and paraeducators under the direction of physical therapists or assistants must be clearly documented.

Informal Communication

The informal communication among related service providers and all of the teachers involved in a particular student's IEP has been facilitated by the availability of e-mail. Because the therapists may move among several schools, there may be little downtime in a particular school for informal, face-to-face interactions. Therefore, to enhance communication, managers must assure that there is time for staff to represent rehabilitation services at formally scheduled meetings of the special education team. Emphasizing the importance of accurate documentation of the services provided and filing that documentation in a centralized location for timely access by all members of the IEP team is also critical for communication among the team.

Conclusions

The management of school-based physical therapy services offers unique challenges and rewards. It provides the satisfaction that comes from being a respected, indispensable part of a transdisciplinary special education program. Managers are responsible for staff who must be effective team players, communicators, and documenters throughout a school system.

Because there is a higher legal standard of care expected when people are less able to take care of themselves, managers must be vigilant in addressing the legal and ethical issues confronting physical therapists who care for children. The reward for establishing long-term professional relationships with children and their families often outweighs the system requirements that must be addressed. The financial support of special education programs, personnel shortages, and government mandates may demand as much of the attention of managers as their responsibility for the quality of care provided through the related services.

The team approach to solving complex problems helps to focus on the big picture of least restrictive learning environments. School-based practice presents many opportunities to take pride in contributing to the accomplishments of many children who might otherwise not have a chance if not for the combined efforts of many health and education professionals. Activities 15.1 to 15.14 provide the opportunity to address school-based management decision-making.

ACTIVITY 15.1
IN YOUR AREA

Find exceptional education services in your state's board of education's webpages. Find information on the special education program in your local school district. What useful resources are available at the American Physical Therapy Association for managers?

Example:

http://www.pediatricapta.org/special-interest-groups/school-based-therapy/index.cfm)
What are five key points gleaned from these resources that are of most value to managers?

ACTIVITY 15.2
A PLACE TO SIT

Marsha Miller is the new director of rehab services for pre-K–12 schools in Hamilton County. An important issue is the lack of space in the school for the rehab teams. Each school needs at least a place for staff to keep their personal things and prepare documentation. At best, an area for all disciplines to share with basic therapeutic equipment and a space for student privacy would be welcomed.

How should Marsha address this problem? Consider: Where are they now? Where do they want to be? What does Marsha have to work with? How will she get there?

ACTIVITY 15.3
COMMUNITY RESOURCES

Larry Eubanks has moved to Uniontown to become the Coordinator of Rehabilitation Services for Union County Schools. He wants to develop a link on the school board's webpage for community resources that parents, students, and staff alike may access. He wants the list of resources to be as comprehensive and relevant as possible.

How should he go about implementing this idea? Note: It may be helpful to develop an actual list from your own school district. Consider: Where are they now? Where do they want to be? What does Larry have to work with? How will he get there?

ACTIVITY 15.4
UNSATISFACTORY PERFORMANCE

Larry Eubanks spent one day within the past year, unannounced, in each school to observe clinical performance and interactions of his staff with school personnel. He was impressed with everyone's efforts and felt confident that he had inherited a good team doing a good job. He was surprised by a call from Fred Fielding, the teacher who is the orthopedic program coordinator at Jackson Middle School. Fred is demanding that Sonja Sammons, the physical therapist, not return to the school because of her disruptive behavior, and expects Larry to replace her as soon as possible. Fred reports that Sonja spends more time socializing and provoking student conflicts than doing her job. Larry's observations of her clinical interventions with three students were acceptable.

What should Larry do? Consider: Where are they now? Where do they want to be? What does Larry have to work with? How will he get there?

ACTIVITY 15.5
SCHOOL-BASED VERSUS COMMUNITY-BASED

Larry Eubanks has been working closely with Total Therapy Care to coordinate the care of several students with disabilities in Union County Schools over the past year. He negotiated a contract between Union County and Total Therapy Care to provide services in one of the county's special education centers. That contract has been working well with no issues. However, Larry has received calls from two different parents of children who are being treated by Tanya Vargas, a full-time physical therapist employed by the school board for K–12 schools in the northern half of the county. The parents report that they are very concerned because their children also receive therapy three times/week at Total Therapy Care, and the physical therapist there tells them that what Tanya is doing is undermining what they are trying to do with their children.

What should Larry do? Consider: Where are they now? Where do they want to be? What does Larry have to work with? How will he get there?

ACTIVITY 15.6
STAFF SHORTAGE

The good news is that Union County is the fastest growing county in the state. The bad news is that the school board is having difficulty meeting the educational demands of the additional students who have moved to the area. Larry Eubanks has been Rehabilitation Coordinator for Union County Schools for 5 years now. He received a memo from the Sarah Chiles, County Director for Special Education, requesting a meeting next week. She asked that Larry be prepared to identify at least three ways to control costs other than staffing and three strategies for recruiting staff to meet the needs of 120 new special education students next year.

What are some ideas that Larry may present? Consider: Where are they now? Where do they want to be? What do they have to work with? How will they get there?

ACTIVITY 15.7
CLINICAL EDUCATION IN SPECIAL EDUCATION

One of the recruitment strategies that Larry Eubanks suggested during his meeting with Sarah (see Activity 15.6) was to establish clinical education agreements with the local university's physical therapy program and the community college's physical therapist assistant program. This also may relieve his personnel shortage to have professional students helping with care. He reported to Sarah that the program coordinators have approached him in the past but he did not feel that his staff was ready.

What are the issues that Larry and Sarah need to consider before they meet with the coordinators of clinical education from the university and community college? Consider: Where are they now? Where do they want to be? What does Larry have to work with? How will he get there?

ACTIVITY 15.8
ADAPTIVE PHYSICAL EDUCATION

Larry Eubanks has received his third message from Melissa Quintos, one of the adaptive physical education teachers in Union County. She has been insistent in her requests for him to devise a countywide plan to integrate therapy more effectively into adaptive physical education. Larry is hesitant because he feels Melissa often oversteps the boundary between physical therapy and physical education. She sees herself as a therapist rather than a teacher collaborating with therapy.

What should Larry do? Consider: Where are they now? Where do they want to be? What do they have to work with? How will they get there?

ACTIVITY 15.9
SUPERVISION OF PHYICAL THERAPIST ASSISTANT

Clarice Montiago has recently called Larry Eubanks regarding her son Charlie to request that Sally Simmons, the physical therapist assistant, not work with her son. She just learned that Sally is not a licensed physical therapist. Clarice states that she knows her son's rights and he must be treated by a physical therapist.

What should Larry do? Consider: Where are they now? Where do they want to be? What do they have to work with? How will they get there?

ACTIVITY 15.10
TO WALK OR NOT TO WALK

There is only one item on the agenda for the fall physical therapy staff meeting. Larry Eubanks has sent a memo stating the meeting will be a workshop to develop recommendations for policies and procedures about determining which children are to incorporate walking during school hours as part of their IEPs. This issue has been a source of contention between the therapists, who strongly feel that students who are able to walk to and from class should walk. Teachers and administrators insist that only students who can perform within the demands of schedules should be walking between classes and to and from activities. Their argument is that it is disruptive for students to be excused early or to be late for every class and lunch because of the extra time needed to walk.

What should the policy and procedure state? Consider: Where are they now? Where do they want to be? What do they have to work with? How will they get there?

ACTIVITY 15.11
MAINSTREAMING VERSUS INCLUSION

Larry Eubanks just realized that the communication problem that he has been having with some of his staff is because of a difference of opinion about least-restrictive environment. Some of his therapists believe that their job is to adapt the child to the school as much as possible and that they should only be in classes and activities in which they can succeed. Other staff members believe that the school should make all efforts to adapt classrooms, and the school as a whole, to meet the needs of all the children.

Which view is right? What difference does it make? What should Larry do? Consider: Where are they now? Where do they want to be? What do they have to work with? How will they get there?

ACTIVITY 15.12
PARENTAL DEMANDS

Joe and Anne Lee have asked for a meeting with Larry Eubanks, Rehabilitation Coordinator for Union County Schools, and Joyce McCullen, Principal at Pretty Lake Elementary School. They are very unhappy with the decision made at the last IEP meeting that their daughter Lulu will not be receiving physical therapy in school. Lulu had been receiving physical therapy two times/week at Kids-R-Great Rehab in town, but the Lees' health insurance no longer covers these services. They believe that she has not reached a plateau and can improve only with more physical therapy. Although they attended the IEP meeting and heard that all accommodations have been made for Lulu to meet her learning goals, they are not satisfied. The Lees have advised Mrs. McCullen that they have contacted a lawyer and know their rights.

How should Larry prepare for the meeting? Consider: Where are they now? Where do they want to be? What do they have to work with? How will they get there?

ACTIVITY 15.13
DIRECTION AND SUPERVISION

Terri Edmundson, physical therapist at Pretty Lake Elementary School, has established the method that Timmy Fletcher is to use to ascend and descend the school bus steps. She has directed Jake Ortiz, the physical therapist assistant, to have Timmy practice on the steps three or four more times in the next week. Terri also tells Jake that when he is satisfied that Timmy can perform the stairclimb, he is to instruct Debra, the orthopedic aide assigned to Timmy, to meet him at the bus every day to supervise him getting on and off the bus until further notice. Timmy's mother calls Larry Eubanks, rehabilitation coordinator, at the end of the week to ask whether she should be helping Timmy on and off the bus at home every day since he is doing it at school, or whether he should continue to use the wheelchair lift on the bus at the home end.

What should Larry say? Consider: Where are they now? Where do they want to be? What do they have to work with? How will they get there?

ACTIVITY 15.14
PRODUCTIVITY

Based on the analysis of time logs submitted for four random weeks by 12 physical therapists, Larry Eubanks is faced with the following results based on 37.5 hours/week of work:

ACTIVITY	MEAN PERCENTAGE OF TIME SPENT BY PTS TRAVELING AMONG SCHOOLS	MEAN PERCENTAGE OF TIME SPENT BY PTS ASSIGNED TO ONE SCHOOL
Student contact	44%	46%
Paperwork	19%	20%
Meetings, including IEPs	16%	28%
Lunch	6%	6%
Travel	15%	0%

What should Larry conclude about the work of his staff? Should the percentages for the distribution of work of physical therapist assistants be the same? Consider: Where are they now? Where do they want to be? What do they have to work with? How will they get there?

REFERENCES

1. U.S. Department of Education, Office of Special Education Programs. Part B Child Count, Fall, 2011. http://www.ideadata .org/arc_toc13.asp#partbCC. Accessed May 16, 2013.

2. U.S. Department of Education, Office of Special Education Programs. Part C Child Count, Fall, 2011. http://www.ideadata .org/arc_toc13.asp#partcCC. Accessed May 16, 2013.

3. United States Congress. Individuals With Disabilities Education Improvement Act 2004. Sec 101, Part AA, Subpart 4, Sec 602 (3)(A) Definitions. http://thomas.loc.gov/cgi-bin /query/z?c108:h.1350.enr. Accessed May 16, 2013.

4. United States Congress. *Related Services in IDEIA 2005*. Sec 101, Part A, Subpart 4, Sec 02 (26)(A). http://thomas.loc .gov/cgi-bin/query/z?c108:h.1350.enr. Accessed May 16, 2013.

5. McConlogue A, Quinn L. Analysis of physical therapy goals in a school-based setting: a pilot study. *Physical and Occupational Therapy in Pediatrics*. 2009;29(2):154-169.

6. Osgood RL. *The History of Inclusion in the United States*. Washington, DC: Gallaudet University Press; 2005.

7. Siegel LM. *The Complete IEP Guide: How to Advocate for Your Special Ed Child*. 4th ed. Berkeley, CA: Nolo; 2005.

8. U.S. Department of Justice. *A Guide to Disability Rights Laws*. September 2005. http://www.ada.gov/cguide.htm.

9. U.S. Department of Education. Recovery Act. http:// www.ed.gov/recovery. Accessed May 16, 2013.

10. Rosenfeld SJ. *Section 504 and IDEA: Basic Similarities and Differences*. http://www.wrightslaw.com/advoc/articles/504 IDEA Rosenfled.html. Accessed September 21, 2007.

11. Kaminker MK, Chiarello LA, O'Neil ME, et al. Decision making for physical therapy service delivery in schools: a nationwide survey of pediatric physical therapists. *Physical Therapy*. 2004;84:919-933.

12. McEwen I, ed. *Providing Physical Therapy Services Under Parts B & C of the Individuals With Disabilities Education Act (IDEA)*. Alexandria, VA: Section on Pediatrics, American Physical Therapy Association; 2000.

CHAPTER 16

Management Issues in Home-Care Organizations

LEARNING OBJECTIVES

● Discuss the characteristics of the range of contemporary home-care services and hospice.
● Analyze licensure, certification, and accreditation demands in home care.
● Discuss contemporary home-care practice issues.
● Analyze the work of physical therapists in home-care settings.
● Determine the managerial roles and challenges to managerial responsibilities.
● Analyze managerial decision-making in given home-care situations.

PART 1   The Contemporary Setting

Overview of Home Care

Home care is that broad array of professional and paraprofessional services, post-acute and long-term care, with medical and social services provided in nonmedical, residential settings that include two broad parallel and interrelated functions: [1]

- Social and supportive services: Their purpose is to keep the person in the home and as functional as possible by providing personal care. This type of home care is often uncompensated care provided by family and friends. If additional supportive assistance is needed, it is more often than not paid for out of pocket. These paid services do not require a high level of skill. Contrary to popular impressions, it may be more expensive than institutional care if it is needed 24/7 and the client is severely dependent.

- Post-acute services: These services may be episodes of care of varying lengths, which include intermittent, short-term visits by health professionals. They are professional, skilled services; therefore, reimbursement by Medicare, Medicaid, and other health insurance policies applies.

Although care of the sick and elderly in their homes is not new, it is only recently that home care became an important part of the business of healthcare. People of all ages who have a wide range of physical and mental impairments receive home care. For example, working-age adults who are commonly receiving Medicaid benefits and children make up 40% of home-care patients.[1]

Based on 2009 statistical data prepared by the National Association for Home Care & Hospice, there are an estimated 33,000 home health provider organizations—10,500 are Medicare certified and 9,000 of them are freestanding organizations. Home health provider organizations deliver care to 12 million people in the United States and employ about 1 million people. Physical therapy staffs make up 26,000 of these employees,

and they average 5.39 patient visits per day. These organizations supplement rather than replace the informal, unpaid care that families, neighbors, and friends provide in the home. One in three households has informal caregivers (66 million people caring for both children and adults). Eighty-six percent of informal caregivers provide care to a relative, and 14% of them are caring for their own child.[2]

The purpose of home care is to maximize health and functioning in people with long-term needs so that they may remain in the community in the least restrictive environment. This includes providing support for families who care for them. The needs of patients and their caregivers in the home have increased as changes in hospital reimbursement policies have led to earlier hospital discharges. New portable technologies have been developed to allow sicker patients to be cared for in the home. Services, such as intravenous nutrition, chemotherapy, respiratory therapy, dialysis care, fetal monitoring, telemonitoring, and other high-tech therapies, have moved into the home setting. The resultant rapid growth in home-care services has become a major issue in the provision of healthcare.[3]

These technological advances have skewed the home-care population to clients who are frailer and more medically compromised yet who seek to remain safely in their homes. Meeting the needs of this population involves creative and complex discharge planning from hospitals and long-term care organizations. After all, the return to home is a time-honored goal of hospitalizations and an important stage of rehabilitation. Shifting from the dependency of inpatient care to independence at home requires the serious planning of many people. The planning must be taken seriously because the control of one's environment is the major criterion for a person's independence. The unique circumstances of each patient make it difficult to anticipate every potential problem related to the return to home after an episode of inpatient (hospital or nursing home) care. At the least, the discharge plan needs to include the determination of:[4]

- Safety and accessibility of the home environment
- Willingness of the patient to receive home services
- Availability of willing and able family or caregiver to assist the patient in activities of daily living (ADLs) and instrumental activities of daily living (IADLs)
- Additional resources available to supplement family caregiving

For more information on home care go to the webpages of the National Association for Home Care and Hospice and links to its partner organizations found in Web Resources.

Types of Home Care

Terms used to name and discuss the care provided in the home may be used inconsistently and result in confusion. Assumptions should not be made about the legal or certification status of a business based on its name. For instance, *home health* and *home care* may be used interchangeably, or *home health* may refer to nursing services with home care reserved for the broader context of all services, or *home health* may mean Medicare certification of an agency and *home care* may refer to private pay services. Table 16.1 summarizes the differences among the three broad types of home care and the role of physical therapy services in each. Any of these services may exist as part of an integrated healthcare delivery system; a franchise (unit of a national

TABLE 16.1   Characteristics of home health agencies, hospices, and home-care aide agencies and the role of physical therapy in each

TYPE OF HOME CARE	PURPOSE	PATIENT ELIGIBILITY REQUIREMENTS	ROLE OF PHYSICAL THERAPY
Home Health (Care) Agencies	Skilled intermittent care that includes disease state management	Typically certified as Medicare agency. To be eligible for home care as a Medicare beneficiary: Must be homebound, MD certification of need, require skilled intermittent or part-time care. Must be medically necessary. Continues until outcomes reached or maintenance program established and can be turned over to less technical provider (custodial care).[1]	Integral component of an integrated, interdisciplinary approach to skilled care
Hospices	Professional (medical) and volunteer (social) services for those at the end of life (77% of hospice patients die at home)	Certified as Medicare agency. To be eligible for hospice services, need documented proof of only 6 months to live but can live longer and continue to receive care. Agree to palliative rather than curative or life-prolonging care.[5]	May range from a more consultative role with a focus on assisting caregivers as a patient's condition declines, to a strong interdisciplinary team approach to palliative care at the end of life.
Home-Care Aide Agencies	Homemaker, personal care services to assist with activities of daily living	No certification requirements because it is not a covered skilled service. Licensure rules vary from state to state.[2]	May have consultative or teaching role in the agency in preparing home care aides for their duties with complex, dependent patients. The coordination of skilled services with home-care aides occurs when both skilled services and home health aides are provided concurrently.

Note: Organizations that provide private duty nursing, home medical equipment, infusion therapy, and home pharmacy may be included in an "other" category.

company); a joint venture; or a freestanding, privately owned organization.

The Family and Home Care

For many people with acute and chronic conditions living at home, assistance from family, benevolent volunteers, or paid caregivers is generally required (although not always available). These needs for assistance and issues related to them transcend class, race, ethnicity, age, gender, place, and time. Uncertainty about the length of time support will be needed is a common concern for many families involved in the care of loved ones at home. This uncertainty influences their willingness to begin to engage in the care of a person. More important, new family structures complicate the provision of unpaid home care. These new kinship roles have changed the traditional family model of informal caregiving arrangements required to keep the ill and elderly in their homes.[6]

Family members assume four roles when involved in home care regardless of the type of disability the loved one has, the funding source for care, and the amount or the types of services required:[7]

- *Providers of direct care.* Most family members believe that this care is their responsibility or obligation. They may be reluctant to have "outsiders" in their homes, but must agree to outside help because they lack specialized skills to care for the very sick.

- *Task sharers.* Family members perform special tasks that are unique to meeting the particular needs of an individual that only family members can meet. Family sharing of these responsibilities requires clarification of normal household duties. Meeting these patient needs supplements and complements rather than substitutes for outside services that are provided.

- *Brokers.* Arranging home-care services for a patient among the myriad of fragmented services, eligibility requirements, and funding requires family members to develop organization and coordination skills to meet this role.

- *Monitors.* Determining the quality of the task-related skills and the interpersonal relationships of healthcare workers with the patient becomes a family responsibility. It is a critical component of assessing the effectiveness of care often provided by several people.

Even if family members are comfortable assuming these roles, the advantages of home care—convenience, more independence and control for the patient, and personalized attention—must be weighed against the disruption to the order of the home as it moves from a place of refuge and privacy to a healthcare setting. For informal caregivers, who are predominantly spouses and female adult children, "caring" remains inconvenient, challenging, and disruptive to the daily patterns of living and working. In U.S. culture, the demands of home care are grossly undervalued and codified as housework, family obligation, or perhaps a voluntary charitable responsibility.[3] Policy makers see care provided in the home as a potentially less expensive care setting; however, for patients and their families home-care services provide relief from direct caregiving and the management of care.

Home Care and Public Policy

Home care is full of dichotomies for healthcare policy makers. For instance, home care is both formal professional services provided by paid staff as well as unpaid assistance furnished by such informal supporters as families and neighbors. It is both acute and long-term care with medical and/or social components. It is a service with merits of its own while also valued in terms of reductions in institutional care. Depending on the viewpoint, the determination of the goals and components of home care and its place in the continuum of healthcare can be complex.

Because of these complexities, policy makers consistently revisit the costs and benefits of home care. Professional providers of home care are continually adapting and adjusting case mixes and patterns of care to match available reimbursement without reducing the home services needed or desired by the sick and vulnerable. Given ongoing adjustments to meet these complex needs, it is no surprise that home care is not always the anticipated thrifty substitute for costly institutional care that policy makers desire.

Some tough political questions are yet to be addressed effectively, such as:[3]

- Is caring for the sick at home a private family obligation or a responsibility shared with a caring society?

- Should home care be provided only under the most restrictive of circumstances, or whenever it can help?
- When will the fundamental question of how to determine the appropriate recipients and payers of home care be resolved?
- How can payers overcome an unwillingness to pay for home care because of lack of trust that services provided in private patient homes are legitimate?

Licensure, Certification, Regulation, and Accreditation

Generally, all home-care organizations are licensed in accordance with state statutes. Requirements for licensure may include assurance of financial stability and liability insurance, lease agreements, compliance with background screening checks of employees, qualifications of the administrator and director of nursing, and corporation documents.

To provide services to patients insured by Medicare and Medicaid, a home-care organization is required to be certified by the Centers for Medicare & Medicaid Services (CMS). Accreditation of the organization is a voluntary process that federal, state, and other reimbursement models are dependent on in their certifications of providers of home care.

The Community Health Accreditation Program (CHAP) of the National League for Nursing is one of the accrediting bodies for home health organizations. Since 1965, CHAP has taken a lead in developing mechanisms for recognizing excellence in community health. CMS granted CHAP authority for home health and hospice organizations, which means that CHAP, not state agencies, may have responsibility for surveys of these organizations to determine that an organization meets Medicare's conditions of participation for reimbursement of the services they provide.[8]

The CHAP accreditation process is based on standards of excellence for management, quality, client outcomes, adequate resources, and long-term viability. The goal of this process is to assist all types of community-based healthcare organizations to do the following:[9]

- Strengthen internal operations.
- Promote continuous quality improvement.

- Promote consumer satisfaction.
- Promote positive client outcomes.
- Meet community health needs in a cost-effective and efficient manner.
- Maintain the viability of community health practice nationwide.
- Assure public trust in community-based services and products.

Like most accrediting bodies, CHAP provides guidance and criteria to be met as evidence of efforts to accomplish these goals. Their criteria are based on four key underlying principles that drive their standards:[9]

1. The organization's structure and function consistently support its consumer-oriented philosophy, mission, and purpose.
2. The organization consistently provides high-quality services and products.
3. The organization has adequate human, financial, and physical resources to accomplish its stated mission and purpose.
4. The organization is positioned for long-term viability.

Another, more recent, home-care organization accrediting body is The Joint Commission.[10] Its seal of approval is nationally recognized as an indication that an organization meets certain quality standards. Unlike CHAP, The Joint Commission accredits a wide range of healthcare organizations. In its home-care accreditation decisions, The Joint Commission uses data generated through Medicare's Outcome and Assessment Information Set (OASIS). OASIS is the documentation/reimbursement system required by Medicare to assess outcomes in home-care organizations. Like CHAP, The Joint Commission surveys can be approved as a substitute for federal and state agency surveys of home-care organizations for certification or licensure.[11]

Hospice and Rehabilitation

Management of physical therapy and other rehabilitation services in hospice requires a broader view of quality of life to address the dignity of people in death and dying. Managers need to begin the orientation of staff to their roles in hospice with the concept that hospice is an environment and attitude of care rather than a place.

For many people, dying is a lingering process of difficulties, with each stage resulting in a little more loss of the capacity to bounce back. Rehabilitation in hospice has been called "rehabilitation in reverse" because a team addresses the patient's deterioration rather than instituting changes that would improve the patient's condition. Optimizing function at each stage must be discussed with the patient and family so that expectations are not threatening.[12]

Using the same skills that they bring to all settings, therapists in hospice care may need to deal with their own feelings about death and dying. Accepting the following classic premises underlying hospice helps to address new adaptations or skills required to maximize function and safety for the patient and family:[13]

- Basic regard for the recipient of care
- Acceptance of death as a natural part of living
- Consideration of the entire family as the unit of care
- Maintenance of the patient at home for as long as possible
- Assistance for the patient attempting to assume control over his or her own life
- Instructions for patient self-care
- Relief of pain and other distressing symptoms
- Comprehensive provision of services by an interdisciplinary team
- Total, not fragmented, care

Although every Medicare-certified hospice is mandated to have an occupational, physical, and speech therapist under contract and available to provide services, the actual use of those services is not required in plans of care. Managers responsible for rehabilitation staff in hospice may need to develop strategies for educating other members of the hospice team about the role of the rehabilitation team, particularly if there is concern that receiving rehabilitation may raise false hopes of recovery. The care provided in hospice tends to be more holistic and the roles of members of the team become blurred and overlap as a result. As the predominant health professional, the nurse often determines the involvement of other professionals on an as-needed basis.[12] For additional information on hospices, go to the three organizations. Web pages listed in Web Resources: American Academy of Hospice and Palliative Medicine (AAHPM), Hospice Foundation of America (HFA), and American Physical Therapy Association (APTA) Hospice and Palliative Care.

Unique Features of Physical Therapy Practice in Home Care

Although physical therapists may work full-time in any type of home-care agency (see Table 16.1), they are most likely to be employed by, or contract their services with, home-care agencies that provide skilled services to people across the life span. For some therapists, home-care assignments may be a part of their responsibilities as staff therapists in inpatient or outpatient settings. The following list includes examples of potential models of organizations in which physical therapists may manage home-care services:

- Pediatric private practice that provides services to children in the home and office
- Home-care agency providing pediatric services only
- Private, nationwide home-care corporation with many locations
- Skilled nursing facility that has rehabilitation staff who provide home-care services within the retirement community of which it is a part
- Home-care agency that is a preferred provider for an adult congregate living facility or retirement community Note: These arrangements do not override patient choice of provider.
- Home-care unit whose staff is employed by a hospital organization and who provides services only to patients discharged from that hospital
- Freestanding home-care agency that forms a legal relationship with a hospital that then becomes a unit of service in that healthcare system—accountable care organization (ACO)
- Physical therapy company that provides per diem staff to several home-care agencies
- Registry of healthcare professionals that provides staff either locally or as travelers typically through short-term contracts with agencies
- Physical therapist who is an independent contractor accepting cases from a variety of home-care organizations. Note: Medicare patients requiring more than one home-care service must receive those services through

a Medicare-certified home-care agency rather than from individual providers.

- Hospice programs

Home-care services that physical therapists provide seems to present the same universal challenges and rewards of work found in any other setting. Most of the unique aspects of home care are present because the care is provided in the home, and they are presented in Sidebar 16.1.

To achieve their full potential at home, the rehabilitation team needs to get patients and their families to agree about their home-care plans and goals. This often requires a delicate balancing of the eccentricities of all the parties, which may include extended family members, household staff (e.g., housekeeper, cook), home-care aides, or private duty nurses. Home-care physical therapists and other professionals often need to encourage patients to set aside the enjoyment of secondary gains, such as being cared for, having reduced family responsibilities, or simply taking pleasure in the attention they receive in their new situations.

SIDEBAR 16.1

Characteristics of Work in Home-Care Settings[14]

- Care is patient focused, occurring for approximately 45 minutes with one patient (and his or her family) at a time who is typically highly motivated to participate. Goals are shifted to the relevant, immediate function needed to achieve the maximum level of independence in the home environment.

- Perceptions about the functional ability of the very ill and increased need to understand comorbidities and medication interactions are key to goal setting in home care.

- There is involvement with comprehensive care in an interdisciplinary team that focuses on activities of daily living, assessing and instructing in the use of durable medical equipment, and providing caregiver training so the patient remains functional at home.

- Creative and professional challenges may arise in devising relevant care plans and obtaining measurable clinical outcomes with minimal equipment and assistance in less-than-ideal treatment areas because of the physical layout of homes and/or the size and type of furniture present.

- Providing interventions for strengthening specific muscle groups that are important for a particular functional activity may shift to performing functional activities as exercise. Exercise is uniquely tailored and highly individualized to meet specific patient needs and address unique functional deficits.

- Productivity goals are affected by factors beyond one's control: traffic congestion, road conditions, weather conditions, patients' own time commitments, coordinating the presence of caregivers, and coordinating schedules of other team members.

- There may be difficulty scheduling visits because of the patient's own commitments, such as physician appointments. Coordinating the presence of the caregiver for teaching and the visiting schedules of other members of the care team may occur. There may be decreased professional control because patients are in their own residences.

- Independence in structuring therapist work time and travel breaks that allow "breathing time" rather than continuous patient care may need to be provided.

- Addressing safety concerns is a top priority, including driving in various weather conditions, travel in unfamiliar neighborhoods, unkempt homes that are less-than-ideal circumstances for treatment and comfort, and a layout of a home that is often confining and so requires more maneuvering.

- More emphasis should be placed on problem-solving *with* the patients who must be true partners and follow through on instructions on their own when other activities compete for a patient's time.

- Opportunities may be limited for face-to-face communication and interaction with other team members for patient care discussions and peer support because of the short time spent in the office of the organization.

- There may be a need for a more comprehensive 24-hour assessment of the patient and his or her environment.

At the other extreme, there are the challenges presented by less fortunate patients with limited, unreliable, or unpredictable support systems who insist on staying in their homes even if the risks to their safety and well-being are very high.

Physical therapists in home-care settings also must make a shift in their plans of care and goals to reflect the importance of social and cultural influences in home care. Unlike other settings, where these factors are considered in terms of adaptations to the culture of the organization, home-care physical therapists find themselves enmeshed in the culture and psychosocial dynamics of *each* family they work with. A broader understanding of all the factors affecting the outcomes of rehabilitation at home is required. Because these influences are more pronounced and hard to avoid when on the patient's turf, physical therapists may need to develop a series of questions to be better prepared to identify, at least, the cultural influences that are important to the patient. Some suggestions for questions to ask are:[15]

- How would you describe yourself?
- Tell me about your cultural heritage or background (i.e., ethnicity, racial identification, language). How important is this to you?
- What was your religious upbringing? How important is this to you?
- What was your family's socioeconomic status growing up? How did this affect you?
- Do you have any experience with disability or being a caregiver?
- What did it mean to grow up as a girl (boy) in your culture/family?

PART 2   Managing in Home Care

Overview of Management in Home Care

Managers in home care may assume a wide range of responsibilities depending primarily on the structure of the home-care organization. The following list includes some examples of potential managerial roles in home care:

- **Director of Nursing:** The director of nursing or some other assigned person in a small, developing home-care agency assumes responsibility for nursing services and for hiring and assigning patients to physical therapists.
- **Regional Managers:** Regional managers of physical therapy in a large national chain of home-care agencies recruit, orient, and supervise the overall care provided by physical therapists in several different locations in their assigned region. As part of the management team, they contribute to decisions related to the organization as a whole and interpretation of outcomes and other data. Each office in the region may have a person who assigns patients and supervises other patient-related care duties of the physical therapists.
- **Director or Supervisor of Rehabilitation:** The director or supervisor of rehabilitation in a free-standing or hospital-based home-care agency supervises all members of the rehabilitation team regardless of their disciplines. The director of rehabilitation in a large teaching hospital handles all aspects of physical therapy services provided in various inpatient, outpatient, and home-care units. The larger the organization is, the more likely it will be that unit supervisors manage the day-to-day operations of these units. They may have some flexibility in shifting staff among units as staffing needs demand.
- **Private Practice:** The owner of a private practice, particularly a pediatric practice, coordinates assignments of physical therapists that include a mix of outpatient and home-care patients.
- **Contract Managers:** Managers of contract therapy companies negotiate contracts for assignment of physical therapists in any of the above home-care settings.

- **Solo Practitioner:** A solo practitioner is a physical therapist who provides home-care services only to patients who pay the therapist directly out of pocket. Typically, the solo practitioner works in isolation without collaboration with nurses or other providers. This practitioner may not require a physician referral in some jurisdictions.

In all of these scenarios, managers face the same challenges in the delivery of high-quality physical therapy services in home care. These managers are presented with the same management challenges found in other healthcare settings, but they are compounded by the fact that home care is a field operation. The "field" that is managed in home care may encompass several counties or a large metropolitan area. This off-site arrangement may make face-to-face contact with other staff at a central home office impractical on a daily basis because of distances that they must travel and productivity goals they must meet.

Management Responsibilities

Mission, Vision, and Goals

Gathering support from the staff in the field to carry out the mission, vision, and goals of a home-care organization may be difficult to structure because interactions with coworkers and supervisors are limited. Opportunities to convey the big picture of home care may not easily present themselves. Because this lack of cohesiveness may contribute to staff turnover, managers may need to identify a variety of means for transforming the mission and vision into action, and for demonstrating the link between the goals of the organization and their day-to-day responsibilities. For instance, expecting *all* providers of care in the organization to participate in regularly scheduled staff meetings is a strategy to reinforce the vision and mission and update everyone on the big picture of the organization.

At the same time, managers need to participate in the creation, or regular review, of the mission and vision of a home-care organization so that they reflect the role of contemporary rehabilitation practice. As healthcare policy changes, opportunities for identifying and clarifying the role of rehabilitation in the goals of home-care agencies lie with managers. CMS's Home Health Agency (HHA),

CMS's Home Health Prospective Payment System Regulations and Notices (PPS), and the APTA's Home Health Section include important resources (see Web Resources).

Policies and Procedures

Federal and state regulatory demands dictate many of the policies and procedures in home care because of the long lists of "musts" that are in their regulations. Managers are responsible for the review of these regulations and for their coordination with the goals and performance of the staff they supervise. They may prepare a mini rehabilitation version of the policies and procedures manual to accomplish this review of the key policies and procedures and to update information that may assist staff in the performance of their duties. For instance, specific application of ethical principles and legal responsibilities in home care may need to be included. Clinical guidelines, either adopted or created by the home-care agency staff, may be coordinated with policies and procedures. A modified version of policies and procedures is likely to be adopted by staff who find the information more useful and user friendly.

Marketing

As in other large healthcare settings, managers in large, national home-care corporations are, on the one hand, more likely to be presented with the tools for organization-wide program development and marketing plans for implementation than they are to be responsible for their development. On the other hand, managers in freestanding agencies may have more input into this overall planning for an agency, or they may be assigned to program development for physical therapy or interdisciplinary rehabilitation services. The trend toward niche markets and disease management programs presents opportunities for the inclusion of physical therapy in marketing plans.

Managers need to be diligent in championing physical therapy in home-care organizations that are historically dominated by nursing care–driven goals and programs. Because nurses are typically the designated case managers of patients in home care, physical therapists have been dependent on the nurses for referrals to physical therapy. Recently, a shift to a rehabilitation model in home care because of changes in Medicare-reimbursement expectations has helped to increase the utilization of physical therapy services. Encouraging nurses to have broader perspectives of the role of rehabilitation in hospice and in the care of patients who have acute and chronic conditions of multiple systems is an important managerial role.

Staffing

Most jurisdictions require and home-care agencies prefer that physical therapists who work in home care generally have experience in other clinical settings. Because home care is a field operation involving complex, clinical decision-making, managers prefer people who have already demonstrated skill and confidence in settings that permit interaction with other professionals on a regular basis for at least 2 or 3 years. Guiding the successful transition of physical therapists to the world of home care may require careful selection of employees. A formal, structured orientation is essential because home care is an atypical setting with a shift in the patient/therapist relationship that may be difficult or uncomfortable for some therapists.

Therapists who have previous acute hospital experience are accustomed to heavy caseloads and short treatment sessions. These therapists may need guidance to adjust to the slower pace of home care and longer one-on-one treatment sessions with patients. However, home-care physical therapists who have also worked in outpatient settings may be reluctant to set high goals for patients who appear very ill compared with the level of function observed in outpatients. Addressing the characteristics of home care listed earlier and anticipating needs of therapists as they transition to home-care work are management priorities. Managers must also attend to staffing patterns that support the continuity of care (provider continuity) to increase the patient's satisfaction through consistent communication, which may also decrease adverse events and improve patient outcomes.[16]

Ride-Alongs

Managers should not underestimate the need for ride-alongs—making visits with other staff—as part of the orientation process. Typically, the clinical expertise needed for direct patient care is not problematic for therapists new to home care. Rather, it is learning the formal regulation requirements of a home-care system, planning a daily schedule, and finding strategies for care within the limited space and minimal resources of a person's home that must be addressed. These issues may be included during ride-along orientation sessions, which also identify commonly used neighborhood shortcuts and other timesaving strategies. Managers who implement such orientations help new employees develop a sense of *esprit de corps* in their new positions.

Managers in home care face the same issues as managers in other settings in managing a mix of physical therapists who are full-time employees with those who work part-time or on a per diem, as-needed basis. Per diem positions in home care may be more desirable than in other settings for people who seek less than full-time work. Home care is probably the setting that offers the most flexibility for work schedules that accommodate personal needs of staff.

Although not considered good management practice for staff assignments, some managers may allow per diem employees to accept or reject new assignments, limit their service area, or schedule vacations with short notice. Because they are paid a flat fee per visit, allowing them to "cherry-pick" is often seen as a way to encourage them to accept more patients. This practice may be good for per diem staff but often leads to resentment among full-time staff who may not be at liberty to refuse assignments because they have productivity expectations to meet. Allowing unfair practices may create further problems if full-time salaried employees become dissatisfied and leave because they perceive that they are at a disadvantage when expected to care for more patients, those that are most difficult, or those farthest away.

Avoiding a sense of unfairness among full-time employees who see per diem staff as being at an advantage, while concurrently encouraging per diem staff to "belong," is a compounded problem in home care because it is a field operation. Careful control of these factors can require intricate balancing because a manager's need to supplement full-time staff with per diem workers may fluctuate. Without much notice, managers may eliminate or significantly reduce the number of assignments to a per diem pool of therapists because of reduced referrals for physical therapy. Just as quickly, the demand for services may increase unexpectedly. To shift from one circumstance to the other, establishment and enforcement of consistent policies and procedures for *all* employees become critical.

The flexibility and freedom in home-care work that make it attractive for therapists create a major challenge for managers. For instance, if an agency seeks to develop interdisciplinary teams in certain geographic areas, staff may be reluctant to travel for meetings or to spend more time communicating with one another. It may be difficult to get staff to commit non–patient care time to the development and implementation of disease management programs. This development work is perceived as unpaid labor, particularly if physical therapist productivity is based on the number of visits, or if upper management discourages any activity that is non–revenue generating.

Physical Therapist Assistants

Statutes that control licensure rules in each state may determine whether physical therapist assistants are employed in home-care agencies. Should physical therapist assistants be permitted to practice in home care, managers need to determine their role and the supervisory role of the physical therapists with whom they work.

As the complexity and acuity of patients in home care continue to increase, managers need to question whether physical therapist assistants are prepared for making immediate clinical decisions for *every* patient. After all, many patients present serious, unexpected decision-making challenges, even for the physical therapists who care for them.

It is critical that managers avoid making blanket policies and procedures regarding the roles of physical therapists and physical therapist assistants, including the assignment of patients to assistants. The ability of physical therapists to make individual judgments about directions to a physical therapist assistant regarding *each* patient's care must be preserved by managers to deter potential legal and ethical issues.

A physical therapist must weigh the condition and needs of the patients against the experience and skills of assistants, who may require different levels of direction and supervision for each patient and for the same patient over time. A necessary starting point for managers is to clearly define these professional supervisory relationships and responsibilities for patient care. Verbal and written communication and formal reporting expectations must be specific and followed.

Patient Care

Medicare's OASIS is a group of data elements that drive the clinical work of home care across all disciplines. The data generated forms the basis for measurement of outcome-based quality improvement (OBQI). Its use is part of Medicare's Conditions of Participation for Medicare certification—in other words, it is not an option. In addition to sociodemographic data, health and functional status data are emphasized. Although designed for aggregate outcome measures, OASIS data also are used for patient assessment and care planning for individuals. At the agency level data are used for case mix reports including patient status at the start of care and the identification of areas for improvement within the agency. The expectation is that documentation of care integrates OASIS terminology and concepts.[17] See Web Resources for detailed information on the components of OASIS.

The orientation of physical therapists to their responsibilities in the generation of OASIS data must include the importance of this information. An agency's management decisions about the amount of care required and provided to each patient is critical in the delivery of effective, cost-effective patient care that is consistent with evidence-based practice and professional duty. A systematic approach to comparing key factors at the start of care, at 60 days, and on discharge provides opportunities for analysis of physical therapy effectiveness at a variety of levels. Physical therapy managers in home care may look at OASIS outcomes to answer questions, such as:

- What was the change in a particular patient's status from admission to discharge?
- What was the value of physical therapy for an individual?
- Was physical therapy included appropriately (not underutilized and not overutilized) for patients in a selected diagnostic or case mix group?
- How do physical therapists compare with each other in their care of similar patients?
- In the aggregate scores, what can physical therapists do to improve patient outcomes across the board?

This system, although time consuming and detailed, may serve as an important management tool to answer questions that go beyond required reporting. As with other settings, the CMS also provides Home Health Compare as a resource (see Web Resources). Managers in agencies that provide services to patients with private insurance policies need to consider adoption of similar, relevant outcome measures for these patients. If the home-care agency is in a state that participates in a Medicaid Comprehensive Assessment and Review for Long-Term Care Services (CARES) program that determines the least restrictive setting appropriate for adults, or the similar Children's Multidisciplinary Assessment Team (CMAT) program for children, managers may identify opportunities for analysis of their data related to physical therapy and other rehabilitation disciplines.

Durable Medical Equipment

Physical therapy managers also may play an important decision-making role in home care involving the provision of durable medical equipment and the incorporation of new technology into patient care and patients' homes. Identifying and informing physical therapists of the impact of medical devices and communication technology available to monitor or improve the functional ability of patients form an important role for home-care managers.

Physical therapists need to be prepared to understand and instruct patients in new technology from ergonomic devices for safety to medical devices for monitoring physiological status. Preparing home-care physical therapists for teaching and persuading patients and their families to handle new technology may be more important in home care than in any other setting. Managerial support to assure the comfort level of the staff with technology may be necessary if they are expected to make clinical decisions about selection and funding.

Fiscal

Although rehabilitation services have always played an important role in home care, the introduction of the Medicare prospective payment system for rehabilitation benefits in home care has directed even more attention to its management. Payment is based on categorizing patients in one of the 153 Home Health Resource Groups (HHRP) for a home-care episode of care. This potential for increased reimbursement and the shift to the rehabilitation model rather than the medical model for the determination of outcomes of care have resulted in a greater demand for physical therapy services in the past few years. For example, recent reimbursement changes include payment for physical therapy to establish maintenance programs to prevent a decline in the functional status after a patient is discharged from rehabilitation. For more information on prospective payment, go to the APTA and CMS Web pages found at Web Resources.

Fiscal responsibilities of middle managers in home-care agencies typically include the need for:

- Understanding Medicare and Medicaid reimbursement and monitoring changes in rules
- Educating the staff assigned to them regarding accurate patient assessment, clinical decision-making, case management, and documentation in compliance with the regulations within these payment systems
- Advising upper management of the effect of their administrative decisions on the professional standards of care, legal rules, and ethical obligations of their staffs
- Coordinating productivity standards, staff schedules, and patient assignments

Managers of therapy services are in a pivotal position to decrease the potential for misuse of physical therapy services while contributing to the profitability of an agency. It may be dependent on incentives to the home-care agencies for using these services. Correcting agency policies (formal or "understood") that may undermine the professional responsibilities of their staff is as important as the generation of revenue. Physical therapists should be able to turn to their managers for guidance and for advocacy with upper management when conflicts between agency expectations and professional duties occur.

Physical therapy managers may have other fiscal responsibilities that commonly arise during strategic planning and budgeting cycles. At the least, their contributions to these processes are important to the identification of, and commitment to, the resources required to provide physical therapy and other rehabilitation services in a home-care agency. Accountability for utilization of resources, achievement of budgeted revenue expectations, and achievement of productivity goals lies with these managers.

One certainty in today's unpredictable healthcare environment is that managers will continue to do more with less. As a result, controlling costs becomes a focus of managerial energy. The expense of technology compared with its contribution to increased communication and efficiency of work as well as to the quality of care often requires convincing arguments. The responsibility of managers to identify potential resources and to justify their requests may be intensive. Persuading physical therapists who are reluctant to change or to learn new technology may be another hurdle. Perhaps looking at field operations in non-healthcare businesses such as UPS or FedEx may identify existing means for addressing communication, scheduling, training, and quality issues.[18]

Legal, Ethical, and Risk

Assisting physical therapists in resolving legal and ethical issues in home care may present unique managerial challenges because the settings are patients' homes. Each home is the private domain of the patient who invites, or permits, the healthcare team to enter as an agent of the home-care agency. As such, the agency is answerable for all the actions of those employees within the scope of their work and for all foreseeable consequences of that work.

Supervision

Home-care managers have a responsibility for finding a reasonable means to supervise the actions of employees although they occur over a wide geographic range. Supervising strategies include follow-up calls to patients to ask how therapy is going, random scheduling of reporting by the therapists to the manager, or conducting unannounced on-site visits. The determination of reasonable supervision depends on the risks each of the physical therapists presents. Experienced physical therapists with unsolicited positive compliments from their patients may require less supervision than physical therapists who are new to home care or about whom patient or coworker complaints have been made. Managers decide which therapists they can trust to seek help when needed, and which assigned patients are potential risks at the time of admission and demand careful monitoring of their care.

Moreover, supervision is important because home care is a high-risk environment for physical therapists. They have less control of the treatment setting and less authority in the home environment. At the same time, they have direct observation not only of a patient's clinical status but also of their social and family situation. It becomes more difficult for therapists to distinguish their job responsibilities from professional responsibilities and their moral duty. Managers may provide guidance on, or at least discussion of, these important issues and their influence on decision-making in home-based care.

Safety

It is difficult for any type of home-care provider to avoid action concerning unsafe or abusive conditions because they are often direct observers of the situation. If they are unable to effect change directly, reporting and seeking help are critical actions. Attending only to physical therapy goals and interventions is much more difficult in home care. Environmental, socioeconomic, cultural, and family relationship issues often overshadow the immediacy of the patient's therapy needs. The one-on-one interactions and real-life problem-solving that make home care so attractive to many people are also what increases its complexity and its risks.

Because of these risks, managers must demand careful documentation as a paramount responsibility of therapists. Regardless of OASIS requirements, documentation of home care also must specifically address risks identified and actions taken. Because patients may decline to accept the advice or to comply with the suggested action, especially in their homes, documentation of what is said and what is done is obligatory.

Fraud

Like all healthcare settings, the potential for fraud exists in home care, but because it is a field operation, managers have a more difficult job of monitoring the potential for and the occurrence of fraud, which includes:[19]

- The provision of unnecessary services
- Billing for services not provided
- Overcharging
- Forgery

- Negative charting (only document the problems, excluding improvements)
- Substitution of lesser qualified providers
- Double billing
- Kickbacks

Managers may find themselves responsible for protecting their staff from fraud committed by higher management and for protecting higher management from fraud committed by their staffs. The nature of home care may require managers to exert a higher level of diligence to prevent and expose fraud.

Underuse

Underuse of care presents another risk for managers to monitor. If patients do not receive the amount of care they need, particularly to live safely at home, managers have to investigate the reasons and take action accordingly. Underutilization also is a factor if therapists prematurely discharge a patient who may be difficult or unpleasant or whose home situation makes the physical therapist uncomfortable. Managers need to be alert for discharge trends that may be an indication of this "dumping" of patients.

The delegation of skilled care to family members and other nonskilled paid helpers may also lead to potential underutilization of skilled services. Although teaching caregivers is a critical intervention in home care because skilled visits are intermittent, reductions in visits should reflect the accomplishment of patient goals rather than the increased availability of caregivers. Managers need to develop a strategy to avoid the latter.

Admissions and Discharge

Risks to patient safety in home care are increased because "discharge to the community" is a quality indicator for hospitals. To achieve their quality goals, a hospital's decision to send patients to their homes rather than to long-term care facilities may inadvertently place the patient in unsafe conditions once at home.[20]

Managers of home care need to prepare their staffs for the effects of these hospital decisions on their plans of care for patients who may be medically unstable because they may have been discharged too soon. Given a choice, patients usually choose discharge to home, without a full understanding of the efforts that will be necessary to accomplish their goals. Once they are home, it becomes more difficult to persuade them that an alternative placement may have been more appropriate. Hospital readmissions become another indicator for managers to analyze as they develop strategies to address this issue.

Communication

Having all staff in the same building at the same time may be an infrequent occurrence in home care. The manager's interaction with staff is more often one-on-one, which may become burdensome for the manager unless electronic modes of communication become routine and interactive. In smaller organizations, managers may get to know staff members better because of these individual interactions, but in larger organizations, it may be impossible to know the staff whom they supervise because of the limited contact time with each person on a regular basis. It may be that a manager meets with new employees for orientation and rarely sees them after that unless accreditation standards demand formal, systematic review of performance and competency.

Communication limitations also affect the availability of managers to troubleshoot specific clinical decision-making and other practice problems that may be more urgent and complex in a patient's home. The ability to handle broad problems across several staff members is compounded by the fact that each staff member is working in isolation. If formal efforts to develop professional and social interactions among staff, beyond the required patient conferencing, are not made successfully, the manager may be a home-care physical therapist's only formal connection to the agency and the only source of one-on-one professional advice.

Should the manager of rehabilitation in a home-care agency not be of the same discipline as a therapist, the importance of establishing a networking and mentoring program increases dramatically. The sharing of experiences, identifying similar practice problems, and informal socializing may contribute to the improvement of quality services. The ability of managers to provide these opportunities, perhaps at monthly staff meetings, in field organizations is an important responsibility.

In addition to informal feedback, formal evaluation of work performance by managers may include written data from patient satisfaction surveys, employee self-assessments, and outcome reports combined with direct observation of performance. Regardless of accreditation requirements, without mechanisms for feedback and evaluation, managers only assume what the level of work performance is. *Satisfactory* often means "no complaints," but it also may mean substandard care provided by physical therapists who may not meet competency expectations.

Conclusions

The management of home-care physical therapy requires a very different set of skills from management in other healthcare settings. The skills that make managers effective in another healthcare organization do not necessarily transfer to home care. Attention to the unique aspects of field operations and the special work of caring for people who are often very sick in their homes requires additional preparation.

Because the home-care environment poses greater risks and the work performance of employees is minimally supervised, managers in home care must have a high level of trust in the people they hire. Careful screening of the credentials and attitudes of potential employees followed by detailed orientation to the home-care setting are essential to reduce risks and assure quality care.

Managers must develop therapists with strong patient skills to work with complex patients who may have few resources in their homes to contribute to the rehabilitation process. They must prepare staff for the greater influence that cultural and social factors have on care in the home. Managers must develop skills in their therapists that lead to positive patient care experiences so that both patient *and* employee dissatisfaction is diminished. Activities 16.1 to 16.13 provide the opportunity to address home-care management issues.

ACTIVITY 16.1
PERSONNEL DIFFERENCES

John Anderson is Director of Rehabilitation for Central Home Health. He has received an application for one of his full-time therapist positions from Judith Marquez. Judith came to the United States from the Philippines through a recruitment agency that arranges placement of health professionals trained in other countries. She was assigned to work in several nursing homes during her 5-year contract, which has now expired. Her references are excellent.

John's experience with another foreign-trained physical therapist was negative. That person was shy, had a heavy accent, and required assistance because of her small size. He is also concerned that the patients treated through Central Home Health might make staff from other countries uncomfortable or even resist care from them.

What should John consider in his interview with Judith? Should he hire her? Consider: Where is he now? Where does he want to be? What does John have to work with? How will he get there?

ACTIVITY 16.2
THE BIG PICTURE

Pleasant Valley Regional Home Health Services has all three components of home care in its organization—Pleasant Valley Home-Care Agency (a provider of skilled care), Pleasant Valley Hospice, and Pleasant Valley Home-Care Aides (a provider of private care). The role of physical therapy in the hospice and home-care aide organizations is very informal. Occasionally, a particular patient's needs or problems arise and the physical therapy manager is called on to address them.

The board of directors of Pleasant Valley Regional Home Health Services has asked the physical therapy manager to investigate the need for a more formal rehabilitation presence in their hospice and home-care aide businesses. What should the manager's report to the board be?

ACTIVITY 16.3
SCHEDULING

Sally Sanchez has asked to meet with Joanna Gilbert, the new rehabilitation manager of the home-care agency where she has worked for the past 4 years. Sally is very upset to learn that her vacation request for 2 weeks during the holidays has been denied. She thought the policy was that staff rotated every other year for holiday coverage and this is her off year. She and her family have already made reservations for their holiday trip. Joanna apologizes but says she had no choice because there is no one to replace her. The temporary pool (on-call staff) has been eliminated because of budget cuts and the three per diem staff members have told her they also are taking their vacations at that time.

What are their choices for the next step? Consider: Where are they now? Where do they want to be? What do they have to work with? How will they get there?

ACTIVITY 16.4
HIRING A PHYSICAL THERAPIST ASSISTANT

Although permitted by statute, Comfort Home Care has not hired physical therapist assistants to provide care. Because of growth, the much-needed three new positions for physical therapists have not been filled for more than 6 months. Delilah Deavon, the manager of rehabilitation, receives an application from Jonathan Wiley, a physical therapist assistant with 20 years of experience including 3 years most recently in home care in another state. She has mixed feelings—excited finally to have an applicant and disappointed that it is not from a physical therapist.

What should Delilah do next? Consider: Where is she now? Where does she want to be? What does Delilah have to work with? How will she get there?

ACTIVITY 16.5
A STAFF SHORTAGE

Adam Anderson has been the manager of rehabilitation services at No Place Like Home, a Medicare home-care agency, for 3 years. For the first time, the administrator of the agency, Sally Simmons, has demanded that Adam begin direct patient care duties full-time because recruitment efforts have been unsuccessful in filling the two open physical therapy positions. The agency is at risk of losing referrals because of limited therapy services, and the nurses are becoming angry that the shortage of therapists is affecting their outcomes. Adam reluctantly agrees and voices his concern about

losing ground on the great progress he has made on program development, boosting staff morale, and improving quality outcome scores, which he was hired to do. Sally agrees with him but insists more patients need to be seen. She asks for suggestions to maintain his positive work efforts while meeting patient care demands.

If you were Adam, what would you suggest? Consider: Where is Adam now? Where does he want to be? What does he have to work with? How will he get there?

ACTIVITY 16.6
A PATIENT CALLS

Rose Rodriquez, physical therapy manager at We Come to You Home Care, receives a call from the Maude Morgan, the daughter of Frank Fabrizi. She tells Rose that a physical therapist has not made a visit to Frank in more than a week. She is wondering why therapy suddenly stopped. When Rose investigates, she finds Frank's signature on four treatment slips for the days in question and reports it to Maude. When Maude insists that this cannot be so, Rose and Guy

Trujack, the administrator of the agency, go to the Fabrizi home to show Frank the signed treatment slips. They become convinced that the physical therapist, Ruthie Myers, forged Frank's signature and did not provide treatment on those 4 days.

What should happen next? Consider: Where are they now? Where do they want to be? What do they have to work with? How will they get there?

ACTIVITY 16.7
A DANGEROUS SITUATION

Betsy Petersen, Rehabilitation Manager for Best Home Care, receives a call from Charlotte Goldman, who is one of her full-time staff therapists. Charlotte reports that she has just left a patient's home and is too afraid to go back. She asks Betsy to reassign the patient to another therapist and suggests that a male therapist may be a good idea.

When Betsy asks for details, Charlotte reports that although the home is in one of the better neighborhoods with expensive furnishings, it was in shambles. Except for the bedroom where the patient was, the house was cluttered and there was foul-smelling garbage. More important, however, the patient had a gun on the table next to the hospital

bed and she suspects that he may have been under the influence of drugs. He appeared anxious when Charlotte asked him about family members who might be able to help him. He told her she should not worry about the gun, because he only has it to protect himself when he is alone in the house. The patient is unable to leave his bed without assistance, and he requires intensive nursing care and rehabilitation to improve his functional status. She also is concerned about the other members of the team currently assigned to him.

What should Betsy do? Consider: Where are Charlotte and Betsy now? Where do they want to be? What does Betsy have to work with? How will she get there?

ACTIVITY 16.8
A NEW OPPORTUNITY

Barbara Bradley has been the rehabilitation manager for a home-care agency for adults for 2 years. She has been approached by a new agency, Kids at Home, to become their rehabilitation manager in developing programs for home-care services to children and young adults who are homebound.

What questions should Barbara ask Kids at Home? What should she ask herself? Consider: Where is Barbara now? Where does she want to be? What does she have to work with? How will she get there?

ACTIVITY 16.9
ROLE OF REHABILITATION IN HOSPICE

Dr. Brooks just received a request from the nurse to have a physical therapist evaluate his patient in hospice, Mr. Clark. She told him that Mr. Clark is still ambulatory but spending more time in bed, and his ability to use the bedside commode is declining. The doctor questions how a physical therapist can help in what is the expected declining progression of Mr. Clark's disease and functional abilities.

The director of nursing asks physical therapist Sam Solomon to call the doctor to explain his role as therapist in this case and in hospice in general.

What should Sam include in his discussions with Dr. Brooks? Consider: Where is Sam now? Where does he want to be? What does Sam have to work with? How will he get there?

ACTIVITY 16.10
MANAGING PERFORMANCE

Sam Solomon, Director of Rehabilitation in a home-care agency, is concerned about Leslie McDonald, one of the staff physical therapists who continues to have significant overtime on most days. Her caseload is no heavier than that of the other therapists and her driving miles are not excessive. She appears to remain in each home a long time yet does not complete her documentation in that time. These extended visits and completion of her documentation at the end of the day are adding to her hours. The agency encourages staff to document at the point of care.

What should Sam do? What suggestions might Sam have for Leslie? He is considering a field visit or ride-along with Leslie. Is that a good decision? Consider: Where are Leslie and Sam now? Where does Sam want Leslie to be? What does Sam have to work with? How will he get there?

ACTIVITY 16.11
SAFETY OF STAFF

Barbara Bronski, the Director of Rehabilitation at National Home-Care Services at Sunset Lake, has been appointed to a corporate task force to develop policies and procedures to guide managers in decisions about assignments that may place employees at risk in patients' homes. Particularly, three recent issues need to be addressed:

- Lack of assistance in handling obese patients

- Lack of assistance rearranging furniture for patient safety
- Hands must be washed before and after treatment sessions

What suggestions do you have? Consider: Where are they now? Where do they want to be? What does the task force have to work with? How will they get there?

ACTIVITY 16.12
A MEETING OF THE MINDS

Joanna Gilbert is the Director of Home-Care Rehabilitation. Her home-care staff's concerns about the transitioning of discharged patients from the hospitals to home continue to grow. She has had minimal contact with three other rehabilitation managers in the same healthcare system, two in the general hospital and one in the rehabilitation hospital. She must ask for a meeting to discuss some issues. She plans to begin with her two top agenda items:

- Inappropriate therapist recommendations for equipment to be delivered to the patients' homes

- Inpatient documentation that the family has been instructed in exercise or transfers when the family reports that they only observed and were not really trained

How might they resolve these issues? Consider: Where are they now? Where do they want to be? What do they have to work with? How will they get there?

ACTIVITY 16.13
DOWNSIZING

Carl Cutbertson's position as the home health rehabilitation coordinator has been eliminated as part of the downsizing of staff because of the merger of two healthcare systems. It has been decided that the nursing supervisor of each district in the reorganized home health division will be responsible for the rehabilitation services in each district. The nurse supervisor will be assigning therapists to patients and evaluating their performance as therapy services are

decentralized throughout the system. His staff has asked to meet with him before he leaves his position to help them strategize what they need to do to continue to provide quality services in this new model.

What should Carl recommend? Consider: Where are they now? Where do they want to be? What do they have to work with? How will they get there?

REFERENCES

1. Cox DM, Ory MG. The changing health and social environments of home care. In: Binstock RH, Cluff LE, eds. *Home Care Advances: Essential Research and Policy Issues.* New York, NY: Springer Publishing; 2000.
2. National Association for Home Care & Hospice. Basic statistics about home care. http://www.nahc.org/assets/1/7/10HC_Stats.pdf. Accessed September 10, 2013.
3. Buhler-Wilkerson K. *No Place Like Home: A History of Nursing and Home Care in the United States.* Baltimore, MD: Johns Hopkins University Press; 2001.
4. Crossen-Sills J, Bilton W, Bickford M, et al. Home care today: showcasing interdisciplinary management in home care. *Home Health Nurse.* 2007;25:245-252.
5. Moore PC, McCollough RH. Hospice: end-of-life care at home. In: Binstock RH, Cluff LE, eds. *Home Care Advances: Essential Research and Policy Issues.* New York, NY: Springer Publishing; 2000.
6. Binstock RH, Cluff LE. Issues and challenges in home care. In: Binstock RH, Cluff LE, eds. *Home Care Advances: Essential Research and Policy Issues.* New York, NY: Springer Publishing; 2000.
7. Miller B. Families and paid workers: the complexities of home care roles. In: Binstock RH, Cluff LE, eds. *Home Care Advances: Essential Research and Policy Issues.* New York, NY: Springer Publishing; 2000.
8. The Community Health Accreditation Program, Inc. (CHAP). History. http://www.chapinc.org/AboutCHAP/History. Accessed September 10, 2013.
9. The Community Health Accreditation Program, Inc. (CHAP). CHAP accreditation. http://www.chapinc.org/Accreditation. Accessed September 10, 2013.
10. The Joint Commission. Mission and vision statement. http://www.jointcommission.org/about_us/about_the_joint_commission_main.aspx. Accessed September 10, 2013.
11. The Joint Commission. Seeking home care accreditation. http://www.jointcommission.org/accreditation/home_care.aspx. Accessed September 10, 2013.
12. Pizzi MA, Briggs R. Occupational and physical therapy in hospice: the facilitation of meaning, quality of life, and well-being. *Topics in Geriatric Rehabilitation.* 2004;20:120-130.
13. Koff T, ed. *Hospice: A Caring Community.* Cambridge, MA: Winthrop; 1980.
14. Coke T, Alday R, Biala K, et al. The new role of physical therapy in home care. *Home Healthcare Nurse.* 2005;23:594-599.
15. Hays PA. Addressing the complexities of culture and gender in counseling. *Journal of Counseling and Development.* 1996;74:332-338.
16. Russell D, Rosati RJ, Andreopoulos E. Continuity in the provider of home-based physical therapy services and its implications for outcomes of patients. *Physical Therapist.* 2012;92:227-235.
17. Centers for Medicaid & Medicare Services. Outcome and Assessment Information Set (OASIS). http://www.cms.hhs.gov/OASIS/Downloads/maincomponentsandgeneralapplication.pdf. Accessed September 10, 2013.
18. Cluff LE, Brennan PF. The use of technology in home care. In: Binstock RH, Cluff LE, eds. *Home Care Advances: Essential Research and Policy Issues.* New York, NY: Springer Publishing; 2000.
19. Payne BK. *Crime in the Home Health Care Field: Workplace Violence, Fraud, and Abuse.* Springfield, IL: Charles C Thomas; 2003.
20. Polzien G. Promoting safety and security at home. *Home Healthcare Nurse.* 2007;25:218-222.

WEB RESOURCES

American Academy of Hospice and Palliative Medicine. http://www.aahpm.org/about/default/index.html. Accessed November 29, 2013.

American Physical Therapy Association. Comprehensive summary of Medicare Home Prospective Payment System (HHPPS) for 2013. http://www.homehealthsection.org/associations/9809/files/Comprehensive_Summary_Home%20Health%20PPS%202013%20Final%20Rule.pdf. Accessed November 29, 2013.

American Physical Therapy Association. Home health section. http://www.homehealthsection.org/. Accessed November 29, 2013.

American Physical Therapy Association. Hospice and palliative care. http://www.apta.org/PatientCare/HospicePalliativeCare/. Accessed November 29, 2013.

Centers for Medicare & Medicaid Services. Home care prospective payment system. http://www.cms.gov/Outreach-and-Education/Medicare-Learning-Network-MLN/MLNProducts/downloads/HomeHlthProspaymt.pdf. Accessed November 29, 2013.

Centers for Medicare & Medicaid Services. Home Health Agency. http://www.cms.gov/Center/Provider-Type/Home-Health-Agency-HHA-Center.html?redirect=/center/hospice.asp. Accessed November 29, 2013.

Centers for Medicare & Medicaid Services. Home Health Prospective Payment System Regulations and Notices (PPS). http://www.cms.gov/Medicare/Medicare-Fee-for-Service-Payment/HomeHealthPPS/Home-Health-Prospective-Payment-System-Regulations-and-Notices.html. Accessed November 29, 2013.

Hospice Foundation of America. http://www.hospicefoundation.org/. Accessed November 29, 2013.

National Association for Home Care and Hospice. http://www.nahc.org/. Accessed November 29, 2013.

The Official U.S. Government Website for Medicare. Home Health Compare. http://www.medicare.gov/homehealthcompare/. Accessed November 29, 2013.

The Official U.S. Government Website for Medicare. Process of care measures. http://www.medicare.gov/HomeHealthCompare/Data/Quality-Measures/Quality-Measures-List.aspx. Accessed November 29, 2013.

Management Issues in Hospitals and Health Systems

LEARNING OBJECTIVES

- Discuss the characteristics of the types of contemporary hospitals.
- Analyze licensure, certification, and accreditation demands in hospitals.
- Discuss contemporary hospital practice issues.
- Analyze the work of physical therapists in hospitals.
- Determine the managerial roles and challenges to managerial responsibilities.
- Analyze managerial decision-making in given hospital situations.

PART 1   The Contemporary Setting

Brief Overview of Hospitals and Health Systems

In the past 25 years, the organizational changes that have occurred in hospitals may have had more of an effect on the actual practice of physical therapy than any other factor in any other setting. Rehabilitation services in acute care moved from major revenue-generating centers in the fee-for-service model of reimbursement in the early years of Medicare to a cost center (not direct profit producers) in the current prospective payment system of Medicare. The focus of management has become reducing the cost of care per patient and making physical therapy a value-added service—providing something beyond standard expectations that does not add to costs.

Once the gold standard of physical therapy practice, and often the preferred work setting of many physical therapists, large acute-care hospitals were where new graduates were encouraged to take their first jobs because those hospitals were perceived to be the foundation for all other practice settings. Most physical therapists sought to work in acute care at the beginning of their careers because that was where the majority of patients were cared for when they needed rehabilitation services. The variety of clinical experiences presented by patients with a wide range of diagnoses in acute care settings, opportunities to follow patients for extended periods in the early stages of their recovery, and the availability of experienced mentors were perceived as important to professional development of novice physical therapists.

Many of these factors continue to affect the career choices of physical therapists. The current high patient turnover in hospitals provides therapists with a large variety of patient experiences, many of which are often unique or at least rarely seen. Therapists remain challenged by complex, immediate clinical decision-making and constant communication with other members of the care team required in hospital-based practices.[1] What has changed is that patients no longer reach their optimal rehabilitation goals before discharge to home. Instead, physical therapists set specific, limited functional goals that prepare patients for discharge as soon as possible.

Because of these shorter lengths of stays, therapists have assumed two important roles. First, they are consultants who make discharge recommendations based on their determination of a patient's rehabilitation potential and identification of the safest post-acute care setting. Second, they are educators who, for example, conduct classes to prepare patients for elective surgeries, and training sessions for hospital personnel to develop safe patient handling techniques.

Selected Issues in Inpatient Hospital Care

Freestanding community hospitals may soon be outdated if mergers and acquisitions continue on their current course and the Affordable Care Act promotes accountable care organizations (ACOs). These ACOs are formed for increased efficiency and effectiveness among the healthcare organizations that provide the spectrum of care for patients (see Chapter 3 for more information on ACOs). Instead, this chapter focuses on selected contemporary issues among general hospitals and healthcare systems, academic health centers, specialty hospitals, subacute, and long-term acute care centers (which may occur in a variety of organizations) that demand the attention of mid-level managers in each setting.

Growth of Hospitals

Another trend of importance to inpatient managers is that, despite all of the concerns about lack of funding and increased regulations, constant growth appears to be the actual state of the hospital industry. Hospitals seem to be constantly under construction or renovating. This expansion suggests that healthcare continues to be insulated from actual market forces that negatively affect the growth of other large businesses, such as retail sales, home construction, and manufacturing.

Healthcare systems do not seem to lack the assets needed to back these large projects. Mergers have contributed to this growth because they have allowed hospitals to shed redundancy, eliminate waste, and streamline staffing models while building on the strengths of several organizations to enrich a single bottom line. Managers who embrace the challenges of these growth organizations as they continue to evolve find many unexpected upward career opportunities. Their experiences may involve an ever-increasing separation from the roles of a healthcare professional to the new roles as a management professional. Because these positions in hospitals do not require licensure, it takes only desire and determination to climb up managerial career ladders in hospital systems.

Healthcare Systems and Hospitalists

One of the emerging trends important to acute care managers is the role of hospitalists in acute care medical practice. Although inpatient medicine specialists have been common in hospitals in other countries, hospitalists are a relatively new branch of medicine in the United States. The term was first introduced in 1996 to identify physicians who serve as the physicians-of-record for inpatients, returning them back to the care of their primary care providers at the time of hospital discharge.[2] Assignment of patients to hospitalists means quicker responses to their daily medical demands, which results in shorter lengths of stay with fewer complications and risks. Decreased costs through this increased efficiency result. For more information on the influence that hospitalists have had on acute healthcare, go to the Society of Hospital Medicine in Web Resources.

Patients admitted to a hospital without a primary care physician may be assigned to a hospitalist without a choice in the matter. Patients with primary care physicians may continue to receive care directly from them, or they may be cared for by a hospitalist with little notification or explanation from their primary care physician. Because the hospitalist position is a new specialty in medicine, many patients may not even know the role of the hospitalist in supervising their care, or even care about that role, particularly when they also are under the care

of one or more surgeons or other medical specialists. For other patients with chronic, complex medical conditions, unless they are repeatedly assigned to the same hospitalist with each admission, beginning all over with a different hospitalist each time may be frustrating. Patients may be unhappy or fearful if the continuity of care that their primary care physician had provided is lost.

As reimbursement rates continued to drop, primary care physicians discovered that hospitalists saved them both time and money. Interrupting their office practices for quick visits to attend to their patients in the hospital was no longer needed, and frequent phone call interruptions during patient visits in their offices from hospital nurses seeking orders decreased.

For hospital managers, communication with the broader cadre of primary care physicians often resulted in treatment delays and miscommunication because discussions were not always face-to-face, or nurses served as intermediaries in communications. The immediate availability of hospitalists generally improved communication and decision-making because they are more consistently available to members of frontline care teams who continue to provide important clinical details for medical decisions.

Academic Health Centers

The Institute of Medicine has identified the unique role and challenges that academic health centers (AHCs) face in healthcare. They concurrently train health professionals, conduct research that advances health, and provide care—often to the most ill and poorest populations. Their integration of these three responsibilities produces the knowledge and evidence that are the foundations for treating illness and improving health. Go to the Institute of Medicine in Web Resources for more information.

Academic health centers are degree-granting institutions with a medical school and at least one other health professional academic program that owns, or has an affiliation with, a teaching hospital, health system, or other organized healthcare provider. They may be private or public organizations. Some are based in universities while others are freestanding institutions. One type of AHC organization is an integrated model with teaching, research, and patient care the responsibility of one board of directors. A second type is the split model in which, typically, there is a chief executive officer for teaching and research who reports to a board in an academic institution and another chief executive officer who is responsible for patient care in an affiliating healthcare system who reports to a different board of directors. Variations of these two models occur as AHCs react to local factors and politics that affect their organizations.[3]

Academic health centers are complex business enterprises that continue to move toward corporate models of integrated operations to more effectively encompass research, education, and patient care. Upper-management positions have been transformed to reflect these organizational changes with increased accountability and broader responsibility for resource allocation among these competing priorities. Funding of patient care is commonly at the mercy of state legislatures or city and county boards through Medicaid and other public funding.

Physical therapy managers in AHCs must balance these new corporate paradigms with traditional academic models that emphasize creativity and academic freedom. These organizations accomplish this balance without losing sight of their greater responsibility for societal missions that cannot be overshadowed by the business of research, teaching, and patient care.[3] They frequently provide services that are not available in other healthcare organizations for the care of patients with complex medical conditions and severe trauma. While competing with other healthcare organizations, they must also cooperate and coordinate with them so that patients who require specialized care are moved among them as their conditions demand. Like all healthcare organizations, AHCs face the same legislative and market pressures to survive economic upheavals in competitive healthcare markets.

All managers in AHCs face even more complexity in their assigned roles because internal competition for resources is spread over teaching, research, and patient care. Particularly for managers who aspire to academic roles, these settings may offer attractive career opportunities because they offer exposure to these interrelated facets of AHCs. Managers may also face more pressure to include clinical educational opportunities for students within an AHC than they would in other

types of healthcare systems. Accommodating the requests of universities for student placements may be considered an important recruitment tool, but it has to be balanced against productivity goals and available staff with experience and willingness to be clinical instructors.

Specialty Hospitals

Specialty hospital is an umbrella term that includes a wide range of nonprofit or for-profit, public or private organizations whose purpose is to provide either short-term or long-term care for particular populations such as people who:

- Need alcohol and drug abuse rehabilitation
- Need physical rehabilitation
- Have tuberculosis
- Have cancer
- Are women (and their infants)
- Are children
- Are veterans or military personnel
- Have ear, nose, and throat impairments
- Have cardiac disease
- Require orthopedic surgery
- Have other chronic diseases (e.g., respiratory)
- Need long-term acute care

Although some of these specialty hospitals have had a long history, including those for children and veterans, maternity or tuberculosis hospitals, and rehabilitation centers, a recent surge in the numbers and different types of organizations has raised some concerns. In certain areas of the country, collaborations between specialty hospitals and physician groups have raised suspicions about the financial arrangements they have made with one another. These arrangements have been perceived to have a negative effect on funding for neighboring general hospitals.

Supporters of specialty hospitals see them as providing financial incentives for hospitals and for physicians to produce higher quality outcomes more efficiently. Because they are smaller with more focused patient-centered care, they argue that they challenge other hospitals to innovate and improve. Detractors believe that physicians compete unfairly by referring patients to their own specialty hospitals and that these hospitals focus only on the most lucrative procedures for the healthiest and best-insured patients.

The counterargument is that many general hospitals have policies that demand physicians refer patients only to their hospitals. They often purchase physician practices and direct those physicians to refer to that hospital exclusively, and they operate health plans that include network referral requirements. These general hospitals may really be no different from specialty hospitals in terms of their dependency on relationships with physicians.

The effect of physician-owned cardiac, orthopedic, and surgical specialty hospitals on the Medicare program led to a report to Congress in 2005. Highlights of that report, based on analysis of only a few hospitals with the data available at the time, included the following facts:[4]

- Costs for Medicare patients are not lower but their patients have shorter lengths of stay.
- They do treat patients who are generally less severe cases (with expectations for more profits), and they concentrate on particular diagnosis-related groups (DRGs), some of which are relatively more profitable.
- They tend to have a lower share of Medicaid patients than do community hospitals.
- The financial effect on community hospitals in the same markets has been limited.
- Their objective is to gain greater control over how the hospital is run, to increase their productivity, and to provide greater satisfaction for them and their patients.

In a more recent study of Medicare data on 10,478 patients who underwent total hip replacement and 15,312 patients who had total knee replacements from 1999–2003, they determined that fewer Medicare-reimbursed surgeries and more privately insured surgeries were conducted in physician-owned specialty hospitals than in non-physician owned. The patients in the physician-owned hospitals had lower rates of the common comorbid conditions of obesity and heart failure, and fewer of the patients were African American although they were situated in neighborhoods with a higher proportion of African American residents.[5] Controversy surrounding these physician-ownership issues is expected to continue to receive the attention of policy makers.

Rehabilitation Hospitals

Other specialty hospitals that are not physician owned also may face challenges. Of particular interest to physical therapists are inpatient rehabilitation hospitals, which have undergone changes to adjust to a Medicare prospective system that became effective in 2002. The system is based on a patient assessment instrument similar to that used in skilled nursing facilities and home-care agencies for data collection. Medicare defines a rehabilitation hospital as one in which a certain percentage of patients (the 75% rule) require intensive rehabilitation with diagnoses that fall into this recently revised list of 13 diagnostic groups that include stroke, spinal cord injury, and amputation. For an update on the 75% rule (now at 60%), a list of the remaining diagnostic groups, admission formula, and the like, see Web Resources for Inpatient Rehabilitation Payment.

The major struggles with Medicare reimbursement for inpatient rehabilitation managers have been the steady and dramatic decline in patient volume attributed to these policy changes and the related concern of limiting patient access to inpatient rehabilitation services.[6] Another ongoing issue is related to patient ability to participate in intensive rehabilitation. Because patients are discharged sicker and quicker from acute care settings, they may not be able to meet the requirement of participating in 3 hours of therapy a day. Others may not need 3 hours of therapy to meet their goals. Failure to predict patient outcomes may have negative financial consequences. Lack of, or limited, coverage for both inpatient and outpatient rehabilitation in many new models of health insurance may also contribute to a decline in inpatient rehabilitation volume for patients who are not Medicare recipients. As these policy and reimbursement issues continue, managers in rehabilitation hospitals can continue to expect organizational adjustments to remain profitable with more limited patient populations to draw on.

Another management responsibility in inpatient rehabilitation is the admissions committee. Physical therapists in acute care hospitals are predicting each patient's ability to meet the requirements for inpatient rehabilitation in their discharge planning recommendations. At the same time, admission committees of rehabilitation hospitals are reviewing these same plans to determine acceptance of patients for admission. Generally, patients need to have a medical condition that cannot be managed at a lower level of care. Complex criteria and the results of the evaluations of the members of the team determine reimbursement for each patient in the prospective payment system imposed on rehabilitation centers that has shifted to addressing medical necessity rather than medical stability in these admission decisions.

Managers in rehabilitation hospitals are responsible for patient care that now happens within reduced lengths of stays for patients with more complex medical conditions that must still achieve optimal outcomes for safe discharge back to the community. These factors require therapists to focus on functional training, early involvement of caregivers in discharge planning, and motivation of patients to participate to their maximum potential in treatment. This patient management requires a team approach for consistency in care, excellent communication skills, and good clinical decision-making that includes the patients' points of view. Organizing staff into specialty teams to care for patients with the same diagnosis such as stroke or spinal cord injury is now common in rehabilitation centers as a result.

There is less focus on traditional nursing care and diagnostic testing in rehabilitation hospitals. The management of interdisciplinary services for the coordination of interventions among all members of the team—rehabilitation and nursing—is the focus instead. Managers shift their efforts to the development and performance of staff, who establish longer-term professional relationships with patients than do therapists working in acute care hospitals. Preparing staff with the skills to establish viable discharge plans based on family support and resources rather than a patient's return to a prior of level of function has been another shift in managerial responsibility for patient care.

Post-acute Care

Post-acute care (PAC) supports patients who require ongoing medical management or therapeutic, rehabilitative, or skilled nursing care. This care is provided in a range of settings already discussed in other chapters—home healthcare in Chapter 16, skilled nursing facilities in Chapter 13, and in the section above on inpatient rehabilitation centers. Long-term acute care hospitals (LTACHs) are the other major type of post-acute care for patients who require intensive, long-term services for complex medical problems such as multi-system organ failure, complex respiratory problems, ventilator dependency, severe postsurgical wounds, renal failure, and complicated infections.

Best thought of as a program rather than a place, LTACH care can be provided in a variety of healthcare settings from freestanding centers devoted entirely to this subacute care or specialized units in nursing homes and hospitals. They provide interdisciplinary services to patients who are admitted for at least 25 days that include frequent physician oversight and advanced nursing care. This group of patients no longer needs the technology and diagnostic services available only in acute care; however, they need more care than can be provided in certified skilled nursing facilities, and they are too sick to tolerate the required hours of therapy in rehabilitation centers.[7]

Although most subacute patients are likely to be elderly, these settings provide care to patients across the life span. It becomes evident why LTACHs are perceived as filling an important gap in the continuum of healthcare. While receiving about the same level and intensity of care that may be found in hospitals, costs may be reduced because the overhead of hospital emergency rooms, surgical suites, and sophisticated diagnostic imaging is avoided.

More information on all of these contemporary hospital issues can be found in Web Resources for the American Hospital Association (AHA), Hospital Connect Search, Association of Academic Health Centers (AAHC), long-term acute care hospitals (LTACHs), and the American Physical Therapy Associate (APTA) Acute Care Section.

Licensure, Certification, Regulation, and Accreditation

Regardless of the type of hospital or hospital system, licensing and accreditation are intertwined. Many jurisdictions defer to The Joint Commission's accreditation of an organization as evidence of meeting state licensure requirements. The Centers for Medicare & Medicaid Services (CMS) also relies on The Joint Commission evaluations of healthcare organizations as a requirement for certification as a Medicare and Medicaid provider.

The Joint Commission has shifted to program accreditation and standardized patient outcome performance measures that can be used for comparison of organizations by interested parties. The heart of their review processes has shifted to unannounced site visits with attention directed to observation of patient care and interviews of patients, family members, students, and all levels of staff in the organization. This accreditation process is based on an on-site survey of the hospital with a consultative partnering rather than an investigative approach to improve the quality of patient care. In all program areas in which accreditation is sought (e.g., stroke, spinal cord injury, traumatic brain injury, pediatrics), the organization is asked to demonstrate to a survey team conformance to standards highlighting the organization's values and approaches in several areas. See Web Resources for more information on The Joint Commission rehabilitation hospitals (and rehabilitation units of hospitals) and also accreditation specifications of the Commission on Accreditation of Rehabilitation Facilities (CARF).

Workforce Issues in Hospitals and Hospital Systems

Downsizing of staff and reducing the number of staffed beds became the hospital management strategy of the 1990s as managers strived to control costs to maintain profits with the prospective payments for the care they delivered. Strategies continue to evolve in both nonprofit and for-profit hospitals as they pool resources, increase purchasing power, and reduce competition through mergers, acquisitions, and other cooperative models.

Staffing Models

Hospital-management models have flattened mid-level positions to reduce the costs associated with wages and benefits for employees who do not contribute directly to the provision of patient services. Smaller hospital units have been combined and many managers, including those who are physical therapists, find themselves responsible for staff from a variety of disciplines and perhaps responsible for some units unfamiliar to them.

Combining physical therapy, occupational therapy, and speech language pathology services (and often psychology, electromyography, and other

units) under one manager is a commonly used strategy. The clinical manager of the new unit is likely to be a rehabilitation professional, but nurses or other health professionals may also have responsibility for rehabilitation units. Even with these efforts, many newly formed multidisciplinary managerial units are small compared with the total number of nursing personnel or nonclinical support staff (i.e., housekeeping, maintenance, kitchen).

Because the major responsibility of clinical managers has changed from discipline-specific revenue generation to interdisciplinary program cost management, the skills required for these positions have less to do with one's clinical expertise than they have to do with the skills needed to control and reduce costs while maintaining the quality of patient care to achieve expected patient outcomes. Managers have shifted from discipline-specific experts to efficiency and cost-reduction experts, regardless of the initials behind their names in these new, complex matrix models of management.

Doing more with less has become, perhaps, the most important skill for these managers as they seek to achieve more stringent patient outcome expectations and sustain the quality of patient care. All mid-level managers in healthcare organizations share duties and responsibilities that are blurred rather than clearly and consistently delineated so that staff can be more quickly and effectively reorganized as organizational demands change. To manage these "big picture" responsibilities, mid-level managers divide staff into smaller units under the direction of team leaders. Team leaders carry at least a partial patient load and handle the details of daily operations such as staffing levels and problem-solving. Another staffing strategy is to rotate staff among units of the hospital for 3 months or so. Particularly for novice therapists, this rotation allows the breakdown of acute care skills into more manageable blocks while building rapport with nursing staff and enhancing consistency of patient care. Therapists become more confident in each unit that then allows assignment to any unit as staffing needs arise.

Program Management

Another staffing issue has arisen with regrouping services into programs. Interdisciplinary teams are assigned to programs to meet the needs of particular populations more efficiently and effectively.

Clinical decision-making becomes decentralized as responsibility in programs falls to a smaller focused group of frontline providers. The roles of physicians in these programs may vary from ultimate authority to consultative. Program managers in this model typically are responsible for all fiscal and human resources needed to implement the program. The nonclinical hospital support services typically remain centralized in this model.

Program management models may take on a variety of modifications depending on several factors, such as the number of different populations to be served, availability of staff to be distributed among programs, and the size of the organization. For instance, a large teaching hospital may have rehabilitation, pharmacy, and nursing managers with responsibility for staffing and assignments. These individuals work with program managers who are responsible for the care and outcomes for the stroke, organ transplant, oncology, or cardiac program.

Another mixed model example is one in which a program manager is responsible for inpatients and outpatients across the continuum of their care in a particular program (e.g., oncology). Other programs have managers who are responsible for each inpatient unit, with another manager responsible for all combined outpatient services. Coordination of the responsibilities and the distribution of accountability in these mixed models can be confusing and subject to frequent changes because they are often the result of trial-and-error decisions or the flux in available personnel.

Support for program management is driven by the knowledge that groups whose members devote a higher percentage of their time to working with a particular patient population tend to develop stronger relationships (i.e., shared goals, shared knowledge, and mutual respect) and more effective patterns of interaction. These interactions are believed to result in increased quality of care for the patient *and* reduced hospitalization costs for the payer.[8]

Program Management and Physical Therapists

Several themes were identified in interviews with physical therapists deployed to different programs when discipline-based departments such as physical therapy were disbanded as a result of a merger of several hospitals and other units in a large healthcare system. Among the conclusions were that the physical therapists experienced:[9]

- A sense of loss of professional identity because the collegiality and informal friendships that were part of departmental interactions were gone. No longer having a department head felt as if professional representation in the organization was lost as well.

- Low morale, which was expressed as a sense of giving up, lack of enjoyment, no job satisfaction, and expectations to do more with no change in salaries.

- Additional management and administrative responsibilities without preparation to assume them. The need for strong communication skills became more important because there was no one person to rely on, forcing the therapists to speak for themselves. The tasks and work of the physical therapy director did not go away; rather, it was redistributed with each physical therapist assuming those tasks within his or her program teams. Standards of practice were no longer monitored as a result, creating a potential negative effect on the quality of care.

- Less support for educational funds and opportunities, including curtailment of in-services

- Inconsistent mentoring and orientation of new employees

Professional advantages to program management also were identified. They include increased interdisciplinary work, which increased the visibility of physical therapists, expansion of the scope of physical therapy responsibilities, and more opportunities to learn from other disciplines.[9]

Whether or not the same themes are prevalent among hospital employees today requires further investigation. New graduates may now be better prepared for program responsibilities. Comparison of a physical therapist who is the only physical therapist in a program with physical therapists who are assigned to several programs simultaneously may also be needed.

Perceptions of both informal (effective relationships with others on the program team) and formal (contributions to organizational goals) power are equally important predictors of the empowerment of physical therapists in an organization. Sources of formal empowerment disappear as professional networks in organizations are disbanded, support from peers is reduced, and discipline-specific leadership positions as a researcher, department head, or clinical education coordinator are less available. However, in the program model, program-specific and patient-specific information is enhanced and opportunities for informal power may be improved within a coordinated interdisciplinary team approach to care.[10]

Inpatient Acute Care and Physical Therapy

The dramatic changes that have occurred in hospitals in response to the many economic and policy changes that have transformed healthcare in the past 25 years have affected the delivery of rehabilitation services in hospitals in several important ways. Some strategies for controlling costs of rehabilitation services in acute care settings have been:

- Eliminating centralized therapeutic gyms and treatment areas to reduce space and equipment costs and the need for staff to transport patients
- Conducting therapy sessions at the patient bedside for increased efficiency (transporting patients to a therapy department has essentially been eliminated) and effectiveness (functional training provided where hospital function occurs)
- Creating smaller, centralized staff offices for documentation and coordination of services
- Shifting as much inpatient service as possible to outpatient settings (e.g., presurgical physicals, laboratory tests, intake interviews completed as outpatient services before the patient is admitted to the hospital for other than a medical emergency)
- Shifting the provision of durable medical equipment and other supplies to patients postdischarge to reduce the inpatient cost/patient
- Discharging patients as soon as possible to less intensive and less costly settings

Many older physical therapists have been surprised about the professional role they now play in acute care settings because care has shifted to meeting the immediate functional needs of patients and facilitating discharge, typically in a few days. Currently, patients are moving in and out of hospitals faster, and their therapy sessions are shorter and more focused on function at the bedside. This approach meets the demand of caring for more patients with fewer staff. Providing interventions other than functional training has become more of an exception rather than the rule for many patients. Teaching other caregivers and making recommendations about the coordination of care become important professional roles in hospital settings.

It may be difficult for some novice therapists to predict the ability of the patient to function safely in the least restrictive setting when there is limited time to gather the data to reach those decisions. Other new graduates thrive on these expectations. They enjoy the fast pace of decision-making in acute care. They relish the excitement of positively affecting the function of people who are critically ill or who have suffered traumatic injuries, and delight in being at the cutting edge of new medical advances.

In most hospitals, rehab services function as a field operation. Therapists are scattered about the hospital to take care of patients at the bedside with little interaction with one another during the day. This lack of ongoing peer interaction creates another issue for managing the new graduate. More experienced staff may find mentoring disruptive and time-consuming in their daily routines. Although important for all new graduates in any setting, formalizing mentoring may be key to success in acute care. Having someone to turn to as they develop clinical decision-making skills in the fast-paced, unpredictable acute care setting may be essential because of the profound effect these decisions have on a patient's recovery and discharge placement.

Physical Therapy in Other Types of Hospitals

Physical therapy in long-term acute care is primarily influenced by the longer times that therapists work with patients and each patient's potential for improvement. Therapists need a wide range of skills as members of interdisciplinary teams caring for patients with a wide range of complex medical problems that may or may not improve in functional status. Managers may need to assure that staff are prepared for the emotional reactions to patients with very low levels of function.

Physical therapy practice in rehabilitation hospitals has probably changed the least over the years. Although reimbursement regulations have resulted in the standards requiring intensive one-on-one care and more need for staff as a result, the model of patient care remains the same. The teamwork in neurological rehabilitation units has been investigated and may be applicable to all of inpatient rehabilitation units. Benefits of working on these teams were related to sharing of knowledge and expertise across disciplines, integrated work that is coordinated to address common patient goals, decreased repetition and increased efficiency of care.[11]

Sidebar 17.1 and Figure 17.1 summarize some of the differences in physical therapy practice across the three levels of inpatient care. The work in long-term acute care is a mix of the two other settings and falls somewhere between them on each continuum in the figure.

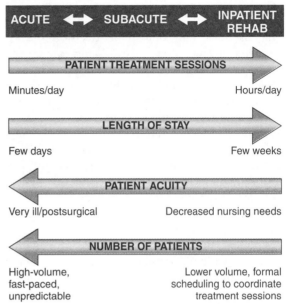

FIGURE 17.1 Comparison of physical therapy in different acute care settings.

SIDEBAR 17.1

Characteristics of the Work in Acute Care and Rehabilitation Hospitals

Acute Care:

- Experience with a variety of patients with complex problems if able to rotate among hospital units, or an opportunity to specialize clinical practice with assignment to a single program or unit

- Decreased interaction with other physical therapists in larger hospitals and systems unless deliberate efforts are made for meetings and the like, and less opportunity for informal mentoring

- Interactions with multidisciplinary team members including case managers, social workers, doctors, nurses, respiratory therapists, orthotists

- Fast-paced and unpredictable schedule that is individually controlled by each therapist

- Independence in the content of work and solving problems

- Opportunities for interaction with specialists on the cutting edge of practice, researchers in large medical centers, and the newest technology

- Decreased opportunity for establishing professional relationships with patients

- Possibility of assignment to specialty units that is not consistent with professional goals or interests

- Patients too ill or unwilling to participate in rehabilitation sessions

- Develop ability to think quickly for important patient care decisions

Rehabilitation Hospitals:

- Central gym and patient care conferences allow constant interaction with other physical therapists and rehabilitation providers that leads to joint team decision-making

- Establishment of longer term professional relationships with patients

- Work schedule is assigned or negotiated with other members of the team

- Typically assigned to a specialty team. Opportunity to develop specialty practice, but risk of assignment within an area of practice that is of less interest

- Little interaction with referring or specialty physicians. Team led by physician who chairs meetings

Discharge Planning

The fast pace and immediate decision-making required to meet productivity and quality of care goals in hospitals has raised the question of whether it is the most suitable setting for new graduates. Planning for discharge as they are conducting their initial examination and evaluation, often with limited information, has become a new challenge for physical therapists. Rather than determining appropriate goals for a patient and establishing a plan of care to reach them, physical therapists are faced with meeting pre-established discharge days within the limits set by prospective payments for patients.

Physical therapists share their information about the patient's current status and potential for rehabilitation with other members of the clinical team (hospital case managers, discharge planners, and admission screeners from potential facilities for patient placement) who contribute information on social and financial resources affecting discharge decisions. Representatives from post-acute care settings are sent to hospitals to recruit patients ready for discharge who are most appropriate for admission to their facilities. These liaisons are important to maintaining the competitive edge and financial viability of their institutions.

For many patients, physical therapists with the knowledge and skills to contribute to this multidisciplinary, consultative discharge process may be more important than those who provide direct interventions to improve their functional status. These role changes have raised broader practice questions about acute care physical therapy within the profession. Answers to these questions, which include the following, will continue to evolve as healthcare policies impact the management of care in hospitals:

- Is physical therapy a core or supplemental service in general acute care settings?
- What is it that physical therapists do in acute care that no other professional can do?
- Are the typical patient care services provided by physical therapists in acute care considered skilled services?
- Should physical therapy practice in acute care be reinvented? If so, how?
- Is discharge planning in acute care an advanced skill?

PART 2   Overview of Management in Hospital-Based Practices

Contemporary Hospital Management and Physical Therapy

The size of the hospital or healthcare system is the key factor in determining the role of rehabilitation managers and their responsibilities. Some potential models include the following:

- In a relatively small community hospital, the physical therapy manager may also be the primary provider of patient care—both inpatient and outpatient—using support staff or other therapists as necessary.
- The physical therapist may be the manager of an interdisciplinary program or programs.

- In larger hospitals, several unit supervisors and/or program managers may report to a rehabilitation manager or director.
- In a large healthcare system that includes several hospitals and outpatient centers, there may be several managers who may function relatively independently of one another, or they may function as a team that coordinates personnel assignments and other management decisions for consistency throughout the system.
- There may be a systemwide vice president of rehabilitation services, who centralizes the efforts of supervisors in several centers who have less responsibility for management

decisions and more responsibility for implementation of policies.

- A national chain of hospitals may have a regional manager of rehabilitation services with directors in several freestanding hospitals who report to him or her with little interaction with one another.

Management Responsibilities

Mission, Vision, and Goals

Probably more than in any other healthcare setting, mid-level managers may struggle with decisions made by upper management that may seem contradictory to the missions of many hospitals—to be of service to the community. Offering an acceptable level of quality at the least cost, in a more transparent system, first requires agreement among the members of an organization on what their goals mean and how they are to be put into operation and measured.

Although individual therapists may have a great deal of independence in their patient care decisions, managers may feel more limited in their ability to try new approaches or ideas without the permission of upper management. With decreased time and effort for orientation and mentoring of employees, managers may need to be alert to employees who find themselves in program boxes rather than disciplinary silos. Employees' relationships to the organization may be limited to an assignment to a particular team. Managers may take extra effort to assure employee understanding or commitment to the larger organization and its goals. Managers may be redefining the mission, vision, and goals or reasserting and reassuring staff that they have not changed as mergers and acquisitions take place.

Policies and Procedures

The larger the organization, the more likely managers are to be responsible for the implementation of, rather than the creation of, policies and procedures that may be "packaged" to comply with accreditation and regulatory requirements. There may be specific professional issues affecting the quality of care that require additional policies and procedures. Evidence-based practice may be one example.

Evidence

A survey of physical therapists revealed that about 70% of all physical therapists said they read professional literature at least monthly. Only 26% reported searching online databases for new information and about the same percentage of people critically appraised research reports. Other findings showed that the respondents had a positive attitude toward evidence-based practice (EBP), but barriers, including time, access, and search skills, reduced their actual implementation of EBP.[12]

Evidence-based practice may be implied (or assumed) in accreditation and other regulatory requirements, and even in policies and procedures that may address an individual's efforts to practice based on evidence as part of job descriptions and evaluation of performance. However, managers may find that EBP may not serve as the foundation of actual patient care. The information mastery model is a tool to answer clinical questions that seems more comfortable and useful than the traditional evidence-based medicine (EBM) process.[13] This approach may be valuable in all healthcare settings, but it is especially useful in hospitals because it provides managers an opportunity to bring together their staffs who are scattered throughout a hospital-based practice. This process of information mastery relies on a search of secondary online databases in which original resources have already been screened for validity and relevance. This bypasses the EBM process to answer a clinical question that has been posed. For example, a clinical question might be: What is the effect of early mobility on patients in intensive care units? Answers to questions about the information gathered are then directed to the specific intensive care patients that a therapist or group of therapists actually cares for. The specific questions are:

- Are the results of the review of the literature relevant to the patients I see?
- Is the new information valid for my patients?
- If it were true, would the new information require a change in my/our practice?

The information mastery model answers questions that make evidence-based practice seem more practical and applicable for many professionals. Because the process directs attention to practical clinical questions in terms of patients actually cared for, physical therapists may be more eager and willing to invest time and thought in gathering and applying new information. Managers who recognize and reward staff efforts to improve care and follow through with formal changes in response to findings promote positive encouragement to staff by identifying problems and seeking solutions.

Electronic Health Records

The other information issue important to managers is ensuring that staff members have the technical skills to interact with electronic health records effectively, accurately, and legally. Spurred by the Health Insurance Portability and Accountability Act (HIPAA) of 1996 and The Joint Commission requirements, the electronic health record provides data to support operations, research, healthcare policy, regulation, performance improvement, and patient care.

The use of the electronic health record in a variety of healthcare settings by physical therapists has been investigated.[14] Based on this review of the literature, some conclusions were drawn. For instance, one of the advantages of electronic documentation is standardization of terminology and formats. A potential drawback is a system that does not reflect the workflow and practice demands of therapists. Efforts to develop a national physical therapy databank that merges with a health organization's existing system may not be possible because of confidentiality regulations and reluctance of competitors to share information with one another.

Policies and procedures related to implementation of HIPAA guidelines are a given. Managers also may need policies and procedures to assure the technical skills of therapists for the management of patient databases. Acquired skills must be adequate for accurate and thorough documentation. Providing information to software and systems developers so that the electronic health record reflects the work of physical therapists is also important.

Marketing

The trend in hospitals and healthcare systems seems to be a customer focus that identifies the expectations of key stakeholder groups (customers) and regularly determines their level of satisfaction with the organization. This approach means that marketing efforts focus on finding out what people want and design the service to meet it, rather than

creating a service and then selling it. Collecting data through patient satisfaction surveys, focus groups, follow-up telephone calls after discharge, and community surveys is now common. Many hospitals collect data on discharged patients through participation in the Hospital Consumer Assessment of Healthcare Providers and Systems (HCAHPS) survey. The Centers for Medicare & Medicaid Services (CMS) publishes HCAHPS results on its Hospital Compare website. See Web Resources for HCAPHS and Hospital Compare.

Managers need to assure that the information gathered by hospital marketing departments includes not only the patient's experience but also the need for rehabilitation services. Without the traditional department head as the voice for physical therapy or rehabilitation, there is a risk that these services may get lost if the selective information focuses on nursing and physician interactions.

Community Interactions

Hospitals and healthcare systems are often the largest employer in an area. Managers need to consider the effect of their decisions not only on the health of the community but also on its economy. For instance, downsizing staff, mergers, eliminating competition, relocating hospitals, and negotiating third-party payer contracts all have an effect on the community that goes beyond measurement of health outcomes. Conversely, community businesses that change their healthcare insurance contracts and coverage options for employees affect hospital finances. City and county development often depends on the reputation of its hospitals to attract new businesses and for those businesses to attract new employees.

Representing the hospital on the boards of corporations and community service organizations is an important role for hospital managers to monitor the current state of the community. This community service becomes another source of information on a different set of customers—community leaders and organizations. Informal conversations and relationships that occur at board meetings are often the basis of trust and cooperation that is vital to the growth of the hospital and the community so that trends and developments can be anticipated. Hearing what community leaders are really saying about a hospital may be as important as the impressions of particular patients.

Staffing

Perhaps more than any other staffing issue, hospital-based rehabilitation managers need to consider the effect of nursing staff shortages on the provision of rehabilitation services. Therapists rely on cooperation and coordination with nursing personnel so that all components of patients' care are addressed. When nursing services are not working efficiently and effectively, it is difficult for therapy to work. Rehabilitation and program managers need to work with nursing in the development of staffing patterns and schedules that work best for everyone. Assuring that therapy sessions are included in a patient's busy schedule of diagnostic tests and nursing interventions may require a significant amount of a rehabilitation manager's time.

Job Satisfaction

Job satisfaction and burnout of physical therapists have received some attention because of the turmoil that has occurred in hospitals in recent years. It appears that physical therapists who see their work as controllable, with choices, and who can develop workable strategies to meet their productivity standards, not only survive but thrive in hospital-based practices. Seeing options and opportunities lays the foundation for developing time-management, assertive communication, delegation, discharge, and task-prioritizing skills.[15]

Regardless of the discipline of the immediate supervisor or manager, attention to reinforcing and maintaining the strong sense of professional identity of physical therapists may be important to their recruitment and retention. Physical therapists may be willing to accommodate organizational changes and demands as long as their ability to interact with other professionals and patients is preserved.[16]

Contingency Workers

The importance of commitment of employees to an organization cannot be underestimated. Low absenteeism, less turnover of staff, higher job satisfaction, and high performance levels may be the result of commitment of full-time employees. The power of committed employees may be at risk with the rise in contingent employment arrangements, which include in-house temporaries, float staff who are moved among units as needed, direct-hire or seasonal workers, lease workers, consultants, and independent contractors.[17]

Both employers and employees are attracted to the flexibility offered in contingency work. Hospitals see an opportunity to cut costs associated with employee benefit packages. They are able to manage the absences of regular staff and patient load fluctuations that may be seasonal. Health professionals may see contingency work as improving their employment opportunities with a variety of short-term work experiences that give them more flexibility. They may choose the work they engage in at any point in time, they have the opportunity to try out a variety of employment settings or even locations before making permanent career decisions, and their hourly fees are higher than the wages per hour performing the same job.

When cost and flexibility are the primary reasons for managerial decisions to hire workers to meet short-term specific needs (a contingency situation), the use of temporary workers (temps) appears to be good business. It may not be such good business as a stopgap staffing measure when temps are hired to fill ongoing personnel shortages. As the demand for particular workers increases, so do their employment opportunities. During these times, health professionals may prefer contingency work because of the freedom to select work assignments that are most attractive to them. This preference further contributes to shortages in full-time, traditional employees.

Physical Therapist Assistants

Managerial decisions about the utilization of physical therapist assistants and other support personnel are important in hospitals because the patients are medically unstable with complex conditions. Having professionals who are prepared to meet the demands of quick turnaround discharge planning that begins with the initial evaluations of patients is vital. This need often excludes physical therapist assistants in the care of many patients.

However, when the actual physical therapy interventions for acute patients are routine and straightforward, physical therapist assistants may be directed to assume responsibility for established plans of care. Clinical pathways and other guidelines used to standardize plans of care also make the assignment of many patients to physical therapist assistants appropriate.

Managers must be aware of state statutes that regulate practice of physical therapist assistants in acute care settings. They may not be permitted to work without the direct supervision of physical therapists in hospitals. Unlicensed technicians may face the same statutory limitations. In addition to these practice regulations, reimbursement requirements may define skilled care in such a way that unlicensed personnel may not be utilized in direct patient care at all. This may be particularly true in rehabilitation hospitals.

Managers must be cautious in implementing blanket policies and procedures, such as the automatic turnover of patients to assistants after the initial session is conducted by the physical therapist. The judgment of the physical therapist about tasks and duties that are assigned to others should be made on a patient-by-patient basis, particularly in hospitals where a patient's medical condition may be fragile or unpredictable. A physical therapist assistant who is assigned specifically to one physical therapist may significantly improve the quality of therapeutic time they each spend with patients. By either working alone with a patient or with the therapist when a patient demands the support of two people to participate in a therapy session, physical therapist assistants have an important role to play. When they are working as partners on the same caseload, there is more opportunity to dovetail direct patient care and administrative tasks. While physical therapists are performing tasks that cannot be delegated, the physical therapist assistant can contribute to direct patient care and perform many support tasks such as scheduling, preparing patients for treatment, documentation, or arranging for equipment delivery.

Contrast this physical therapist and physical therapist assistant pairing with a model in which the physical therapist assistant is assigned a caseload composed of patients previously examined and evaluated by several therapists or with a physical therapist who has assigned patients to more than one physical therapist assistant. Direction and supervision by whom and when become much less clear and riskier. Hospital managers also may consider physical therapist assistants in hospitals as the glue that holds contingency workers and students together as they address their nonpatient care responsibilities. Full-time physical therapist assistants with long work histories in a hospital may have a great deal of knowledge about the idiosyncrasies of the organization. Physical therapist assistants are invaluable as the first point of contact as new staff and students navigate their new surroundings and learn to manage their time. Remembering that physical therapist assistants are extenders of all of the roles of physical therapists increases their value to organizations.

Weekend and Holiday Staff

Supervision issues are particularly important during holidays and weekends when reduced staffing of rehabilitation services may occur. Identifying the physical therapist responsible for supportive staff becomes challenging because everyone working on holidays and weekends is typically very busy with a patient who *must* be treated for one reason or another. This work dynamic is complicated by the fact that everyone working on a weekend or holiday may be a contingency worker. The weekend team members may not know one another, which may further complicate the communication and establishment of a supervisory relationship. Particularly when the work schedule and patient assignments are pre-established for the weekend staff, it is easy for them to become so involved in direct patient care that there is little interaction with coworkers, let alone time for supervision of others. Managers need to be alert to the risks inherent in these situations. Orientation to policies and procedures for these special days may be crucial in deterring risks and maintaining the quality of services. See Australia's OSSIE Guide to Clinical Handover Improvement in Web Resources.

Patient Care

Anecdotal reports have always suggested that the more physical and occupational therapy a patient receives, the better are the outcomes of care. Two studies confirmed the relationship between, and the frequency and duration of, therapy services and outcomes such as discharge to home.[18,19] The challenge for managers is achieving the same results with fewer staff to provide the service and decreased contact time with each patient. These studies suggest that with more physical therapy, both the mobility scores of patients may have been improved and the discharge placement from hospitals may have been less restrictive for many patients. How managers may affect other decision makers who are eager for early discharge of patients and rely on general guidelines rather than individual patient data in discharge planning is a major management concern.

Although conducted more than 10 years ago, one study identified perceptions of physical therapists about factors that affected acute care practice. They included:[20]

- Discomfort with patient medical complications, behaviors, and pain
- Lack of patient motivation and cooperation
- Ability to integrate a great deal of information—pathology, pharmacology, radiological and diagnostic reports—to assess their patients' needs, and project realistic, achievable goals to effectively prepare the patients for the next level of care
- Difficulty in adding to or changing a patient's orders and receiving appropriate referrals
- Scheduling of multiple required medical tests
- Inadequate time to work with patients to accomplish goals
- Preparation for treatment sessions and failed attempts to see patients is time consuming
- Patient discharge frequently occurring within 1 or 2 days of referral without opportunity to coordinate with the family and with postdischarge providers
- Distinguishing between patients who require high-level, ongoing care by the physical therapist and those who could be seen by support personnel for treatment
- Increasing numbers of part-time and per diem staff and new graduates who may not be prepared to function effectively in the acute care setting

It is hoped that during the past 10 years new graduates have been better prepared for the acute care practice and current employees continue to demonstrate the expertise required to manage very complex, sick patients. Managers have opportunities to advocate for patients and their staff as they address factors such as people who are too sick to participate in physical therapy and scheduling conflicts that often place diagnostic tests and other procedures ahead of physical therapy. Managers who develop positive relationships with hospitalists also may reduce some of the tensions related to fulfilling physician orders in a timely manner rather than immediately.

Managers also may need to do a detailed job analysis to identify, at least, the direct patient care skills that therapists must have in acute care. Even a simple checklist of specific things to know and things to do during treatment sessions may be helpful, particularly for new graduates, new employees, and contingency workers who are coping with the complexity of hospital-based care. Updating this list as new technology and new procedures are introduced is an important management responsibility. Orientation to the nonpatient-care duties and responsibilities is equally important particularly because physical therapists often work independently of one another in hospitals.

Although physical therapists in acute care establish their own daily work schedules, managers who are available to assist with scheduling conflicts or unexpected tasks that arise contribute significantly to coordination of smooth, efficient patient care.

Asking managers and staff physical therapists to consider how they are spending their time provides valuable insight into assignments, productivity, and roles that may have an important effect on patient care. Opportunities to anticipate the effect of managerial decisions on these roles and to identify which of these factors may be affecting the delivery of quality care and achievement of expected patient outcomes make this a valuable tool, particularly for managers who are not physical therapists.

Fiscal

Mid-level managers in hospitals may be far removed from the complex organizational budgeting and financial planning processes (e.g., borrowing and investing funds) in hospitals and healthcare systems. In the broadest terms, financial information is *one* source of information that is used to accomplish the organization's purposes. Mid-level managers are more likely to rely on accounting (current and prospective) reports to plan and control the services they are responsible for and to report the results of their efforts and decisions. Because this level of information is for internal use only, each organization typically develops a reporting format and process that works for them and uses on-the-job training to prepare managers for these fiscal responsibilities.

Program and department managers are typically held accountable for, at the least, monthly and quarterly reports on staff productivity and the costs of the services provided in their units. Daily review of data may be conducted to assure prompt and responsive managerial decisions. Their responsibility and accountability for the appropriate use of resources in relation to the goals of the organization are typically discussed in terms of accounting reports.

Distinguishing variables that affect the use of resources that are within the control of the manager, as well as those that are not, is an important component of the financial accountability at the program or department level. It includes a strong understanding of reimbursement policies. Depending on the organization's culture (i.e., top-down or bottom-up planning), the ability of mid-level managers to act on or only to report the facts and figures about their units of responsibility is another key way that the roles of managers differ from one hospital to another.

Legal, Ethical, and Risk

Patient safety is perhaps the biggest risk issue for hospitals and healthcare systems. The Joint Commission argues that accreditation itself is a risk-reduction activity because compliance with its standards is intended to reduce the likelihood of bad patient outcomes. With that in mind, The Joint Commission regularly revises its National Patient Safety Goals for each type of healthcare organization. For hospitals in 2013, these goals are:[21]

- Use at least two ways to identify patients.

  This is done to make sure that each patient gets the correct medicine and treatment.

  Make sure that the correct patient gets the correct blood when he or she gets a blood transfusion.

- Improve staff communication.

  Get important test results to the right staff person on time.

- Use medicines safely.

  Before a procedure, label medicines that are not labeled, for example, medicines in syringes, cups, and basins. Do this in the area where medicines and supplies are set up.

  Take extra care with patients who take medicines to thin their blood.

  Record and pass along correct information about a patient's medicines. Find out what medicines the

patient is taking. Compare those medicines with new medicines given to the patient. Make sure the patient knows which medicines to take when he or she returns home. Tell the patient it is important to bring his or her up-to-date list of medicines every time a visit to a doctor is made.

- Prevent infection.

  Use the hand-cleaning guidelines from the Centers for Disease Control and Prevention or the World Health Organization.

  Set goals for improving hand cleaning.

  Use the goals to improve hand cleaning.

  Use proven guidelines to prevent infections that are difficult to treat.

  Use proven guidelines to prevent infection of the blood from central lines.

  Use proven guidelines to prevent infection after surgery.

  Use proven guidelines to prevent infections of the urinary tract that are caused by catheters.

- Identify patient safety risks.

  Find out which patients are most likely to try to commit suicide.

- Prevent mistakes in surgery.

  Make sure that the correct surgery is done on the correct patient and at the correct place on the patient's body.

  Mark the correct place on the patient's body where the surgery is to be done.

  Pause before the surgery to make sure that a mistake is not being made.

The shortage of hospital personnel adds to the risks of negligence and medical errors as fewer people attempt to do more with less for older, more vulnerable patients with complex medical conditions. All managers in hospitals must be constantly alert for hospital-wide opportunities to increase the safety of patients and their employees, while attending to the risks in the provision of services for each patient.

Treatment Cancellations

At the same time, managers need to be certain that staff have guidelines and communication skills necessary to sort out patients who are too ill or unstable to participate in rehabilitation sessions from those who simply prefer not to participate. Understanding that patients have the right to refuse treatment for a life-threatening condition is not the same as patients having the right to refuse therapy because they have visitors or simply do not want to be disturbed. Managers have to analyze cancellation of treatment sessions to determine whether these clinical decisions are appropriate, particularly for staff who may be overwhelmed and inadvertently fail to encourage patient participation.

Communicable Diseases

Another related management issue is assignment of staff to patients who are perceived to place the therapist at risk. Managers may decide to assure that the same therapist does not consistently draw the "short straw" to care for patients with contagious diseases (e.g., severe acute respiratory syndrome, tuberculosis) or uncontrollable behavior. Alternatively, they may decide to prepare some staff to specialize in the care of these patients with special needs to avoid these safety and assignment issues while improving the care of these patients through staff consistency in following isolation and other protective procedures.

Ethical Issues

Rehabilitation managers are often faced with difficult ethical decisions when resources are limited. Deciding whether to see every patient once before treating any patient twice, or establishing a triage system for identifying patients in greatest need of therapy becomes important. This choice is closely related to a manager's relationship with physicians and nurses, who are typically the first providers to identify the needs of patients.

In AHCs, patients who are also subjects in clinical research studies may become priority patients, although those patients with safety risks may require more attention and time. An ethical situation arises when patients do not receive therapy that they need because they are subjects in a study.

Receiving referrals only for patients who are appropriate for rehabilitation services requires that managers educate other professionals about patient goals that therapists can assist in meeting with their skilled services. Reducing inappropriate referrals for therapy increases efficiency and is the best use of limited resources. Failing to be involved in the care of patients who would benefit from rehabilitation interventions is equally disturbing.

Ethical issues occur at every level of management in complex healthcare organizations on a regular basis. It is not unusual to have available full-time in-house legal counsel, a risk-management staff, and an ethics committee to resolve the many possible situations that can go wrong when an organization is responsible for the care of people who are acutely ill or severely injured. Managers must be familiar with the reporting requirements for the hospital to be proactive rather than reactive to legal and ethical dilemmas.

Communication

Sorting out what information needs to be immediately disseminated and what information is better left unshared often leads to difficult decisions in communication with upper management, as well as with staff and managers in similar positions in the organization. Formal policies and procedures for the content, distribution, and approval of both internal and external messages are often in place in large organizations to decrease some of these concerns and to assure consistency in the messages that organizations wish to send.

One-on-one interactions with staff often require managers to be on the move in a hospital. With staff conducting treatment sessions at patient bedsides, managers must go to them for informal meetings. Meeting over lunch breaks may also provide opportunities for chats as long as they do not lead to more work when personnel should be taking a break from their clinical duties.

Conclusions

Hospitals provide many opportunities for professional growth and increased responsibility for people interested in healthcare management careers. It is not unreasonable to suggest that hospital-based rehabilitation may evolve as a specialty practice similar to that of hospitalists that requires knowledge and clinical expertise in a wide range of diseases, trauma, and postsurgical care. New areas of increased value-added rehabilitation include intensive care and emergency room (ER) services.[22,23]

Managers are encouraged to monitor research and policy through the APTA as these and other emerging roles develop, such as their role in emergency rooms and intensive care units. See Web Resources for more information on current issues from the APTA.

Decisions about when and how to intervene with patients who have unstable and unpredictable clinical pictures make this setting demanding and exciting. Managers and the staff they supervise never know what the day will bring. This unexpectedness makes hospitals very attractive to people who seek variety and thrive on work that is never the same from day to day. They interact with a large number of professionals from many disciplines and patients with a range of psychosocial issues and complex diagnoses. Influencing the recovery of people with severe medical problems to achieve what seem to be impossible functional goals contributes to job satisfaction.

Activities 17.1 to 17.20 provide the opportunity to address inpatient hospital and health system management issues.

ACTIVITY 17.1
RELUCTANT PHYSICAL THERAPIST

Annemarie Watson has been a physical therapist at the hospital for more than 20 years. She has not taken well to the series of changes in the hospital's organization. Her favorite expression is "there's nothing new under the sun." She tends to be unimpressed with the progress the hospital has made, and frequently voices her dissatisfaction to anyone who will listen. There has been some concern about her clinical skills, although patients love her and she is effective in meeting their goals. Her documentation is very weak, and she has been resistant to learning the new electronic documentation system.

Rose Evans, the Rehabilitation Manager, is about to meet with Annemarie to share her impressions of her behaviors when Annemarie unexpectedly submits her resignation. She gives being worn out as the reason for resigning. However, she indicates that she is willing to work intermittently for vacation coverage or to provide weekend coverage one or two weekends a month.

What should Rose say? Consider: Where are they now? Where do they want to be? What do they have to work with? How will they get there?

ACTIVITY 17.2
PRIORITY PATIENT LIST

John Butterworth has no choice. The time has come to develop a priority list for rehabilitation patients in the hospital. The resignation of another physical therapist was the last straw. He simply does not have enough staff to treat the number of patients who are referred for physical therapy. He had already announced to the nurses that all patients would be seen only once a day, so referrals to see patients twice a day could not be accepted. He does not want to discourage referrals, which he may never build up again.

What should be his criteria for sorting referrals into a priority list? Patients with orthopedic postsurgical needs before patients who are on the general medical/surgical wing? Patients of a particular physician before those of another? First-come, first-served? Consider: Where are they now? Where do they want to be? What do they have to work with? How will they get there?

ACTIVITY 17.3
GOOD NEWS, BAD NEWS

Helene DuPrise, the Rehabilitation Manager in a large teaching hospital, has good news and bad news. The good news is that referrals for physical therapy are more appropriate and timely because of her efforts to educate hospitalists and nurses about physical therapy. The bad news is that physical therapists often are completing examination and evaluation of patients before diagnostic test results are known and a medical diagnosis has been established. The physical therapists are concerned that they are intervening too soon in many cases. They are making many assumptions about patient status when there may actually be contraindications and precautions that have not been identified because diagnostic reports are not yet available.

Concerned about these risks, what should Helene do? Consider: Where are they now? Where do they want to be? What do they have to work with? How will they get there?

ACTIVITY 17.4
CLINICAL EDUCATION

Antonio Sorranto, Rehabilitation Director for Van Husen Medical Center, has been invited to meet with the vice dean of the School of Physical Therapy and Rehabilitation Sciences and the director of Clinical Education for the school. The only agenda item is to develop a strategic plan to meet one of the mutual goals established by the new dean of the Medical School of Van Husen University and the chief executive officer (CEO) of the medical center. The goal: Beginning with the next class of physical therapy students, every student is to be placed for at least 50% of their required clinical education hours in the units at Van Husen Medical Center (general medical/surgical, orthopedics, neurology, inpatient rehabilitation, outpatient rehabilitation, inpatient/outpatient pediatrics, and a satellite outpatient center).

Each of the 50 students must complete 36 weeks of full-time clinical education, spaced throughout the curriculum as 6 weeks in year one, 12 weeks in year two, and 18 weeks in year three. Antonio has 12 full-time physical therapists and a pool of about 20 contingency staff (who primarily work weekends and as vacation relief). His staff is reluctant to give up their affiliations with other schools, and Antonio feels this plan will decrease recruitment of new graduates from other schools. He also is concerned that the staff will be overburdened.

What should Antonio recommend? Consider: Where are they now? Where do they want to be? What do they have to work with? How will they get there?

ACTIVITY 17.5
A CHILDREN'S HOSPITAL

Ron Fleming, the Director of Rehabilitation at one of the Shriners Hospitals for Children (see http://www.shrinershospitalsforchildren.org/ and click on list of hospitals for more information), is concerned that his small staff of 10 physical, occupational, and speech therapists will be uncertain about their job descriptions because of changes in the hospital's mission of care. The hospital has received several research grants over the years related to the care of children who have congenital limb absences and children who have had amputations. The treatment of children with these conditions is considered the specialty of the hospital.

However, marketing efforts have been directed to building and increasing philanthropic funding for outpatient services. The efforts have been successful.

Ron is concerned, however, that this new outpatient success has resulted in a patient population with a much broader range of diagnoses that are challenging for his highly specialized staff who are experts in amputation. Because the patient census has expanded in the number and the range of problems to be addressed, the current staff members are spending more time treating patients. Time and planning to write proposals to renew grants and progress reports have been compromised. They have already asked for extensions beyond required submission deadlines.

What actions should Ron take? Consider: Where are they now? Where do they want to be? What do they have to work with? How will they get there?

ACTIVITY 17.6
OUTCOMES

Rodney Williams, the Rehabilitation Manager at Osakee Rehabilitation Hospital, is concerned. For the third consecutive quarter, inpatient outcome measures have fallen below the average of outcomes for all 80 hospitals in the Rehabilitation Hospitals of America chain that includes Osakee. He is meeting with the vice president of Osakee and the director of nursing to identify the causes for these disappointing outcomes and to identify action for improvement.

What are the possibilities? Consider: Where are they now? Where do they want to be? What do they have to work with? How will they get there?

ACTIVITY 17.7
STAFFING IN POST-ACUTE CARE

Jerry Weiss is the rehabilitation manager for the newest long-term acute care hospital in the National Hospital Corporation chain. His first task is to staff the six new positions in rehabilitation services. He has a meeting with the director of human resources who wants to brainstorm some recruitment strategies.

What are some ideas Jerry might present? Consider: Where are they now? Where do they want to be? What do they have to work with? How will they get there?

ACTIVITY 17.8
A NEW ASSIGNMENT

For the past 2 years, Jocelyn Ramos has been the supervisor of the inpatient rehabilitation team at Twin Cities Regional Hospital, a 250-bed hospital. In addition to her patient care duties in this position, she has been responsible for scheduling staff and monitoring productivity goals. The position of rehabilitation manager for the 100-bed rehabilitation hospital in the same system has become available. The vice president of clinical services has asked Jocelyn to accept the promotion.

What should she consider in making her decision? Consider: Where is Jocelyn now? Where does she want to be? What does she have to work with? How will she get there?

ACTIVITY 17.9
THE BIG OPPORTUNITY

Their move to the brand-new, state-of-the-art Carrollville Regional Medical Center from the old Carrollville Community Hospital was long awaited by Rosemarie Raddison and her rehabilitation staff. Along with the new hospital came a new upper-management team from the corporate offices of the All American Hospital Corporation that had purchased the old hospital and immediately began construction on the new one. Unhappy with many of the new management team's decisions, Rosemarie, who has been the rehabilitation director at Carrollville for more than 20 years, resigned as soon as the move to the new hospital was completed. The rest of her staff followed and within a month, there was no one left on the rehabilitation staff.

Since then, the hospital has been relying on intermittent services of a few physical therapists who work in other practices in the community. They have been willing to provide a few hours of care to patients in the evenings and on weekends while Carrollville continues to recruit a new rehabilitation director and staff.

After 4 months of searching, none of the rehabilitation positions has been filled despite a state-of-the-art rehabilitation center in the hospital and the attractiveness of Carrollville as one of the fastest growing communities in the state. The fill-in staff are becoming concerned that this is a longer than expected commitment to the hospital.

A recruiter has approached Daniel Steinman, an experienced rehabilitation manager in another state, to consider becoming a candidate for the director position. The salary offer is almost twice what Daniel currently makes, so he is interested in the position and Carrollville is an attractive location.

What list of questions and issues should Daniel prepare in his consideration of this opportunity? Consider: Where is Donald now? Where does he want to be? What does he have to work with? How will he get there?

ACTIVITY 17.10
A SHIFT IN MANAGEMENT

Gaston Martine, a physical therapist, has accepted a new position in a different state. The rehabilitation staff has been advised by the vice president for clinical services that she has taken the opportunity provided by Gaston's resignation to eliminate the rehabilitation manager position. Ron Abelson, the respiratory therapist who is also the cardiopulmonary program manager, will manage all inpatient and outpatient rehabilitation services. Determine the effect of this decision on all stakeholders. Consider: Where are they now? Where do they want to be? What do they have to work with? How will they get there?

ACTIVITY 17.11
INFORMATION MASTERY

Develop a policy and procedure(s) to incorporate a plan for ongoing information mastery for the staff of the rehabilitation services in a large teaching hospital. First, decide whether the policies and procedures will address individuals or the staff as a whole—or both. Consider: Where are they now? Where do they want to be? What do they have to work with? How will they get there?

ACTIVITY 17.12
SAFETY GOALS AND PHYSICAL THERAPY

Discuss which of The Joint Commission's hospital safety goals apply to physical therapists. The safety goals are:

- Use at least two ways to identify patients.
- Improve staff communication.
- Use medicines safely.
- Prevent infection.
- Identify patient safety risks.
- Prevent mistakes in surgery.

What policies and procedures should be in place for physical therapists to contribute to these goals? Consider: Where are they now? Where do they want to be? What do they have to work with? How will they get there?

ACTIVITY 17.13
PRODUCTIVITY

Robyn Latimer, the Rehabilitation Manager for Holy Family Health Center, is distressed to learn that the average productivity rate for her inpatient staff is down. What should be her plan of action? Consider: Where are they now? Where do they want to be? What do they have to work with? How will they get there?

ACTIVITY 17.14
PROMOTION

Phyllis Ames is a physical therapist assistant who has worked at Dellano Community Hospital for almost 20 years—longer than anyone else in the department. She has enjoyed the management responsibilities she has assumed intermittently over the years, particularly when the director's position has been unfilled. She has recently completed a master's degree in health services administration because of these interests. The director's position is again vacant and she is applying for the position.

What should the vice president ponder before offering her the position? Consider: Where are they now? Where do they want to be? What do they have to work with? How will they get there?

ACTIVITY 17.15
WEEKEND STAFFING

Riverside Rehabilitation Hospital contracts with Quality Staffing Services to provide rehabilitation services on Saturdays and Sundays. This arrangement is the result of assuring full-time staff that weekend coverage was not an expectation. This promise has been a great recruitment tool to fill full-time positions.

However, recently, several of the physical therapy and occupational therapy staff who are full-time employees of Riverside are also contracting with Quality Staffing Services for additional income, much to the surprise of Debra Watson, Riverside's Rehabilitation Manager. Sometimes the physical therapists are assigned to other organizations in the area, and, more surprisingly to Debra, they have reported to work at Riverside on weekends as employees of Quality Staffing Services. Quality Staffing Services has also been inconsistent in the people assigned and unpredictable in the numbers who appear to work each weekend.

Debra had already voiced her concerns about her lack of input into the staff that Quality Staffing Services assigns to Riverside to Rhonda Smith, the Human Resources Director at Riverside. During the meeting, Rhonda advises Debra that there is no policy about concurrent employment with other companies. She would obviously prefer that Debra arrange for overtime pay for Riverside staff who work weekends at Riverside rather than paying the very high rates that Quality Staffing Services charges for weekend services.

What should they do? Consider: Where are they now? Where do they want to be? What do they have to work with? How will they get there?

ACTIVITY 17.16
WORKING IN MULTIPLE UNITS

Sanderson Community Hospital has reduced its inpatient staff to just one physical therapist and one physical therapist assistant. There are days when the inpatient census increases unexpectedly. There is also a need for another physical therapist to meet the demands for initial evaluation of several patients within the 24-hour window required. As rehabilitation supervisor, Jonathan Martin's solution to this intermittent staffing need has been to ask the three Sanderson outpatient physical therapists to be on call to help the inpatient staff as outpatient cancellations or patient no-shows create downtime in their schedules. They have refused.

What should Jonathan do? Consider: Where are they now? Where do they want to be? What do they have to work with? How will they get there?

ACTIVITY 17.17
WEEKEND COVERAGE

Tom Bradford is a contract physical therapist who has been working most weekends at Cramwell Rehabilitation Hospital. He is very upset when he meets with Mary Strickland, the Rehabilitation Manager. Tom reports that Bette Shannon, another contract therapist, has been documenting and reporting seeing patients whom she has not seen. Tom learned this yesterday when one of the patients that Bette has been scheduled to see the past few weekends asked Tom why he had not been getting therapy on weekends before. The records show that Bette documented seeing the patient the two previous weekends. Tom was embarrassed by the patient's question and is furious with Bette.

What should Mary do? Consider: Where are they now? Where do they want to be? What do they have to work with? How will they get there?

ACTIVITY 17.18
PATIENT REFUSAL

James Hunter, a rehabilitation manager, is concerned about physical therapist Val Morres. She has significantly more patient cancellations because of patient refusal than any other person does on staff. When James meets with Val to discuss this, Val reports that she strongly believes a person has a right to refuse treatment—it is what she learned in school. Cancellations also give her more time to spend with patients who want therapy, so she really does not understand why it is a problem.

What should James do? Consider: Where are they now? Where do they want to be? What do they have to work with? How will they get there?

ACTIVITY 17.19
PATIENT ASSIGNMENT

Physical therapist Bonnie Bradman feels that Sid Bleekman, the Rehabilitation Manager, has ignored her concerns that she is always assigned the most difficult patients. Although this was flattering at first, she feels these assignments make her look bad because her productivity numbers are down as a result. A memo from Sid advising her to bring up her numbers has angered her. She is meeting with Sid today.

What should Sid do? Consider: Where are they now? Where do they want to be? What do they have to work with? How will they get there?

ACTIVITY 17.20
PRIORITY PATIENT LIST

John Butterworth's plan for developing a priority list for rehabilitation patients has hit a snag. Although he announced that patients could be seen only once a day for therapy, Chris Houseman, the Vice President of Clinical Services, told him he cannot do that. As a matter of fact, Chris wants the policy to be that patients who are uninsured *must* be seen twice a day for therapy to facilitate their discharges because the hospital loses money each day an uninsured patient remains in the hospital.

What should John do? Consider: Where are they now? Where do they want to be? What do they have to work with? How will they get there?

REFERENCES

1. Masley PM, Havrilko C-L, Mahnensmit, MR, et al. Physical therapist practice in the acute care setting: a qualitative study. *Physical Therapy.* 2011;91:906-919.

2. Society of Hospital Medicine. Information about SIM. http://www.hospitalmedicine.org/AM/Template.cfm?Section=About_SHM. Accessed May 21, 2013.

3. Wartman SA, ed. *The Academic Health Center: Evolving Models.* Washington, DC: Association of Academic Health Centers; 2007.

4. Medicare Payment Advisory Commission. *Report to Congress: Physician-Owned Specialty Hospitals.* Washington, DC; 2005. http://www.medpac.gov/documents/Mar05_SpecHospitals.pdf. Accessed May 21, 2013.

5. Cram P, Vaughn-Sarrazin M, Rosenthal GE. Hospital characteristics and patient populations served by physician owned and nonphysician owned orthopedic specialty hospitals. *BMC Health Services Research.* 2007;7:1472. http://www.biomedcentral.com/content/pdf/1472-6963-7-155.pdf. Accessed May 21, 2013.

6. American Hospital Association. Utilization trends in inpatient rehabilitation: Update through Q 2: 2011. https://www.google.com/url?sa=t&rct=j&q=&esrc=s&source=web&cd=1&ved=0CC4QFjAA&url=http%3A%2F%2Fwww.aha.org%2Fcontent%2F11%2F11nov-irfmoranrpt.pdf&ei=3-icUdTGD4Ok9ASQ0oGQDQ&usg=AFQjCNG-blekuaiqmEIuP7xk23IRHE5OG7Q&sig2=R4JJqo5CQzjUze-FanuYT-Q. Accessed May 21, 2013.

7. American Health Care Association. Maximizing the value of post-acute care. https://www.google.com/url?sa=t&rct=j&q=&esrc=s&source=web&cd=1&ved=0CC4QFjAA&url=http%3A%2F%2Fwww.aha.org%2Fresearch%2Freports%2Ftw%2F10nov-tw-postacute.pdf&ei=tOmcUfRUidL0BOXcgNAO&usg=AFQjCNG0UodB1OIa7sS8t-KsOswj5PdNDA&sig2=AeShoMvgOrq2LCV90eBFwQ. Accessed May 21, 2013.

8. Gittell JH. Achieving focus in hospital care: the role of relational coordination. In: Herzlinger RE, ed. *Consumer-Driven Health Care.* San Francisco, CA: John Wiley & Sons; 2004.

9. Miller PA, Solomon P. The influence of a move to program management on physical therapist practice. *Physical Therapy.* 2002;82:449-459.

10. Miller PA, Goddard P, Laschinger Spence HK. Evaluating physical therapists' perception of empowerment using Kanter's theory of structural power in organizations. *Physical Therapy.* 2001;81:1880-1888.

11. Suddick KM, De Souza L. Therapists' experiences and perceptions of teamwork in neurological rehabilitation: reasoning behind the team approach, structure and composition of the team and teamworking processes. *Physiotherapy Research International.* 2006;11:72-83.

12. Iles R, Davidson M. Evidence based practice: a survey of physiotherapists' current practice. *Physiotherapy Research International.* 2006;11:93-103.

13. Geyman JP, Deyo RA, Ramsey SD. *Evidence Based Clinical Practice: Concepts and Approaches.* Woburn, MA: Butterworth-Heinemann; 2000.

14. Vreeman DJ, Taggard SL, Rhine MD, et al. Evidence for electronic health record systems in physical therapy. *Physical Therapy.* 2006;86:434-449.

15. Donohoe E, Nawawi A, Wilker L, et al. Factors associated with burnout of physical therapists in Massachusetts rehabilitation hospitals. *Physical Therapy.* 1993;73:750-761.

16. Lopopolo RB. The relationship of role-related variables to job satisfaction and commitment to the organization in a restructured hospital environment. *Physical Therapy.* 2002;82:984-999.

17. Van Breugel G, Van Olffen W, Olie R. Temporary liaisons: the commitment of "temps" towards their agencies. *Journal of Management Studies.* 2005;42:3.

18. Kirk-Sanchez NJ, Roach KE. Relationship between duration of therapy services in a comprehensive rehabilitation program and mobility at discharge in patients with orthopedic problems. *Physical Therapy.* 2001;81:888-895.

19. Roach KE, Ally D, Finnerty B, et al. The relationship between duration of physical therapy services in the acute care setting and change in functional status in patients with lower-extremity orthopedic problems. *Physical Therapy.* 1998;78:19-24.

20. Curtis KA, Martin T. Perceptions of acute care physical therapy practice: issues for physical therapist preparation. *Physical Therapy.* 1993;73:581-598.

21. The Joint Commission. 2013 Hospital National Patient Safety Goals. http://www.jointcommission.org/assets/1/6/2013_HAP_NPSG_final_10-23.pdf. Accessed May 21, 2013.

22. Rapp J, Paz JC, McCallum C, Cole J, Steffey L. The effects of a physical therapy triage system on the outcomes of the ICU patients with respiratory failure. *Journal of Acute Care Physical Therapy.* 2010(1):21-29.

23. Pawlik AJ, Kress P. Issues affecting the delivery of physical therapy services for individuals with critical illness. *Physical Therapy.* 2013;93(2):256-265. doi:10.2522/ptj.20110445. Epub November 15, 2012.

WEB RESOURCES

Acute Long Term Hospital Association (ALTHA). http://www.altha.org/who-we-are/history.html. Accessed November 29, 2013.

American Physical Therapy Association (APTA). Acute care information. http://www.acutept.org/. Accessed November 29, 2013.

American Physical Therapy Association (APTA). The APTA's series on intensive care. http://www.apta.org/PTinMotion/NewsNow/2012/12/3/2013/DecemberPTJ/. Accessed November 29, 2013.

American Physical Therapy Association (APTA). Physical therapist practice in the emergency department. http://www.apta.org/EmergencyDepartment/. Accessed November 29, 2013.

Association of Academic Health Centers (AAHC). The AAHC's mission is to improve the nation's healthcare system by mobilizing and enhancing the strengths and resources of the academic health center enterprise in health professions education, patient care, and research. http://www.aahcdc.org/. Accessed November 29, 2013.

Australian Commission on Safety and Quality in Healthcare. OSSIE Guide to Clinical Handover Improvement. http://www.safetyandquality.gov.au/wp-content/uploads/2012/01/ossie.pdf. Accessed June 12, 2014.

Centers for Medicare & Medicaid Services. Inpatient rehabilitation facility prospective payment system. http://www.cms.gov /Outreach-and-Education/Medicare-Learning-Network-MLN/MLNProducts/downloads/InpatRehabPaymtfctsht09-508.pdf. Accessed November 29, 2013.

Commission on Accreditation of Rehabilitation Facilities (CARF). CARF is an international and independent, nonprofit accreditor of health and human services. http://www.carf .org/Programs/Medical/. Accessed November 29, 2013.

The HCAHPS (Hospital Consumer Assessment of Healthcare Providers and Systems). First national, standardized, publicly reported survey of patients' perspectives of hospital care. http://www.hcahpsonline.org/files/HCAHPS%20Fact%20Sh eet%20May%202012.pdf. Accessed November 29, 2013.

Hospital Compare. Find a hospital. http://www.medicare.gov /hospitalcompare/search.html. Accessed November 29, 2013.

HospitalConnectSearch. The Hospital Information search engine. http://www.hospitalconnect.com/. Accessed November 29, 2013.

Institute of Medicine of the National Academies. The role of academic health centers in the 21st century. Census study. http://iom.edu/Activities/Quality/AcadmcHealthCentRole .aspx. Accessed November 29, 2013.

The Joint Commission. Hospital accreditation information. http://www.jointcommission.org/accreditation/hospital_seek ing_accreditation.aspx. Accessed November 29, 2013.

Society of Hospital Medicine. http://www.hospitalmedicine .org/AM/Template.cfm?Section=About_SHM

A BRIEF HISTORY OF ORGANIZATIONS, LEADERSHIP, AND MANAGEMENT

Phase One: Early 20th Century

Mass production and large monopolies emerged in this period, which is thought of in terms of some of the giants of the time including Andrew Carnegie, J.P. Morgan, and John D. Rockefeller. Leaders such as these men and innovators such as Thomas Edison were considered to be born and not made. Therefore, the Great Man theory of leadership was generally accepted.

Max Weber (1864–1920) led the thinking about organizations with a rational and mechanical approach that emphasized strict rules to control workers to maximize efficiency. Units of workers needed to mesh and run like the cogs in the machines of large factories and mills. **Henry Fayol** was a pioneer in framing the concept of management in these organizations. He defined the roles of managers as organizing, leading, planning, controlling, and coordinating. **Frederick Taylor**'s ideas led to the need for experts to determine the one best way to achieve a task. Work became standardized and people received training to perform those tasks.

Mary Parker Follett was a social worker who rejected many of these ideas. She is credited with laying the foundation of the human relations movement of management based on the reciprocal relationships of workers and their supervisors. She believed managers should have power *with* workers rather than power *over* workers, and that the whole was greater than the sum of its parts. She is known for her work on negotiation, dispute resolution, and win-win interactions. Following Follett's lead, **Elton Mayo** also focused on the importance of personal interactions and relationships in work as the Hawthorne Studies (in which work environment factors were manipulated to determine physical and social changes in workers) became the model for the study of work.

Phase Two: Mid-20th Century

Abraham Maslow's psychological theory of the hierarchy of human needs (from basic physiological needs to self-actualization) began to drive organizations to consider factors other than monetary rewards in their management of workers. **Douglas McGregor** was another psychologist whose ideas were consistent with Maslow's model. He identified Theory X as a management model in which employees are viewed as lazy with a dislike for work; therefore, tight controls, coercion, blame, and incentives are needed for work to get done. He balanced that view of people with Theory Y in which managers assume people are ambitious, are self-motivated, and want to do well at their work—which is a strong motivation in itself. By engaging workers in decisions about their work, they can use all of their talents to control and direct their own work.

Between World War I and World War II, healthcare organizations were primarily small, religious-affiliated hospitals that physicians and nurses managed while delivering care. Some large public hospitals, such as insane asylums and tuberculosis sanitoria, were established to care for particular patients. Typically, the management models of Mary Parker Follett were utilized by these not-for-profit and public institutions, but they remained bureaucracies that applied rigid rules to be followed by workers.

After World War II, **Peter Drucker** made several predictions that have come true. He predicted the need for knowledge workers and lifelong learning, the increased privatization of work in public organizations (including hospitals), outsourcing, and the importance of marketing. He believed in the need for academic programs to prepare managers, focused on the role of the middle-level managers, and developed a widely used tool for their use—Management by Objectives.

During this period, the **Macy Foundation** funded a series of conferences that brought together scholars from a wide range of disciplines. This work laid the foundation for systems theory and cybernetics. The concepts of open and closed systems that arose from this group became the foundation of contingency theorists such as **Fred Fiedler**. These models were based on the convention that there is no best way to manage or make decisions because of constantly changing internal and external situations. Organizations became organisms that could adapt to their external environment through the interaction of the internal processes of its subsystems.

Herbert Simon coined the word *satisficing* to describe decision-making that satisfies an acceptable threshold but sacrifices the optimal possible outcome. Satisficing is necessary because managers do not have the ability or resources (bounded rationality) to accurately predict the outcomes of their decisions. The relationship between an organization and its workers came to be viewed as an exchange with these competing coalitions pursuing their own self-interests. Standard operating procedures became the subtle ways for managers to control the work of others and the flow of information.

The focus of healthcare during this period shifted to the care of children with poliomyelitis and adults with war-related and industrial-accident injuries until the passage of the entitlement legislation that created Medicare and Medicaid. Dramatic changes resulted from this generous government funding that included dollars for hospital expansion and the training of healthcare professionals. Hospitals, for the first time, had to meld the needs of patients and the work of professionals with their business goals.

Phase Three: Late 20th Century

In this period, a strong interest in the role of leadership began to rise with the pioneering work of **Warren Bennis** and **Chris Argyris** who developed the concept of learning organizations. The Managerial Grid Model of **Robert Blake** and **Jane Mouton**, which intersected an organization's concern for people with their concern for production, gained popularity. **William Ouchi**'s Theory Z focused on employee loyalty, morale, and satisfaction by consideration of both on- and off-the-job needs of employees as the means to increase productivity and workforce stability. Ouchi and the Japanese movement in management were influenced by the work of **W. Edward Deming**, who is known as the father of the total quality management movement. He also created the Plan-Do-Check-Act cycle. **George Doran** developed the SMART and SMARTER approach to setting work objectives as interest in strategic planning and problem-solving evolved in this period. The interest in quality led to Six Sigma, a process improvement program that identifies and removes production defects to achieve 99.99966% error-free results.

The expectancy theory of **Victor Vroom** led to the path-goal theory based on the work of **Martin Evans**. In this model, leaders are flexible in their approach to followers who can reach the organization's goals by some combination of direction, challenges, inclusion in decision-making, and relief of stresses that impact performance. Over the years, this work was reinforced by the development of Vertical-Dyad Linkage Theory and the resulting Leader-Member

Exchange (LMX) Theory in which high-quality relationships (based on trust and mutual respect) generate more positive outcomes than low-quality relationships (based on satisfying contracts). The idea of in-groups and out-groups sprang from this work. Also, there was renewed interest in the traits of leaders who may be transformational (inspire followers to transcend self-interests for the good of the organization) or transactional (relationship based on exchange of costs and benefits through rules, standard operating procedures).

Peter Senge influenced organizations with his theory of learning organizations and systems thinking that allowed for continuous expansion of the capacity of people working together to see the whole so that organizations can adapt quickly and change directions effectively to accomplish their goals. **Robert Greenleaf** contributed the concept of servant leadership for both individuals and organizations that embodied the importance of putting the needs of others before one's self.

Phase Four: 21st Century

The evolution of strategic management perspectives brings theories into the 21st century. **Michael Hannan** and **John Freeman** developed the theory of organizational ecology. They suggest that the environment selects and retains the organizational models that survive because of their ability to compete, acquire scarce resources, and rely on a wide diversity of forces to change as needed. This model has proved useful for understanding many aspects of contemporary healthcare systems such as competition for specialized services and integrated delivery systems.

New social network perspectives are adding to the understanding of formal and informal work groups in large organizations and of teams that arise from projects involving people who may be geographically separated and unknown to each other except in regard to the project. Systems theories have evolved to address the need to understand complex, adaptive systems. These are systems capable of learning from experience and changing, just as people do. This understanding of complexity becomes important to healthcare systems as they seek innovation in patient care delivery to respond to crises such as medical errors and new epidemiology such as SARS and Ebola.

GUIDELINES FOR PREPARING PROGRAM PROPOSALS, FEASIBILITY STUDIES, AND BUSINESS PLANS

Program Proposal Guidelines

I. **Introduction: Summary Statement**

One-paragraph description of the program. Who? What? When? Where? Why? How?

II. **Statement of Need**

What purpose does the program serve? Provide data to support the need. Relate to vision, mission, or goals of the organization. What are the projected benefits and whom do they benefit?

III. **Detailed Description of the Program**

Target audience?

Scope of work?

Goals?

Systematic approach to tasks and processes?

Resources required?

Personnel and their responsibilities?

Timetable?

Expected patient (client, other) outcomes?

IV. **Financial Justification**

How much will the program cost?

How much revenue will it generate?

V. **Larger Context**

How does the program relate to (impact) other units in the organization?

VI. **Program Outcomes and Assessment**

What will the program accomplish? How will it be measured?

VII. Conclusion

One paragraph. In summary, why should this program be implemented?

Feasibility Study Guidelines

I. General Description

One paragraph that answers the following:

What is the idea?

What are the possible scenarios or business models that might be considered for this type of project?

Why was this one selected for further study?

If implemented, what product or service will be marketed?

How will the business make money?

Where will it be?

What would be the time span from initiation to the time the door is opened for the business to run at full capacity?

What is its potential impact on the community?

What is the expected vision and mission?

II. Market Feasibility

A. *Size and scope of the industry, market, market segments (e.g., physical therapy = industry, orthopedic physical therapy = market, and sports-related injured patients = market segment)*

B. *The market (stability? growth? changing?)*

C. *Competition (Who? How many? Where are they?)*

D. *Emerging opportunities (New populations? Potential for new brand? Healthcare policy changes?)*

E. *Demand (What is the need?)*

F. *Potential market share and/or market segment (Expanding to meet needs competition cannot meet or taking away from competitors?)*

G. *Potential buyers (Insurers? Employers? Patients?)*

H. *Projected units of services (Visits/month? Gym memberships?)*

I. *Potential market barriers (Insurance contracts? New competition?)*

III. Technical Feasibility

A. *Facility needs (Size and type? Related services? Build-out?)*

B. *Location (Access? Transportation? Regulatory requirements? Workforce availability?)*

C. *Equipment (Purchase? Lease? Delivery? Set up?)*

IV. Financial Feasibility

A. *Estimate of the total capital requirements (Start-up funds to cover expenses until revenue is realized? Facilities, equipment, and supplies needed to open the doors? Working capital? Contingency capital?)*

B. *Estimate of equity and credit needs (Family? Investors? Banks? Government?)*

C. *Budget (Expected revenue and costs? Profit margin? Expected net profit? Breakeven? Cash flow? Best- and worst-case scenarios?)*

D. *Fully operational balance sheet*

E. *Underlying assumptions and summary*

V. Organizational/Managerial Feasibility

A. *Legal structure (Corporation, Limited partnership, Other?)*

B. *Staffing and governance (Lines of authority? Decision-making structure?)*

C. *Important stakeholders (Joint venture partners? Alliances? Other?)*

D. *Availability of key personnel (Business managers? Consultants? Legal? Accounting? Other?)*

E. *Key leaders and/or founders (Character? Skills? Past experience?)*

VI. Summary and Recommendations

One paragraph: Summary of recommended project, issues/assumptions for further study, Recommendations for action and next steps

Business Plan Guidelines

The U.S. Small Business Administration has a model for how to write a business plan that provides step-by-step detailed instructions. Go to http://www.sba.gov/category/navigation-structure/starting-managing-business/starting-business/how-write-business-plan.

Index

Note: page numbers followed by b, f, and t refer to Side Bars, Figures, and Tables, respectively.